Accession no.
36159713

KT-500-871

Qualitative Research in Nursing

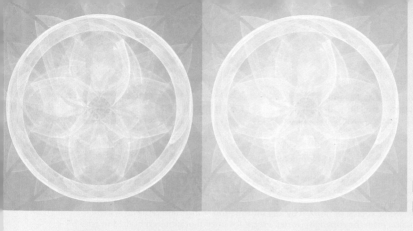

FIFTH
EDITION

Qualitative Research in Nursing

Advancing the Humanistic Imperative

HELEN J. STREUBERT, EDD, RN, ANEF
Vice President for Academic Affairs
Our Lady of the Lake University
San Antonio, Texas

DONA RINALDI CARPENTER, EDD, RN
Professor
Department of Nursing
University of Scranton
Scranton, Pennsylvania

LIS - LIBRARY

Date 28/3/12	Fund nm-Riv

Order No.
2284704

University of Chester

Wolters Kluwer | Lippincott Williams & Wilkins
Health
Philadelphia · Baltimore · New York · London
Buenos Aires · Hong Kong · Sydney · Tokyo

Acquisitions Editor: Hilarie Surrena
Product Manager: Mary Kinsella
Design Coordinator: Holly Reid McLaughlin
Manufacturing Coordinator: Karin Duffield
Prepress Vendor: MPS Limited, A Macmillan Company

Fifth edition

Copyright © 2011 Wolters Kluwer Health | Lippincott Williams & Wilkins.

Copyright © 2007, 2003, 1999 Lippincott Williams & Wilkins. Copyright © 1995
J. B. Lippincott Company. All rights reserved. This book is protected by copyright. No part of this book may be reproduced or transmitted in any form or by any means, including as photocopies or scanned-in or other electronic copies, or utilized by any information storage and retrieval system without written permission from the copyright owner, except for brief quotations embodied in critical articles and reviews. Materials appearing in this book prepared by individuals as part of their official duties as U.S. government employees are not covered by the above-mentioned copyright. To request permission, please contact Lippincott Williams & Wilkins at 530 Walnut Street, Philadelphia, PA 19106, via email at permissions@lww.com, or via our website at lww.com (products and services).

9 8 7 6 5 4 3 2

Printed in China

Library of Congress Cataloging-in-Publication Data

Helen J. Streubert.
 Qualitative research in nursing : advancing the humanistic imperative / Helen J. Streubert, Dona Rinaldi Carpenter. — 5th ed.
     p. ; cm.
 Includes bibliographical references and index.
 Summary: "Qualitative Research in Nursing is a user-friendly text that systematically provides a sound foundation for understanding a wide range of qualitative research methodologies, including triangulation. It approaches nursing education, administration, and practice and gives step-by-step details to instruct students on how to implement each approach. Features include emphasis on ethical considerations and methodological triangulation, instrument development and software usage; critiquing guidelines and questions to ask when evaluating aspects of published research; and tables of published research that offer resources for further reading"—Provided by publisher.
 ISBN 978-0-7817-9600-2 (pbk.)
 1. Nursing—Research—Methodology. 2. Qualitative research—Methodology. I. Carpenter, Dona Rinaldi. II. Title.
 [DNLM: 1. Nursing Research—methods. 2. Qualitative Research. 3. Quality Assurance, Health Care. 4. Research Design. WY 20.5 S752q 2011]
 RT81.5.S78 2011
 610.73072—dc22
                             2010024213

Care has been taken to confirm the accuracy of the information presented and to describe generally accepted practices. However, the authors, editors, and publisher are not responsible for errors or omissions or for any consequences from application of the information in this book and make no warranty, expressed or implied, with respect to the currency, completeness, or accuracy of the contents of the publication. Application of this information in a particular situation remains the professional responsibility of the practitioner; the clinical treatments described and recommended may not be considered absolute and universal recommendations.

 The authors, editors, and publisher have exerted every effort to ensure that drug selection and dosage set forth in this text are in accordance with the current recommendations and practice at the time of publication. However, in view of ongoing research, changes in government regulations, and the constant flow of information relating to drug therapy and drug reactions, the reader is urged to check the package insert for each drug for any change in indications and dosage and for added warnings and precautions. This is particularly important when the recommended agent is a new or infrequently employed drug.

 Some drugs and medical devices presented in this publication have Food and Drug Administration (FDA) clearance for limited use in restricted research settings. It is the responsibility of the health care provider to ascertain the FDA status of each drug or device planned for use in his or her clinical practice.

CCS0411

This book is dedicated to my family, especially to my children, Michael, Linda, Matthew, Kenny, Pamela, Shannon, Samantha, and Andy. As adults, they have protected me, loved me, and most importantly encouraged me when I needed it most. They have also blessed me with my grandchildren, Enrique, Anna, and Matty. As they know, there is no greater gift than the gift of family and they offer that gift selflessly every day. I also dedicate this edition to my sister, Theresa and to my Dad, who provide me with strength and a courage to face uncertainty. Finally to my "sister" Sue who listens to me always with an open heart and a loving spirit.

HJS

This 5th edition is dedicated to the memory of my father Vito Salvatore Rinaldi, who taught me by the way he lived about the importance of hard work, determination, strength of character, kindness, and unconditional love.

DRC

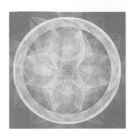

About the Authors

*H*elen J. Streubert EdD, RN, ANEF, is Vice President of Academic Affairs at Our Lady of the Lake University, San Antonio, Texas, where she leads the academic programs. She has authored and coauthored articles and book chapters on qualitative research and nursing education. In addition, she has presented her work nationally and internationally.

Dona Rinaldi Carpenter, EdD, RN, is Professor of Nursing at the University of Scranton, Pennsylvania, where she teaches medical-surgical nursing and nursing research to undergraduate and graduate students. Her research interests focus on nursing education and professional commitment. She has authored and coauthored several articles and book chapters and has presented her work at national and international meetings.

Contributors

Sandra Beth Lewenson, EdD, RN, FAAN, is Associate Dean of Academic Affairs at the Lienhard School of Nursing at Pace University, Pleasantville, New York. She teaches in both the undergraduate and graduate programs. Her areas of expertise include community health and the history of nursing. Her research focus is nursing's historical relationship with the women's suffrage movement at the beginning of the 20th century. She has published several books and articles on the topic.

Barbara K. Buxton, PhD, RN, is Assistant Professor of Nursing at the University of Scranton, Pennsylvania, where she teaches in the undergraduate and graduate programs. Her clinical background is in mental health nursing. She has conducted research on women with obesity, stigma, and health care. Her doctoral dissertation was a phenomenological study that described the experiences and perceptions of large women with regard to health care.

Patricia Moyle Wright, PhD, RN, ACNS-BC, is Assistant Professor of Nursing at the University of Scranton, Pennsylvania, where she teaches in the undergraduate and graduate programs. Her clinical background includes community health, hospice, and medical-surgical nursing. She has conducted research on maternal bereavement and has published several articles on end-of-life care, hospice nursing, and grief.

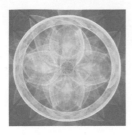

Reviewers

Diane M. Breckenridge, RN, MSN, PhD
Associate Professor
La Salle University
Philadelphia, Pennsylvania

Laurie Nagelsmith, MS, RN
Assistant Dean, School of Nursing
Excelsior College School of Nursing
Albany, New York

Tracie Risling, BA, BSN, MN, RN
Faculty—Nursing Education Program of
    Saskatchewan
SIAST Kelsey Campus
Saskatoon, Saskatchewan

Jane Greene Ryan, MSN, CNM
Clinical Assistant Professor
College of Nursing and Health Professions
Drexel University
Philadelphia, Pennsylvania

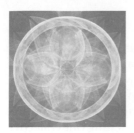

Preface

*T*he fifth edition of *Qualitative Research in Nursing: Advancing the Humanistic Imperative* presents major revisions and updated material essential to qualitative research methods and publications. A new and expansive look at the actual process of conducting a qualitative research study, writing a qualitative research proposal, and clinical application of qualitative methods are also included. Each companion chapter has been completely revised and includes a new research article applicable to the method addressed with accompanying critiques. Further, a new peer-reviewed research proposal and critique follows Chapter 16. These are included as examples for readers preparing qualitative grant proposals. We continue to work diligently to bring to the reader the latest in qualitative thinking by nurses and those who have supported nurses' work. Therefore, major revisions and updates have been included, as they were available during the preparation of this fifth edition. Finally, this edition continues to include the same strong philosophical and methodological principles that have been important to our readers over the years.

The purpose of this book has, from it's inception, been to assist those new to qualitative inquiry to discover the fundamental characteristics of a set of methods that have been critical to the advancement of nursing's scientific body of knowledge. The text provides a strong and organized reference for understanding qualitative methodology. We continue to believe strongly, however, that it is only through engagement in the methods that those new to qualitative inquiry will begin to appreciate the value of the methods (approaches) for studying the human condition as it is revealed in nursing practice.

Clearly qualitative research methods have been recognized and valued as legitimate methods of scientific inquiry. This is a major change since the first writing of this text. There is still work to be done, however. Although qualitative research methods have come into their own, with significant numbers of journal pages dedicated to the publication of qualitative work and journals solely dedicated to qualitative research, we continue to be heartened by the fact that more qualitative researchers are able to become panel members of grant review teams and are now securing more research dollars for this exciting and enlightening research paradigm.

Those of you familiar with our text know that our original work arose from our own experiences with trying to develop a qualitative research agenda based on reading the works of, and studying with, those outside of the nursing discipline. This text continues to build on our experiences and shares with the reader the expansion of our own thinking over the years, but also the works of those who have been significant in opening our collective vision in the field of qualitative study. Further, we have added contributors with recent experience in conducting grounded theory and phenomenological investigations. Their new and unique vision adds depth to this content as well as a renewed focus. In particular, the chapter on grounded theory methods has been extensively revised to reflect newer approaches and theoretical foundations of the method.

Our personal lives as nurses, nurse educators, and nurse researchers are built on the common understanding that individuals are integrated wholes who share common experiences with other individuals. It is for this reason that qualitative inquiry supports our commitment to understanding the human condition. We fully believe that we live lives that recognize the interconnectedness of our humanness and we strive to assist others to join in the mutual understanding that we derive from being part of the human experience. The skills for understanding the human experience are found in the pages of this text. We believe that the understanding that is gleaned from participating in qualitative inquiry gives each nurse researcher the opportunity to see his or her practice through a unique lens. To fully realize the skills of a qualitative researcher, we believe that fundamental understanding of the history, elements, context, and outcomes of each approach presented in the text is essential. Further, those who find qualitative inquiry supportive of their personal research philosophy are encouraged to use the primary references documented in the text to explore more deeply the basic ideologies that were responsible for the development of the qualitative research paradigm.

As in our previous editions, the text introduces the historical background of each approach, shares the fundamental elements, how one decides whether to use a particular approach, and the expected outcomes. Knowing these parts will help the reader begin to integrate and synthesize the research paradigm that we have found so successful in bringing about an understanding of a whole and authentic human experience.

Organization

This text is organized to facilitate the reader's comprehension of each approach and to provide examples of how the approaches have been used in nursing practice, education, and administration.

In Chapter 1, Philosophy and Theory: Foundations of Qualitative Research, the reader is introduced to the traditions of science, the interpretations of what constitutes science, perceptions of reality, and the influences of critical and feminist theory on the discipline of qualitative research.

In Chapter 2, The Conduct of Qualitative Research: Common Essential Elements, the development of a qualitative study is examined. The characteristics common to all qualitative studies are offered, including selection of the method, understanding the philosophic underpinnings of the approach selected, and use of a literature review, explicating the researcher's beliefs, choosing a setting, selecting the informant, and achieving saturation.

Chapter 3, Designing Data Generation and Management Strategies, offers the reader ideas about how to select and use specific data collection strategies, including interviews, focus groups, narratives, chat rooms, participant observation, and field notes. In addition, an explanation is provided for managing data including the common elements of data analysis, demonstrating trustworthiness, and presentation of the findings.

Chapter 4, Ethical Consideration in Qualitative Research, represents an expanded revision to the information presented in the last edition. A significant amount of literature has been published with regard to ethical issues in qualitative research. This information is offered to assist the reader in fully understanding the unique and sensitive relationship that occurs in the process of a qualitative study and suggests ways to maximize protection of human subjects while engaged in the relationship.

Chapter 5, Phenomenology as Method offers an in-depth description of philosophy and methodological conceptualizations of this approach to qualitative inquiry. An overview of the phenomenological perspective, with descriptive and interpretive views of the process, is offered. The reader is given an exceptional guide to the process of phenomenological inquiry, including an expansion of previously presented hermeneutics. Table 5-1 lists the procedural step for implementing a phenomenological study from the perspective of six phenomenologists. It is an exceptional reference for the would-be phenomenological researcher.

Chapter 6, Phenomenology in Practice, Education, and Administration, as in previous editions, offers the reader the opportunity to understand the presentation of the method offered in Chapter 5 by giving examples of published phenomenological research from practice, education, and administration. Critique guidelines and formal critique by the chapter author also are provided to assist in understanding the application and quality of the work that is published. To facilitate the integration of the information presented, a reprint of one of the critiqued studies is included. Finally, a table of recently published phenomenological research gives the reader a ready reference of work using this specific approach.

Chapter 7, Grounded Theory as Method; Chapter 9, Ethnography as Method; Chapter 11, Historical Research Method; and Chapter 13, Action Research Method follow the format found in Chapter 5. This includes in-depth discussion of the philosophical and methodological issues specific to the approach. Data generation and treatment as well as ethical issues specific to the particular approach are discussed in detail.

Chapters 8, 10, 12, and 14 repeat the format found in Chapter 6, incorporating a detailed examination of published studies that illustrate a particular approach followed by guidelines for critiquing the approach used. These chapters include tables that offer a substantial resource list of recent studies completed in the areas of education, administration, and practice. Finally, each of these chapters includes a reprinting of a selected study that illustrates the qualitative method discussed in that particular chapter.

Chapter 15, Triangulation as a Qualitative Research Strategy, expands on information related to data, investigator, theory, and methodological triangulation. It is intended to enhance the reader's understanding of the different ways triangulation can be used in a qualitative research study.

Chapter 16, Writing a Qualitative Research Proposal, introduces the reader to the concept of developing a qualitative research agenda, as well as the elements of developing a qualitative research proposal. An example of a peer-reviewed funded grant and critique is included in the chapter.

Chapter 17, A Practical Guide for Sharing Qualitative Research Results, provides a full description of issues related to developing qualitative research projects and dissemination of qualitative research findings. It details for the reader the potential triumphs and the pitfalls in moving qualitative research into a public forum.

Key Features and Benefits
The following features are included in the philosophical and methodological framework.

- Description of the philosophical underpinnings of each approach. This description provides more than the "how" of the approach; it presents the underlying assumptions of the approaches.

- Detailed description of the procedural steps used in each of the approaches. This offers the reader the opportunity to learn step by step how the approach is implemented.

- Completely revised tables profiling studies conducted using each of the approaches. These tables offer the reader an excellent resource for further exploring the existing body of knowledge specific to the approach being discussed.

- In-depth discussion of published research studies that have used the approaches under discussion. This examination shares with the reader not only what has been published but also the strengths and weaknesses of the studies reviewed.

- Specific critiquing guidelines available in all companion chapters for each of the approaches. These guidelines help the reader understand the specific question that should be asked of research studies that have used or will be using the approach.

- Inclusion of completely revised companion chapters. Comparison chapters describing application of each of the approaches included in the text provide strong evidence of the impact these qualitative research methods are having on the discipline of nursing and the potential benefits they will continue to have. These chapters all provide neophyte qualitative researchers with clear descriptions of what is accepted from the researchers who will evaluate their work.
- Inclusion of a sample of a funded qualitative research grant, including the critique offered by the grant review panel.
- Chapters on ethical consideration in qualitative research and triangulation.
- Table highlighting the methods described as they have been used to study nursing practice issues.

We hope that this book will continue to serve as both a starting point for the new researcher and a reference for more experienced nurses. It is expected that each approach detailed will offer the reader a sound understanding of qualitative research methods. Finally, we are grateful for the support of our readership over the years, and hope that the fifth edition of this textbook exceeds your expectations.

Helen J. Streubert
Dona Rinaldi Carpenter

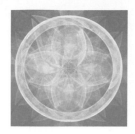

Acknowledgments

The fifth edition of this textbook has been an important undertaking, with major changes since we first began writing about qualitative research methods. As always our life experiences with friends and colleagues who have supported and valued our work continue to influence our writing. We wish to acknowledge all those people who continue to shape our thinking and our way of being in the world . . . our friends, our families, our teachers, our students, and our colleagues.

Specifically, we wish to acknowledge those who have been most closely involved in the production of the fifth edition of this text, and the research assistance of Katherine Harrington, Laura Falzone, and Erin Gilfeather, University of Scranton nursing students.

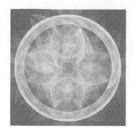

Contents

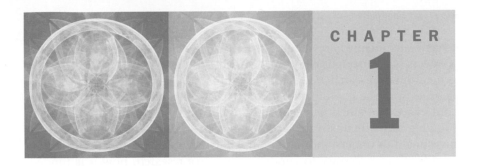

Philosophy and Theory: Foundations of Qualitative Research

Much of the evolution in nursing research over the last decade has been focused on evidence-based (EB) practice. Systemically, these developments have enlivened the debate about what constitutes evidence and reinvigorated the conversation about the merits of qualitative versus quantitative research. Grypdonck (2006) suggests that if qualitative researchers cannot establish or clarify the position of qualitative research within the EB environment, there will be no place for it. Morse (2006a, 2006b) on the other hand argues that qualitative researchers should not seek to gain acceptance in the EB milieu but rather should recognize that the purpose of quantitative and qualitative research represent conflicting agendas. A more moderate position from Mantzoukas (2008) suggests that EB practice shares similar definitions, aims, and procedures with reflective practice. This debate is exciting and offers great potential for the continued development of nursing knowledge. However, it poses some new challenges for qualitative nurse researchers.

In 1995 when the first edition of this text was published, the world of qualitative nursing research looked very different. There were few qualitative studies being published, few qualitative papers being given, and few nurses who called themselves qualitative researchers. Most of the qualitative researchers of that time were trained by sociologists, psychologists, and anthropologists who taught nurses how to use their methods and procedures to generate nursing knowledge. Since that time, qualitative nurse researcher pioneers have adapted what they learned and have helped to create a new generation of researchers. As a result of this early work, nursing knowledge derived from the qualitative paradigm has gained credibility. Journals and conferences are much richer because of the work of those early scholars in bringing to the mainstream a philosophy of science that demonstrates an investment in understanding the human condition. The debates about the qualifications necessary to conduct qualitative research, how it is funded, and its place in advancing nursing science continue. However, today, many of the debates are focused more on evidence than on specific philosophical paradigms. Models such as Cochrane's (1972/1989) model to evaluate research rigor, Haynes' (2007) hierarchy of research studies, and Melnyk and Fineout-Overholt's (2005) levels of evidence rating system challenge the place qualitative research holds in the EB paradigm.

Synthesis of research studies has been touted as critical to advancing the evidence base for nursing practice. Similar statements have been made relative to nursing education. However, synthesis or metasynthesis (the term used in qualitative research) has not been a high priority within the qualitative research tradition because of the challenges it presents. According to Flemming (2007), evidence in qualitative research has been of two primary types: primary studies or synopses of primary studies. Today, in addition to the collection, analysis, and interpretation of primary studies, qualitative nurse researchers are being asked to move beyond reporting of their findings to synthesis of multiple studies.

The presence of the debate about the future development of qualitative research and its place in the development of EB practice illustrates the value placed on the paradigm. The deliberations are important and useful and demonstrate the critical dialogue that continues within the field. The goal of this text is not to resolve the debate regarding the appropriateness of qualitative versus quantitative methods or to resolve the EB debate, but rather to offer nurse researchers an introduction to the philosophies, approaches, strategies, and outcomes that are included in the qualitative research paradigm. This introduction to qualitative research should stimulate its readers to want to learn more about the specific approaches included in the text and facilitate the use of them to discover new nursing knowledge. Appropriate application of qualitative methodologies will make a significant difference in advancing the development of nursing knowledge using these methods, but it will also prepare nurses to engage in the debate about the place that qualitative research holds in the advancement of nursing science within the EB environment.

The tradition of science remains uniquely quantitative. The quantitative approach to research has been justified by its success in measuring, analyzing, replicating, and applying knowledge gained from this paradigm. The inability to quantitatively measure some phenomena and the dissatisfaction with the results of measurement of other phenomena have led to an intense interest in using other approaches to study particularly human phenomena. This interest has led to an acceptance of qualitative research approaches as another way to discover knowledge.

The tradition of using qualitative methods to study human phenomena is grounded in the social sciences. The tradition arose because aspects of human values, culture, and relationships were unable to be described fully using quantitative research methods. Krasner (2000) states that the early philosophers "argued that human phenomena could not and should not be reduced to mathematical formulas" (p. 70). The practice of qualitative research has expanded to clinical settings because "empirical approaches have proven to be of limited service in answering some of the challenging and pressing clinical questions, especially where human subjectivity and interpretation are involved" (Thorne, 1997, p. 288). The appeal for nurses is that qualitative research methods attempt to describe and interpret perplexing human phenomena: phenomena that are not easily quantifiable (Krasner, 2000, p. 70). Nurses and other health care professionals clearly want to grasp the lived experience of their clients, to enter into the world their clients inhabit, and to understand the basic social processes that illuminate human health and illness events (Thorne, 1997).

This chapter shares with the reader the foundations of qualitative research. Its purpose is to present qualitative knowledge structure and generate excitement for the qualitative research approach as an alternative to quantitative inquiry.

PHILOSOPHIC UNDERPINNINGS OF QUALITATIVE RESEARCH

*F*rom a philosophic viewpoint, the study of humans is deeply rooted in descriptive modes of science. Human scientists have been concerned with describing the fundamental patterns of human thought and behavior since early times. Descartes' view of science was long held as the only approach to new knowledge. His ideas were grounded in an objective reality, a position that supported the idea that cause and effect could explain all things. Kant is attributed with questioning the fundamental nature of reality as seen through a Cartesian lens. He opened discussion about human rationality. Kant proposed that perception was more than the act of observation. For him, all reality was not explainable by cause and effect. He raised issues supporting the notion that nature was not independent of thought or reason (Hamilton, 1994). What was observed, therefore, was not the only reality.

The concept of scientific versus practical reason was born of Kant's ideas about nature, specifically as the concept relates to perception (Ermath, 1978; Hamilton, 1994). Later existentialists advanced Kant's ideas to explore reality as it is perceived rather than as an observed phenomenon only. Kant's ideas about freedom and practical reasoning emancipated science.

Scientists questioned whether empiricism was the only way to gain knowledge. Later philosophers such as Husserl furthered Kant's propositions, and, eventually, the German school of philosophy developed and expanded the ideas about self, self-consciousness, reality, and freedom.

The early debates about science and reality established the foundations of the qualitative paradigm that many social scientists use today. Qualitative research offers the opportunity to focus on finding answers to questions centered on social experience, how it is created, and how it gives meaning to human life (Denzin & Lincoln, 1994). Knowing how social experiences construct an individual's reality is an important criterion for developing science. Based on this idea, an exploration of ways of knowing is appropriate.

If one takes the ontologic position that reality is apprehensible, then the positivist or empiricist framework becomes one's reference point. However, it seems inconceivable that individuals can believe they are able to fully apprehend reality. According to Denzin and Lincoln (1994), postpositivists believe there is a reality to be known but have conceded that this reality only will be "imperfectly or probabilistically apprehendable [sic]" (p. 109). Critical theorists and constructivists see reality from a dynamic standpoint. The critical theorist perspective is that reality is "shaped by social, political, cultural, economic, ethnic, and gender values" (Denzin & Lincoln, 1994, p. 109). Further, feminist critical theorists believe that knowledge is cocreated by researcher and those researched. The constructivist, however, sees reality as "relativism—local and specific" (Denzin & Lincoln, 1994, p. 109). Therefore, "reality is actually realities" (Lincoln, 1992, p. 379). Clearly, it is a postpositivist viewpoint that supports the notion of a dynamic reality.

In a human enterprise such as nursing, it is imperative that nurses accept the utility of a research tradition that provides for the most meaningful way to describe and understand human experiences. Recognizing that reality is dynamic is the first step in establishing a truly humanistic perspective of research.

WAYS OF KNOWING

"*T*he term *knowing* refers to ways of perceiving and understanding the self and the world. Knowing is an ontologic, dynamic changing process" (Chinn & Kramer, 2004, p. 2). There are many ways that we come to know information. One way is through experts—someone we view as an authority tells us what to know. As children, this is usually our parent(s). As we grow up, the experts in our lives expand. Additional experts may include teachers, extended family, employers, or formal authority figures such as law enforcement officials. This way of knowing has been called the *received view*.

Trial and error is another way that individuals learn about the world. Through trying out new ideas or actions and determining the value of the response or outcome, we learn what is *correct*. There are other ways that individuals come to know what it is they value. Although it is important to know how it is we come to know, it is equally important to know how what we come to value is created or validated.

For many years, women in particular were told what to know. This limited debate and dialogue about information. Much of what was known and valued was professed by empirical scientists who supported a Cartesian framework that espoused a belief that if objective measurement could not be assigned to a phenomenon, the importance and thus the existence of the phenomenon was in question. Many contemporary scientists and philosophers question the value of this system, particularly in situations that include humans and their interactions with other humans. There is much debate about the relative value of information that is derived from a purely objective standpoint when it comes to human phenomena within a social context. The concepts of objectivity, reduction, and manipulation, which are fundamental to empirical science, defy the authentic fiber of humans and their social interactions. Too many intervening or confounding variables can influence the findings of empirical science when the focus is human social context or interaction.

With the belief that science should inform the lives of people who interact and function in society, researchers need to examine all parts of reality—subjective reality as well as its objective counterpart. Researchers should acknowledge knowing in the subjective sense and value it equally so that scientific knowledge will represent the views of people who experience life. The early phenomenologists believed that the only reality was the one that is perceived. Thus, the measurement of perception challenges the empirical scientist. Perception is not objective; rather, perception is a way of observing and processing those things that are present to the self within the context of one's lived experience. For example, two individuals may observe the same lecture and leave the classroom with different interpretations of what the lecturer said. Each individual's interpretation is based on what that person perceived to be reality—a reality that is developed and constructed over a lifetime of receiving, processing, and interpreting information, as well as engaging in human interaction. The internalization of what becomes known as belief systems comes from perception and construction of what is real for the individual.

WAYS OF KNOWING IN NURSING

Although Carper's (1978) seminal work on ways of knowing in nursing is over 30 years old, it still provides an excellent foundation for understanding knowledge development within the discipline. In this important work, Carper identified four fundamental patterns that emerge as the way nurses come to know—come to understand their world of work: empirical knowing, aesthetic knowing, personal knowing, and moral knowing. *Empirical knowing* represents the traditional, objective, logical, and positivist tradition of science. Empirical knowing and thus empirical science is committed to providing explanations for phenomena and then controlling them. An example of empirical knowing is the knowledge derived from the biologic sciences that describes and explains human function. Biologic scientists have been able to predict and control certain aspects of human structure and function. Treatment of diabetes mellitus is an example of empirical research being applied in the health care field. From their empirical studies, biologic scientists know that providing insulin to individuals with diabetes mellitus controls the symptoms created by the nonfunctioning pancreas. The nursing profession's alignment with empirical knowing and its subsequent pursuit of this mode of inquiry follows the positivist paradigm, which believes that objective data, measurement, and generalizability are essential to the generation and dissemination of knowledge. This type of nursing knowledge is critical in situations in which control and generalizability are important. Chinn and Kramer (2004) expanded our understanding of the traditional meaning of empirics to include theory development and the use of research methods that are not based strictly on hypothesis testing, such as phenomenology and ethnography.

Aesthetic knowing is the art of nursing. The understanding and interpretation of subjective experience and the creative development of nursing care are based on an appreciation of subjective expression. Aesthetic knowing is abstract and defies a formal description and measurement. According to Carper (1978),

> The aesthetic pattern of knowing in nursing involves the perception of abstract particulars as distinguished from the recognition of abstracted universals. It is the knowing of the unique particular rather than an exemplary class. (p. 16)

Aesthetic knowing in nursing provides the framework for the exploration of qualitative research methodologies. Qualitative research calls for recognition of patterns in phenomena rather than the explication of facts that will be controllable and generalizable. An example of aesthetic knowing is the way a nurse would provide care differently for two elderly women who are preparing for cataract surgery, based on the nurse's knowledge of each woman's particular life patterns.

Wainwright (2000) states, "a nursing aesthetic can provide us with an essential set of tools to help answer the question of what amounts to good nursing. It may also provide us with additional insights into the nature of nursing ethics" (p. 755). "Nursing knowledge as defined in nursing theories and when lived by nurses creates the art of nursing" (Mitchell, 2001, p. 207).

Personal knowing requires that the individual—in this case, the nurse—knows the self. The degree to which an individual knows oneself is determined by his or her abilities to self-actualize. Movement toward knowledge of the self and self-actualization requires comfort with ambiguity and a commitment to patience in understanding. Personal knowing is a commitment to authentication of relationships and a *presencing* with others, that is, the enlightenment and sensitization people bring to genuine human inter-actions. Personal knowing deals with the fundamental *existentialism* of hu-mans, that is, the capacity for change and the value placed on becoming.

Personal knowing also supports the qualitative research paradigm. In the conduct of qualitative inquiry, researchers are obligated by the philo-sophic underpinnings of the methodologies they use to accept the self as part of the research enterprise and to approach research participants in a genuine and authentic manner. An awareness of one's beliefs and under-standings is essential to fully discover the phenomena studied in a qualita-tive research inquiry. Furthermore, qualitative researchers believe there is always subjectivity in their pursuit of the truth. The very nature of human in-teractions is based on subjective knowledge. In the most objective research endeavor, subjective realities will affect what is studied. "Scientific research, as a human endeavor to advance knowledge, is influenced by the sociocul-tural and historical context in which it takes place and is considered neither value free, objective, nor neutral" (Henderson, 1995, p. 59).

Moral knowing reflects our ethical obligations in a situation or our ideas about what should be done in a given situation. Through the moral way of knowing, individuals come to a realization of what is right and just. As with personal knowing and aesthetic knowing, moral knowing is another abstract dimension of how it is that individuals come to understand a situation. Moral knowing is based on traditional principles and codes of ethics or con-duct. This type of knowing becomes most important when humans face sit-uations in which decisions of right and wrong are blurred by differences in values or beliefs. Moral knowing requires an openness to differences in philosophic positions. Ethics and logic are required to examine the intrica-cies of human situations that do not fit standard formulas for conduct.

Munhall (2001) states, "all of the foregoing patterns are rich and essen-tial sources of nursing knowledge that can be studied from various perspec-tives of science" (p. 41). The importance of sharing these ways of knowing is to offer the reader a context in which to judge the appropriateness of nurs-ing knowledge and the way that nurses develop that knowledge. It is only through examinations of current belief structures that people are able to achieve their own standards of what will be best in a given situation. Moreover, when we select our research methods, we should choose them based on the questions we are asking (Burnard & Hannigan, 2000) within the context of what is known and what we believe.

May (1994) and Sandelowski (1994) expanded on the idea of knowing as it relates to nursing knowledge. May (1994) used the term *abstract know-ing* to describe the analytic experience of knowing:

> The rigorous implementation and explication of method alone
> never explains the process of abstract knowing, regardless of which
> paradigm the scientist espouses and which method is chosen.
> Method does not produce insight or understanding or the creative

leap that the agile mind makes in the struggle to comprehend observation and to link them together. Regardless of the paradigmatic
perspective held by the scientist, the process of knowing itself cannot
be observed and measured directly, but only by its product. (p. 13)

May (1994) further suggested that knowledge is "shaped *but not completely defined* by the process through which it is created" (p. 14). Based on
her ideas about knowing, she gave credibility to what she called "magic,"
which is similar to the intuitive connections discussed in Benner's (1984)
work on expert clinical judgment. Based on her conversations with and observations of qualitative researchers, May determined that, at a certain point,
pattern recognition creates the insight into the phenomenon under study.
She believes that the ability to see knowledge is a result of intellectual rigor
and readiness (magic). Her ideas support the concept of intuition or, as she
labeled it, "abstract knowing" in nursing research.

Sandelowski (1994) took a position on knowing similar to the aesthetic
knowing described by Carper (1978): We must accept the art as well as the
science of research. Sandelowski believed that the two are not mutually
exclusive.

What differentiates the arts from the sciences is not the search for
truth per se, but rather the kinds of truths that are sought. Science
typically is concerned with propositional truths, or truth about
something. Art is concerned with universal truths, with being true
to: even with being more true to life than life itself. (Hospers, as
cited in Sandelowski, 1994, p. 52)

Both May (1994) and Sandelowski (1994) provide us with an expansion
of the original positions on knowing offered by Carper (1978). These authors provide a validation for knowing other than in the empirical sense.
Most important, they offer nurse researchers a way to discover knowledge
that complements the positivist paradigm and gives voice to other ways of
knowing. In the case of qualitative research and nursing practice, it is only
through examination of the prevailing ideologies that nurses will be able to
decide which ideology most reflects their personal patterns of discovery and
creation of meaning.

MEANING OF SCIENCE

Science is defined in a number of ways. According to Siepmann (1999),
"science is the field of study which attempts to describe and understand
the nature of the universe in whole or part." Aristotle described three types
of science: (1) acquisition of knowledge as a path to truth for its own sake;
(2) practical science, aimed at action based on truth; and (3) productive science that which is aimed at making according to true principles (Guiliano,
2003, p. 45). Guba (1990), in sharing a view of empirical science, articulated
the meaning of science as it is practiced within the premise of value-neutral,

logical, empirical methods that promise "the growth of rational control over ourselves and our worlds" (p. 317). Parse (2001) offers the term *sciencing* to describe "coming to know and understand the meaning of a phenomena [sic] of concern to a discipline" (p. 1). Each of these definitions or descriptions gives a different lens through which to view truth.

Much of what individuals know about science in the nursing profession is based on the empirical view of science, which places significant value on rationality, objectivity, prediction, and control. The question arises: Is this view of science consistent with the phenomena of interest to nurses? The empirical view of science permeates many aspects of human activity. In adopting this view, one adopts a value system. Many empiricists believe that if a phenomenon is not observable, then it is not real. If a particular phenomenon does not conform to reality as it is currently known, empiricists could judge it to be irrational and therefore unimportant. If a phenomenon is studied without controls protecting the objectivity of the study, then it is said to lack rigor or to be "soft" science and therefore results in unusable data. If the findings from an inquiry do not lead to generalization that contributes to prediction and control of the phenomena under study, some empiricists would argue that it is not "good" science. These positions on science are the ones which are currently guiding the adoption of EB practice.

For many years, an empiricist view of science has permeated society and has structured what is valued. Feminist scholars have suggested that the scientific paradigm that focuses on prediction and control has gained wide acceptance because of its roots in a male paradigm. Historically, women have played only a small role in the creation of knowledge. Therefore, male scientists who valued prediction and control over description and understanding have largely created the definitions and values of science. According to Anderson (2004),

> Various practitioners of feminist epistemology and philosophy of science argue that dominant knowledge practices disadvantage women by (1) excluding them from inquiry, (2) denying them epistemic authority, (3) denigrating their "feminine" cognitive styles and modes of knowledge, (4) producing theories of women that represent them as inferior, deviant, or significant only in the ways they serve male interests, (5) producing theories of social phenomena that render women's activities and interests, or gendered power relations, invisible, and (6) producing knowledge (science and technology) that is not useful for people in subordinate positions, or that reinforces gender and other social hierarchies.

An empirical, objective, rational science has significant value when the phenomenon of interest is other than human behavior. However, the goals of this type of science—prediction and control—are less valuable when the subject of the inquiry is unable to be made objective.

As a result of the limitations that come from a positivist view of science, philosophers and social scientists have offered an alternative path to discovery that places value on the study of human experiences. In this model, researchers acknowledge and value subjectivity as part of any scientific inquiry. Human values contribute to scientific knowledge; therefore, neutrality is impossible. Prediction is thought to be limiting and capable of creating a false sense of reality. In a human science framework, the best that the scientists can hope for while creating new knowledge is to provide understanding and interpretation of phenomena within context. Human science and the methods of inquiry that accompany it offer an opportunity to study and create meaning that enriches and informs human life. Burnard and Hannigan (2000) state that regardless of the paradigm, "research is nearly always a searching for patterns, similarities and differences" (p. 5).

Induction Versus Deduction

Knowledge is generated from either an inductive or deductive posture. *Inductive reasoning* is a process that starts with the details of the experience and moves to a more general picture of the phenomenon of interest (Liehr & Smith, 2002, p. 110). For example, a nurse interested in studying the experiences of women during childbirth would interview women who have undergone labor to discover their experiences of it. Within context, the nurse could make statements about the labor experience that might be applicable to understanding the labor experience for women not in the study. Hence, qualitative research methods are inductive.

Deductive reasoning moves from general to specific. A researcher interested in conducting research within a deductive framework would develop a hypothesis about a phenomenon and then would seek to prove it. For example, a nurse wanting to know about the childbirth experience might hypothesize that women in labor experience more pain when they do not use visualization techniques during transition. The researcher's responsibility in such a study would be to identify a pain measure and then collect data on women in the transition phase of labor to determine whether they experience more or less pain based on the use of visualization techniques. Within a deductive framework, the researcher can use the study findings to predict and ultimately attempt to control the pain experience of laboring women. Deductive reasoning is the framework for quantitative research studies.

Both frameworks are important in the development of knowledge. Based on the question being asked, the researcher will select either an inductive or deductive stance.

RELATIONSHIP OF THEORY TO RESEARCH

*I*n addition to understanding the framework from which the researcher enters the research enterprise, it is important to be aware of the relationship of theory to research—specifically, qualitative research. The issue of theory and qualitative research comes up regularly in the literature. The difficulty for the neophyte qualitative researcher is determining what is meant when the statement is made that qualitative research is atheoretical when, on further reading, the researcher discovers debates in the literature that speak to all knowledge being theoretically based. The best way to begin to understand the debate is to understand the language. What exactly is theory? According to Chinn and Kramer (2004), a theory is "a creative and rigorous structuring of ideas that projects a tentative, purposeful, and systematic view of phenomena" (p. 91). The purpose of research is to explain, predict, or control outcomes. In the qualitative research paradigm, the focus is on understanding. Consequently, many qualitative researchers espouse the importance of maintaining an atheoretical stance to their research. The question to be raised is this: Is there a debate, or is there reason to believe that the debate arises from differences in interpretation?

Thomas (2002) offers that the definitional boundaries of the term *theory* have been expanded to the point that any *reasoned* discussion is labeled theory (p. 420). Some would argue that the debate is better described as a conflict of definitions or interpretations. Fawcett (2000) defined *philosophy* as "a statement encompassing ontological claims about the phenomena of central interest to a discipline, epistemic claims about how those phenomena come to be known, and ethical claims about what the members of a discipline value" (p. 6). Fawcett's definition supports philosophy as a higher level of abstraction than theory. Fawcett further shares that the purpose of a philosophy is "to inform the members of disciplines and the general public about the beliefs and values of a particular discipline" (p. 6). One of the ways to manage the interpretive debate is to adopt Fawcett's hierarchical structure regarding philosophy and theory.

Often, to further illustrate the point, qualitative researchers subscribe to a particular school of thought regarding their research based on the specific philosophical position they believe most closely aligns with their personal understanding. For instance, in phenomenology there are two sets of ideas about approaching understanding phenomena: descriptive and hermeneutic. Both of these traditions arise out of a rich history of inquiry into understanding the human phenomena by different phenomenologists. The purpose of subscribing to one school or the other is not to explain, predict, or control particular phenomena but rather to understand the phenomena using a particular set of guiding principles. The purpose of using these principles is to structure the design of the inquiry, not to prove that they are right or wrong.

Chinn and Kramer's (2004) definition of theory is not useful in qualitative research if it is viewed as the "creative and rigorous structuring of ideas that projects a tentative, purposeful, and systematic view of phenomena" (p. 91). Not everything studied by qualitative researchers can be viewed in this systematized way. However, the information discovered as part of a qualitative inquiry may lead to the development of yet unknown theories. Not all qualitative research studies lead to theory development, but certainly specific approaches used in qualitative research can lead to theory development. Grounded theory is an example of such an approach (see Chapter 7). In grounded theory, the researcher's goal is to develop theory to describe a particular social process.

As an example of how a study may lead to theory development, Wuest and Merritt-Gray (2008) used grounded theory methodology to develop a substantive theory of the pattern of abusive control with three subprocesses, counteracting abuse, taking control, and living differently. This study clearly demonstrates the potential use of qualitative research for theory development.

The point of offering the debate about theory to the reader is to place the role of theory development within the context of qualitative research and to help the nurse new to qualitative research begin to understand what on the surface appears to be a contradiction. It is generally accepted that qualitative research findings have the potential to create theory. In the instance of grounded theory, the method is dedicated to the discovery of theory.

With regard to theoretical points of view attributed to specific methods, the reader needs to understand that the term *theory* is used by a variety of authors in many different ways. The term *theory* requires the same degree of scrutiny that many other frequently used and misused terms require. In addition, full disclosure by those using the term is needed so that those interested in understanding the debate have the information required to approach it logically.

Objective Versus Subjective Data Within a Nursing Context

Empirical scientists believe that the study of any phenomena must be devoid of subjectivity (Namenwirth, 1986). Furthermore, they have contended that objectivity is essential in guiding the way to truth. The problem with this position is that no human activity can be performed without subjectivity. Researchers, as well as those being studied, think and act based on their subjective interpretations of the world. It is important in quantitative research to make the study as objective as possible. However, it is critical to understand that no research activity is ever totally without its subjective components.

Based on his reading and interpretation of Hanson (1958), Phillips (1987) suggested that objectivity is impossible: "The theory, hypothesis, framework, or background knowledge held by an investigator can strongly influence what he sees" (p. 9). Kerlinger (1979) also proposed that "the procedures of science are objective and not the scientists. Scientists, like all men and women, are opinionated, dogmatic, and ideological" (p. 264). Therefore, the idea of objectivity loses its meaning. On some level, all research endeavors have the subjective influence of the scientist. Procedural objectivity is the goal; however, even this is biased because the scientist will interpret the findings. Even if the findings of a study are statistical (thought to be an objective measure), the scientist interprets the statistical data through a lens of opinions and biases about what the numbers say (MacKenzie, 1981; Taylor, 1985).

Humanistic scientists value the subjective component of the quest for knowledge. They embrace the idea of subjectivity, recognizing that humans are incapable of total objectivity because they have been situated in a reality constructed by subjective experiences. Meaning, and therefore the search for the truth, is possible only through social observation and interaction. The degree to which the scientist is part of the development of scientific knowledge is debated even by the humanistic scientists. Postempiricists accept the subjective nature of inquiry but still support rigor and objective study through method. The objectivity postempiricists speak of is one of context. For example, postempiricist scientists would acknowledge their subjective realities and then, always being aware of them, seek to keep them apart from data collection but to include them in the analysis and the final report.

Constructivist humanistic scientists believe that "knowledge is the result of a dialogical process between the self-understanding person and that which is encountered—whether a text, a work of art, or the meaningful expression of another person" (Smith, 1990, p. 177). Clearly, subjectivity is acknowledged, but the degree to which it is embraced is based on philosophic beliefs.

Humanistic scientists see objectivity in its empirical definition to be impossible. The degree to which a researcher can be objective, and therefore unbiased, is determined by the philosophic tradition to which the human scientist ascribes. This subjectivity which is included in the discussion of human science conveys an understanding that participation in the world prohibits humans from ever being fully objective.

Nurse researchers engaged in qualitative research recognize the subjective reality inherent in the research process and embrace it. They are bound by method to acknowledge their subjectivity and to place it in a context that permits full examination of the effect of subjectivity on the research endeavor and description of the phenomenon under study.

GROUNDING RESEARCH IN THE REALITIES OF NURSING

Nurse scientists have the responsibility of developing new knowledge. Fawcett (1999) offers that nursing needs three types of research: basic, applied, and clinical. The question that needs answering will drive the research type and paradigm selected. If a nurse scientist is interested in discovering the most effective way to suction a tracheostomy tube, then a quantitative approach will be the appropriate way to study the problem. But, if the nurse scientist is interested in discovering what the experience of suctioning is for people who are suctioned, qualitative research methods are more appropriate. What the nurse scientist must do is clearly define the problem and then identify whether it requires an inductive or deductive approach. Only the researcher can determine what the explicit question is and how best to answer it. As Lincoln (1992) pointed out, the area of health research is open to inquiry, and the qualitative model is a superior choice over conventional methods.

Emancipation

In recent years, much has been written about "emancipatory research" (Henderson, 1995). Two predominant paradigms permeate what is published: critical theory and feminist theory. *Critical theory*, as described by Habermas (1971), is a way to develop knowledge that is free, undistorted, and unconstrained. According to Habermas, the predominant paradigm in science was not reflective of people's reality. He found that empiricism created cognitive dissonance. The goal of critical theory is to "unfreeze lawlike structures and to encourage self reflections for those whom the laws are about" (Wilson-Thomas, 1995, p. 573). "Critical [theorists] . . . sought to expose oppressive relationships among groups and to enlighten those who are oppressed" (Bent, 1993, p. 296).

Similarly, *feminist theory* takes the idea of emancipation further and speaks specifically to women's lives. Feminist theorists value women and women's experiences (Hall & Stevens, 1991). Feminist scholars believe that the traditional laws of science limit and preclude the discovery of what is uniquely feminist. Seibold (2000) identifies feminist research as being focused first and foremost on women's experiences. Feminist researchers attempt to see the world from the view of the women studied and to be critical in examination of the issues and active in improving the condition of those studied.

In both paradigms, the predominant themes are liberating the study participants and making their voices heard. Sigsworth (1995) identified seven fundamental conditions that are necessary for feminist research that, when examined, are appropriate for critical theorist ideas about research as well. These conditions are as follows: (1) the research should be focused on the experiences of the population studied, their perceptions, and their truths; (2) "artificial dichotomies and sharp boundaries are suspect in research involving human beings" (Sigsworth, 1995, p. 897); (3) history and concurrent events are always considered when planning, conducting, analyzing, and interpreting findings; (4) the questions asked are as important as the answers discovered; (5) research should not be hierarchical; (6) researchers' assumptions, biases, and presuppositions are part of the research enterprise; and (7) researchers and research participants are partners whose discoveries lead to understanding.

According to Hall and Stevens (1991), qualitative methods are more in line with the feminist perspective, as well as with critical theorist ideas. The tenets offered earlier are primary in conducting a study regardless of the methodology used. However, by their stated purposes, the methods of qualitative research are far more accommodating to the ideas supported by critical and feminist theorists. Researchers who wish their work to be emancipating and liberating should consider the methods of qualitative research described in this text.

SUMMARY

*I*n this chapter, the fundamentals of qualitative research as a specific research paradigm have been described. Every attempt has been made to offer to the reader varied ideas on each of the topics covered. An explanation of science, philosophy, and theory grounds some of the more rigorously debated ideas in qualitative research. Understanding how individuals acquire knowledge and use their experience to develop their approaches to inquiry helps the reader to value differing research paradigms. Equally important is an understanding that no single paradigm will answer all the questions important to nursing. It is only through use of both qualitative and quantitative research methods that we will come to a better understanding of human beings and their health. The debate about the value of qualitative research in pursuit of EB practice will continue. As such, the qualitative researcher must be comfortable in his/her understanding of the fundamental construction, purpose, and outcomes of the methods included in the qualitative research paradigm.

The information presented in this chapter also included the relationship of historical, practical, and theoretical ideas about qualitative research. It is hoped that these ideas have piqued the reader's interest and will lead to exploration of the specifics of qualitative research as they are developed in this text.

References

Anderson, E. (2004). Feminist epistemology and philosophy of science. In E. N. Zalta (Ed.), *The Stanford encyclopedia of philosophy* (Summer 2004 Edition). Retrieved August 10, 2005, from http://plato.stanford.edu/archives/sum2004/entries/feminism-epistemology/

Benner, P. (1984). *From novice to expert.* Menlo Park, CA: Addison-Wesley.

Bent, K. N. (1993). Perspectives on critical and feminist theory in developing nursing praxis. *Journal of Professional Nursing, 9*(5), 296–303.

Burnard, P., & Hannigan, B. (2000). Qualitative and quantitative approaches in mental health nursing: Moving the debate forward. *Journal of Psychiatric and Mental Health Nursing, 7,* 1–6.

Carper, B. (1978). Fundamental patterns of knowing in nursing. *Advances in Nursing Science, 1*(1), 13–23.

Chinn, P. L., & Kramer, M. K. (2004). *Integrated knowledge development in nursing* (6th ed.). St. Louis: Mosby.

Cochrane, A. L. (1989). *Effectiveness and efficiency: Random reflections on health services.* London: British Medical Journal.

Denzin, N. K., & Lincoln, Y. S. (Eds.). (1994). *Handbook of qualitative research.* Thousand Oaks, CA: Sage.

Ermath, M. (1978). *Wilhelm Dilthey: The critique of historical reason.* Chicago: University of Chicago Press.

Fawcett, J. (1999). The state of nursing science: Hallmarks of the 20th and 21st centuries. *Nursing Science Quarterly, 12*(4), 311–318.

Fawcett, J. (2000). *Analysis and evaluation of contemporary nursing knowledge: Nursing theories and models.* Philadelphia: F. A. Davis.

Flemming, K. (2007). Synthesis of qualitative research and evidence-based nursing. *British Journal of Nursing, 16*(10), 616–620.

Guba, E. G. (1990). *The paradigm dialogue.* Newbury Park, CA: Sage.

Grypdonck, M. H. F. (2006). Qualitative health research in the era of evidence-based practice. *Qualitative Health Research, 16*(10), 1371–1385.

Guiliano, K. K. (2003). Expanding the use of empiricism in nursing: Can we bridge the gap between knowledge and clinical practice? *Nursing Philosophy, 4,* 44–52.

Habermas, J. (1971). *Knowledge and human interests* (J. J. Strapiro, trans.). Boston: Beacon Press..

Hall, J. M., & Stevens, P. E. (1991). Rigour in feminist research. *Advances in Nursing Science, 22*(3), 16–29.

Hamilton, D. (1994). Traditions, preferences, and postures in applied qualitative research. In N. K. Denzin & Y. S. Lincoln (Eds.), *Handbook of qualitative research* (pp. 60–69). Thousand Oaks, CA: Sage.

Hanson, N. R. (1958). *Patterns of discovery.* Cambridge: Cambridge University Press.

Haynes, B. (2007). Of studies, syntheses, synopses, summaries, and systems: The "5S" evolution of services for evidenced-based healthcare decisions. *Evidenced Based Nursing, 10*(1), 6–7.

Henderson, D. J. (1995). Consciousness raising in participatory research: Method and methodology for emancipatory inquiry. *Advances in Nursing Science, 17*(3), 58–69.

Kerlinger, F. N. (1979). *Behavioral research: A conceptual approach.* New York: Holt, Rinehart & Winston.

Krasner, D. L. (2000). Qualitative research: A different paradigm—part 1. *Journal of Wound, Ostomy and Continence Nursing, 28,* 70–72.

Liehr, P., & Smith, M. J. (2002). Theoretical frameworks. In G. LoBiondo-Wood & J. Haber (Eds.), *Nursing research: Methods, critical appraisal, and utilization* (5th ed., pp. 107–120). St. Louis: Mosby.

Lincoln, Y. S. (1992). Sympathetic connections between qualitative methods and health research. *Qualitative Health Research, 2*(4), 375–391.

MacKenzie, D. (1981). *Statistics in Great Britain: 1885–1930.* Edinburgh, UK: Edinburgh University Press.

Mantzoukas, S. (2008). A review of evidence-based practice, nursing research and reflection: Levelling the hierarchy. *Journal of Clinical Nursing, 17*(2), 214–223.

May, K. A. (1994). Abstract knowing: The case for magic in method. In J. Morse (Ed.), *Critical issues in qualitative research methods* (pp. 10–21). Thousand Oaks, CA: Sage.

Melnyk, B. M., & Fineout-Overholt, E. (2005). *Evidence-based practice in nursing and healthcare.* Philadelphia: Lippincott.

Mitchell, G. J. (2001). Prescription, freedom, and participation: Drilling down into theory-based nursing practice. *Nursing Science Quarterly, 14*(3), 205–210.

Morse, J. M. (2006a). The politics of evidence. *Qualitative Health Research, 16*(3), 395–404.

Morse, J. M. (2006b). Reconceptualizing qualitative research. *Qualitative Health Research, 16*(93), 415–422.

Munhall, P. L. (2001). Epistemology in nursing. In P. L. Munhall (Ed.), *Nursing research: A qualitative perspective* (pp. 37–64). Boston: Jones and Bartlett.

Namenwirth, M. (1986). Science seen through a feminist prism. In R. Bleier (Ed.), *Feminist approaches to science* (pp. 18–41). New York: Pergamon Press.

Parse, R. R. (2001). *Qualitative inquiry: The path of sciencing.* Boston: Jones and Bartlett.

Phillips, D. C. (1987). *Philosophy, science, and social inquiry.* New York: Pergamon Press.

Sandelowski, M. (1994). The proof is in the pottery: Toward a poetic for qualitative inquiry. In J. Morse (Ed.), *Critical issues in qualitative research methods* (pp. 44–62). Thousand Oaks, CA: Sage.

Seibold, C. (2000). Qualitative research from a feminist perspective in the postmodern era: Methodological, ethical and reflexive concerns. *Nursing Inquiry, 7*(3), 147–155.

Siepmann, J. P. (1999). What is science? *Journal of Theoretics, 1–3.* Retrieved August 5, 2004, from http://www.journaloftheoretics.com/Editorials/Vol-1/e1-3.htm

Sigsworth, J. (1995). Feminist research: Its relevance to nursing. *Journal of Advanced Nursing, 22,* 896–899.

Smith, J. K. (1990). Alternative research paradigms and the problem of criteria. In E. G. Guba (Ed.), *The paradigm dialogue* (pp. 167–187). Newbury Park, CA: Sage.

Taylor, C. (1985). *Human agency and language.* Cambridge, UK: Cambridge University Press.

Thomas, G. (2002). Theory's spell-on qualitative inquiry and educational research. *British Educational Research Journal, 28*(3), 419–434.

Thorne, S. (1997). Phenomenological positivism and other problematic trends in health science research. *Qualitative Health Research, 7*(2), 287–293.

Wainwright, P. (2000). Towards an aesthetics of nursing. *Journal of Advanced Nursing, 32*(3), 750–756.

Wilson-Thomas, L. (1995). Applying critical social theory in nursing education to bridge the gap between theory, research and practice. *Journal of Advanced Nursing, 21,* 568–575.

Wuest, J., & Merritt-Gray, M. (2008). A theoretical understanding of abusive intimate partner relationships that become non-violent: Shifting the pattern of abusive control. *Journal of Family Violence, 23*(4), 281–293.

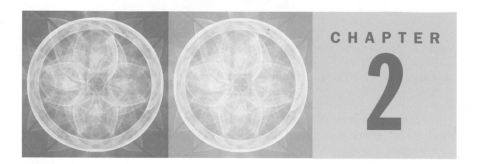

The Conduct of Qualitative Research: Common Essential Elements

*E*videnced-based practice drives much of our health-related inquiry. As the push for evidence increases, questions surface regarding the "fit" of qualitative inquiry in the current era of research. The nurse researcher seeking to use qualitative inquiry must clearly understand the motivation for choosing qualitative research methods. Is the researcher selecting the method to address a political agenda, funding priorities, or to some other externally driven foci? It remains primary that nurses focus on development of nursing knowledge. And because the time and energy required to conduct research are significant, it should be work that nurse researchers are deeply interested in. Therefore, doing qualitative research to advance an important question that has meaning for the researcher is essential. Volante (2008) offers that there is much complexity in nursing and nursing research and that there has been a shift from focusing on individuals to studying the "in-between of the action and interaction of everyday life" which necessitates that researchers reflect and share both their findings and philosophical propositions in an effort to produce evidence (p. 5).

As the conversation regarding best practices and evidence-based interventions continues, it will be important to clearly identify the value of qualitatively derived interventions. Morse (2006) provides six broad areas of qualitative inquiry that can be used to identify, apply, and test interventions (p. 591). These are offered to assist the researcher in understanding the value of qualitative research in developing and testing nursing interventions.

1. Qualitative inquiry provides a theoretical foundation for nursing interventions, so that affective interventions are theory driven.
2. Qualitative inquiry provides a means for identifying covert interventions.
3. Qualitative inquiry is a means for making standard interventions more than a mechanical task.
4. Qualitative inquiry enables increasing the scope of practice by identifying the scope of practice.
5. Qualitative theory expands the definition of "interventions" to include theoretical approaches and qualitatively derived theory.
6. Qualitative methods enable the assessment of interventions (Morse, 2006, pp. 591–593).

Nurse researchers spend significant time developing their research questions and clarifying what it is they are planning to study. It is important that research studies be based on sound rationale and a clear understanding of the research question. Denzin (2000) suggests that in addition to carefully developing the research question, researchers must also examine the political nature of their work. All research represents a political enterprise that carries significant implications. The more nurses understand the motivating factors involved in their work, the more explicit they can be about its benefits.

Once the research question is clearly articulated and the researcher has an understanding of the problem and what impact the research activity will have on those studied, the discipline, and those to whom the results may be meaningful, the researcher will need to decide which research paradigm will most appropriately answer the question. This chapter offers the reasons for choosing a qualitative approach to inquiry, describes the common elements of the qualitative research process, and shares with the reader very practical information regarding how to enter the field. Based on this overview of the important aspects of qualitative research, readers will be able to assess whether qualitative inquiry offers an opportunity to explore the questions that arise from their practice.

Undoubtedly, to fully engage in one of the methods discussed in this book, the reader will need a solid understanding of the method and its assumptions. In addition, it is essential to engage a research mentor (Morse, 1997). As Morse has offered, one cannot learn to drive a car by reading the manual; hence, the researcher should not assume that one could conduct a qualitative study by reading this or any other qualitative research text. A mentor will make "shifting gears" a more effective process.

INITIATING THE STUDY: CHOOSING A QUALITATIVE APPROACH

Exploring the Common Characteristics of Qualitative Research

In the conduct of research, certain attributes are common to the discovery process. This is true of both qualitative and quantitative designs. This section explores those common characteristics of qualitative research. Table 2-1 offers a comparison of qualitative and quantitative methods.

Qualitative researchers emphasize six significant characteristics in their research: (1) a belief in multiple realities; (2) a commitment to identifying an approach to understanding that supports the phenomenon studied; (3) a commitment to the participant's viewpoint; (4) the conduct of inquiry in a way that limits disruption of the natural context of the phenomena of interest; (5) acknowledged participation of the researcher in the research process; and (6) the reporting of the data in a literary style rich with participant commentaries.

The idea that multiple realities exist and create meaning for the individuals studied is a fundamental belief of qualitative researchers. "Qualitative researchers direct their attention to human realities rather than to the concrete realities of objects" (Boyd, 2001, p. 76). Instead of searching for one reality—one truth—researchers committed to qualitative research believe that individuals actively participate in social actions, and through these interactions that occur based on previous experiences, individuals come to know and understand phenomena in different ways. Because people do understand and live experiences differently, qualitative researchers do not subscribe to one truth but, rather, to many truths. Qualitative researchers believe that there are always multiple realities (perspectives) to consider when trying to fully understand a situation (Boyd, 2001).

Table 2-1 • Comparison of Quantitative and Qualitative Research Methods	
Quantitative	*Qualitative*
Objective	Subjectivity valued
One reality	Multiple realities
Reduction, control, prediction	Discovery, description, understanding
Measurable	Interpretative
Mechanistic	Organismic
Parts equal the whole	Whole is greater than the parts
Report statistical analyses	Report rich narrative
Researcher separate	Researcher part of research process
Subjects	Participants
Context free	Context dependent

Qualitative researchers are committed to discovery through the use of multiple ways of understanding. These researchers address questions about particular phenomena by finding an appropriate method or approach to answer the research question. The question leads the choice of method rather than the method leading the question. In some cases, more than one qualitative approach or more than one data collection strategy may be necessary to fully understand a phenomenon. For example, in a study of the culture of Taiwanese nursing homes, Chuang and Abbey (2009) used participant observation, in-depth interviews, and examination of related documents to understand nursing home life for older residents. All the data were recorded in either field notes or verbatim to determine how nursing home residents view their day-to-day living situation. The interviews provided the researcher with individual perceptions of the culture of the nursing home. The participant observations and document review offered additional data to further the understanding of culture of a Taiwanese nursing home. In this instance and in other qualitative research studies, researchers are committed to *discovery*. The discovery process in qualitative research provides the opportunity for variation in the use of data collection strategies. Method and data collection strategies may change as needed, rather than being prescribed before the inquiry begins. As Maggs-Rapport (2000) suggests, "there are benefits to be derived from an approach which combines . . . methods and methodologies, provided that methodological rigor is applied without compromising the underlying value of any one methodology" (p. 224). This process differs from the way traditional or positivist science is developed.

Commitment to participants' viewpoints is another characteristic of qualitative research. Use of unstructured interview, observation, and artifacts grounds researchers in the real life of study participants. Researchers are co-participants in discovery and understanding of the realities of the phenomena studied. Qualitative researchers will conduct extensive interviews and observations, searching documents, and artifacts of importance to fully understand the context of what is researched. Context is critical to authenticating participants' descriptions. As Topping (2006) offers, "to strip the context from the study is to remove the person from the place where the experience was enacted and hence devalue the understanding gained from the experience" (p. 6).

The purpose of the extensive investigation is to provide a view of reality that is important to the study participants, rather than to the researchers. For example, in an ethnography completed by Hunter, Spence, McKenna, & Iedema (2008), the authors were interested in learning how nurses learned from each other in the neonatal intensive care unit (NICU). Hunter et al. (2008) spent 12 months in fieldwork conducting observations and in-depth interviews with nurses, doctors, and allied health clinicians in the 20-bed NICU in order to fully understand the ways that clinicians learn from each other. Their findings offer a perspective on the very complex environment in which nurses practicing in the NICU in Australia find themselves. Their research closely examines social interaction that is so important in understanding the context of learning and the transfer of knowledge that ultimately leads to higher quality nursing practice (p. 664).

Another characteristic of qualitative research is conduct of the inquiry in a way that does not disturb the natural context of the phenomena studied. Researchers are obligated to conduct a study in a manner that least disturbs the natural setting. Using ethnographic research to illustrate this characteristic, the ethnographer would study a particular culture with as little intrusion as possible. Living among study participants is one way to minimize the intrusion and maintain the natural context of the setting. It is unrealistic to believe that the introduction of an unknown individual will not change the nature of the relationships and activities observed; however, the researcher's prolonged presence should minimize the effect of the intrusion.

All research affects the study participants in some way. The addition of any new person or experience changes the way people think or act. The important factor in qualitative research that makes the difference is the serious attention to discovering the *emic view*, that is, the insider's perspective. What is it like for the participant? Qualitative researchers explore the insider's view with utmost respect for the individual's perspective and his or her space. As stated earlier, prolonged engagement by the researcher has the effect of reducing overt changes in behavior of those studied. Therefore, a nurse interested in conducting a qualitative study must provide adequate time for building a trusting relationship and eliminating the distractions created by introducing someone new in the setting.

Researcher as instrument is another characteristic of qualitative research. The use of the researcher as instrument requires an acceptance that the researcher is part of the study. Because the researcher is the observer, interviewer, or the interpreter of various aspects of the inquiry, objectivity serves no purpose. Qualitative investigators accept that all research is conducted with a subjective bias. They further believe that researcher participation in the inquiry has the potential to add to the richness of data collection and analysis. Objectivity is a principle in quantitative research that documents the rigor of the science. In qualitative research, rigor is most often determined by the study participants and consumers of the study. From the participants' points of view: Do they recognize what the researcher has reported to be their culture or experience? From the consumer's perspective: Does the researcher stay true to the participants' expressions of their experience? Is enough evidence provided so that the consumer can assess this? The acknowledgment of the subjective nature of qualitative research and the understanding that researchers affect what is studied are fundamental to the conduct of qualitative inquiry.

Regardless of the approach, qualitative researchers will report the study findings in a rich literary style. Participants' experiences are the findings of qualitative research. Therefore, it is essential these experiences be reported from the perspective of the people who have lived them. Inclusion of quotations, commentaries, and narratives adds to the richness of the report and to the understanding of the experience and context in which they occur. Table 2-1 describes the contrasts between quantitative and qualitative research.

These six characteristics guide qualitative researchers on a journey of exploration and discovery. Doing qualitative research is similar to reading a good novel. When conducted in the spirit of the philosophy that supports it, qualitative research is rich and rewarding, leaving researchers and consumers with a desire to understand more about the phenomena of interest.

Selecting the Method Based on Phenomenon of Interest

Agreement with the basic tenets of qualitative research is the first step in deciding whether to initiate a qualitative research study. Once researchers understand that these essential elements will guide all that they do, they can begin to explore various qualitative methods. It is important to note that all qualitative approaches "share a similar goal in that they seek to arrive at an understanding of a particular phenomenon from the perspective of those experiencing the phenomenon" (Woodgate, 2000, p. 194). What the researcher will need to determine is which approach will answer the research question. The choice of method depends on the question being asked.

Because each method is explained in depth in the following chapters, the examples that follow serve only as an introduction to method selection based on the phenomena of interest. While reading the examples, keep in mind that the qualitative nurse researcher is more concerned with values, beliefs, and meaning attached to health and illness than to aggregates of conditions (Hayes, 2001).

For example, a nurse educator working in the community health setting finds her students reluctant to engage clients despite adequate knowledge of the students' previous successes in communicating with patients. There is something about the individual students' behaviors that has her perplexed. The method she selects is phenomenology. The purpose of phenomenology is to explore the lived experience of individuals. Phenomenology provides researchers with the framework for discovering what it is like to live an experience. Using this method, she can interview each of the students and begin to understand what their lived experience of community health is.

If the nurse researcher is interested in the community health agency in which her students work, given the outstanding community health practiced in the agency as well as its political antecedents, a historical inquiry is the research approach of choice. For a historical study, review of institutional documents such as meeting minutes, policy manuals in addition to community meeting minutes, personal documents, diaries, research papers and proceedings, newspaper articles, commentaries, narratives, and personal interviews will provide the necessary information to chronicle the contribution the agency has made in the care of community.

Another related question that might be important to answer is the following: What is it like to make decisions to improve community health in times of diminishing resources? Based on the preceding comments, phenomenology may be the method of choice; however, assume that it is not the experience of being a nurse in the agency that is of interest to the researcher but, rather, the process that the administration goes through to arrive at the decision about how best to allocate limited resources. In this case, the research method selected would be grounded theory. The researcher is more interested in understanding the process of choosing between multiple, competing demands for resources rather than what the individual nurse experiences as a result of working with limited resources. The purpose of the inquiry is what drives the choice of method. More specifically, the grounded theory researcher interested in the process of choosing among competing priorities in difficult financial times is committed to developing a theory, that being, understanding the process that the agency administration goes through to arrive at that decision.

In a related situation, a nurse might be interested in studying the health practices of one or more neighborhoods served by the agency. The nurse researcher would want to observe and collect information about group members, their activities, values, meaningful artifacts, and life ways, as well as participate in group sessions. In doing so, a full understanding of the culture of the neighborhood's health would become evident. In this case, ethnography would be the method of choice.

If a nurse researcher is interested in social change as it relates to community health and the ability of a selected agency to affect health outcomes for a particular neighborhood, an action research study might be the appropriate choice. By working with agency employees and neighborhood residents to study the interaction between the agency and the neighborhood and how relationship affects health outcomes, the researcher, neighborhood residents and agency employees have the potential to learn from the experiences and build on mutual successes or co-create structures to improve underserved priorities. If the researcher is committed to a collaborative research approach that facilitates participation and action, then action research is an appropriate choice. When researchers choose action research, they serve two masters: theory and practice (Jenks, 1995).

This limited description demonstrates that there are a number of research methods to address specific practice questions. Researchers need to clearly identify the focus of the inquiry and then choose the method that will most effectively answer the question.

Understanding the Philosophic Position

After researchers have identified the research question and have made explicit the approach to studying the question, a thorough understanding of the philosophic assumptions that are foundational to the method is essential. Too frequently, novice qualitative researchers develop and implement research studies without having a solid understanding of the philosophic underpinnings of the chosen method. This lack of understanding has the potential of leading to sloppy science, resulting in misunderstood findings. For instance, phenomenology is an approach that can be used to study lived experience. Based on the philosophic position supported by the researcher, different interpretations might occur. To further illustrate this point, phenomenologists who support Edmund Husserl—a prominent leader of the phenomenological movement—and his followers believe that the purpose of phenomenology is to provide pure understanding. Supporters of the philosophic positions of Martin Heidegger and his colleagues believe that phenomenology is interpretive. Neither group is incorrect; rather, each approaches the study of lived experience with different sets of goals and expectations.

The comments offered here should help the reader develop an appreciation for the importance of understanding the method chosen and its philosophic underpinnings. Making explicit the school of thought that guides an inquiry will help researchers to conduct a credible study and help those people who use the findings to apply the results within the appropriate context.

Using the Literature Review

In the development of a quantitative research study, an interested researcher would begin with an extensive literature search on the topic of interest. This review documents the necessity for the study and provides a discussion of the area of interest and related topics. It helps the researcher determine whether the planned study has been conducted, and if so, whether significant results were discovered. Furthermore, it helps the researcher refine the research question, select a theoretical framework, and build a case for why the topic of interest should be studied and how the researcher will approach the topic.

Qualitative researchers do not generally begin with an *extensive* literature review. Some qualitative researchers would suggest that no literature review should be conducted before the inquiry begins. Others accept that a cursory review of the literature may help focus the study or provide an orienting framework (Creswell, 2003, p. 30). The reason for not conducting the literature review initially is to reduce the likelihood that the investigator will develop suppositions or biases about the topic under consideration. Further, by not developing preconceived ideas about the topic, it is assumed that the researcher will be protected from leading the participants during the interviewing process in the direction of the researcher's beliefs. For instance, if a researcher is interested in developing a theory about the process a client goes through in accepting the necessity of an amputation, a review of the literature before the study might lead to the development of preconceived notions about amputees. The researcher may not have held these beliefs be-fore the review, but, following it, now has information that could affect how he or she collects and analyzes data. Creswell states, "in a qualitative study, use the literature sparingly in the beginning of the plan in order to convey an inductive design, unless the qualitative strategy-type requires a substan-tial literature orientation at the outset" (p. 33).

It is, however, essential to conduct the literature review after analyzing the data. The purpose of reviewing the literature in a qualitative study is to place the findings of the study in the context of what is already known. Generally, qualitative researchers do not use the literature review to estab-lish grounds for the study or to suggest a theoretical or conceptual frame-work. The purpose of the literature review in a qualitative study is to tell the reader how the findings fit into what is already known about the phenom-ena. It is not meant to confirm or argue existing findings.

Explicating the Researcher's Beliefs

Before starting a qualitative study, it is in the researcher's best interest to make clear his or her thoughts, ideas, suppositions, or presuppositions about the topic, as well as personal biases. The purpose of this activity is to bring to consciousness and reveal what is believed about a topic. By bring-ing to consciousness the researcher's beliefs, he or she is in a better position to approach the topic honestly and openly. Explication of personal beliefs makes the investigator more aware of the potential judgments that may occur during data collection and analysis based on the researcher's belief system rather than on the actual data collected from participants. One of the best ways to make one's beliefs known is to write them down. Writing out what one believes before actually conducting the study gives the author a frame of reference. Journaling during the time that one is engaged in the research also helps to keep an open mind and differentiate what the re-searcher's thoughts are versus the ideas, comments, and activities of the par-ticipants. As qualitative researchers conduct their studies, they can use their journal to "reality-test" what is being observed or heard against what they have written down (the researcher's ideas or presuppositions).

As an example, let's say that the topic of interest is quality of life for in-dividuals diagnosed with multiple sclerosis (MS). The researcher has an in-terest in the topic based on a long history of working with individuals with end-stage disease. Based on the researcher's experience, his or her percep-tion is that people with MS live sad, limited existences. If researchers do not explicate these perceptions, they may lead informants to describe their expe-riences in the direction of the researchers' own beliefs about what is real or important. This can occur as a result of the questions asked. In asking ques-tions, the researcher might try to validate his or her ideas about MS without really discovering the meaning of MS for those who live with it. Remember, the way the questions are worded can affect the outcome of the interview and sometimes impose answers on respondents (McDougall, 2000). The act of expressing one's ideas should help remind the researcher to listen and see what is real for the informants rather than what is real for the researcher. Schutz (1970) recommended that researchers follow this process of describing personal beliefs about their assumptions to help them refrain from making judgments about phenomena based on personal experiences.

Once the researcher has explicated his or her thoughts, feelings, and perceptions about phenomena, it is recommended that the researcher bracket those thoughts, feelings, and perceptions. *Bracketing* is the cognitive process of putting aside one's own beliefs, not making judgments about what one has observed or heard, and remaining open to data as they are revealed. Specifically, in descriptive phenomenology, this activity is carried out before the beginning of the study and is repeated throughout data collection and analysis. In ethnographic work, keeping a diary of personal thoughts and feelings is an excellent way to make clear the researcher's ideas. Once revealed, the researcher can set them aside. *Setting them aside* means to be constantly aware of what the researcher believes and trying to keep it separate from what is being shared by the informant. By conducting this self-disclosure, researchers are more likely to be able to keep their eyes open and to remain cognizant of when data collection and analysis reflect their own personal beliefs rather than informants' beliefs.

Ahern (1999) states that the process of bracketing is iterative and part of a reflexive journey. She states that it is important to process your thoughts about the phenomenon of interest. As suggested earlier, writing down your thoughts is one of the best ways to be aware of what you believe. Once they have been written down, you should reflect on what you have written and try to understand why you have written what you have, what values are inherent in your statements, and how do they affect your analysis. It is essential that the researcher be aware of the potential impact that imposing personal agendas can have on the process of data collection and analysis. Bracketing is essential if the researcher is to share the informants' views of the studied phenomena.

Choosing the Setting for Data Collection

The setting for qualitative research is the field. The *field* is the place where individuals of interest live—where they experience life. The inquiry will be conducted in the homes, neighborhoods, classrooms, or sites selected by the study participants. The reason for conducting data collection in the field is to maintain the natural settings where phenomena occur. For instance, if an investigator is interested in studying the culture of an intensive care unit (ICU), he or she will visit an ICU. If a researcher is interested in studying the clinical decision-making skills of nurses, he or she will go to nurses who use this process and ask them where they want to be interviewed or observed.

Being in the field requires reciprocity in decision making. The researcher is not in control of the study setting or those who inform the inquiry. Participants will decide what information they share with the researcher. For instance, if the researcher is interested in studying the experiences of people who live in a nursing home, he or she would need access to people who have this life situation. The researcher will then enter the setting and select appropriate individuals to interview based on specific criteria. However, because of the frailty of the participants they may not wish to share their thoughts or feelings in one sitting or at all. Visiting frequently and building a trusting relationship can help the participant feel more comfortable in sharing sensitive information and provide the element of control that may be very important to the participant. It is essential to remember that using qualitative research methods requires good interpersonal skills and a willingness to relinquish control. The mutual trust that develops based on the reciprocal nature of decision making will enhance the discovery process by allowing access to personal information and private spaces usually reserved for significant people in the lives of informants. The conduct of qualitative research with its requirement of close social interaction may create situations that can either limit or enhance access to information. The close social interaction also has the potential to create ethical dilemmas that need careful attention (see Chapter 4). Only by being aware of the distinctive nature of the interactions and being in the field will the researcher be truly aware of the strengths and potential weaknesses of this form of research.

Selecting Participants

Qualitative researchers generally do not label the individuals who inform their inquiries as *subjects*. The use of the terms *participants* or *informants* illustrates the status those studied play in the research process. "Individuals cooperating in the study play an active rather than a passive role and are therefore referred to as informants or study participants" (Polit, Beck, & Hungler, 2001, p. 31). The participants' active involvement in the inquiry helps those who are interested in their experiences or cultures to better understand their lives and social interactions.

Individuals are selected to participate in qualitative research based on their first-hand experience with a culture, social process, or phenomenon of interest. For instance, if a phenomenologist is interested in studying the culture of women with anorexia, then the informants for the study must be those women who are anorexic. The participants are selected for the purpose of describing an experience in which they have participated. Unlike quantitative research, there is no need to randomly select individuals because manipulation, control, and generalization of findings are not the intent of the inquiry. The outcome of a qualitative study should be greater understanding of the phenomena (Krasner, 2001). Therefore, the researcher interested in women who are anorexic should interview as many anorexic women as necessary to obtain a clear understanding of the culture. This type of sampling has been labeled *purposeful sampling* (Lincoln & Guba, 1985; Patton, 1990). It has also been called *purposive sampling* (Field & Morse, 1985). A similar type of sampling is *theoretical sampling* (Glaser & Strauss, 1967; Patton, 1980). Theoretical sampling, used primarily in grounded theory, is one particular type of purposeful sampling (Coyne, 1997). Theoretical sampling is a complex form of sampling based on concepts that have proven theoretical relevance to the evolving theory (Coyne, 1997; Strauss & Corbin, 1990). More specifically, Glaser (1978) states,

> Theoretical sampling is the process of data collection for generating theory whereby the analyst jointly collects, codes, and analyses his data and decides what data to collect next and where to find them in order to develop his theory as it emerges. (p. 36)

Theoretical sampling "is a valuable way of encouraging studies to develop and build on theory at an early stage" (Thompson, 1999, p. 816).

What both purposeful and theoretical sampling represent is a commitment to observing and interviewing people who have had experience with or are part of the culture or phenomenon of interest. The goal for qualitative researchers is to develop a rich or dense description of the culture or phenomenon, rather than using sampling techniques that support generalizability of the findings. A particular purposeful sampling technique is *snowballing*. Snowballing uses one informant to find another. This technique is especially useful when those you wish to interview are difficult to locate. For example, if you were interested in studying the experience of undocumented workers access to health care, it would be difficult to locate individuals willing to talk to you in one place. However, if you know of one undocumented worker who is willing to talk to you, he/she may be willing to refer you to another. Sixsmith, Boneham, and Goldring (2003) offer that although this strategy may be very helpful, it also has the drawback of potentially limiting those in your study who are from similar backgrounds.

Cohen, Phillips, and Palos (2001) discuss the value of including cultural minorities in qualitative research studies. They share that it is not only valuable to include minorities but also mandated by the National Institutes of Health. Therefore, when studying a particular culture or phenomenon, the qualitative nurse researcher should be aware of the importance and overall benefits of including minorities in the study when appropriate. Cohen and colleagues discuss the potential skepticism that may be encountered when nurses of different cultural backgrounds try to enlist members of other cultures. They suggest that nurse researchers engage diverse populations by using some of the following strategies: (1) seek endorsement and support from community leaders; (2) commit to giving back something to the group you wish to study; (3) develop an ongoing relationship of trust and respect; (4) develop cultural competence and sensitivity; (5) become well acquainted with the group before you approach them; (6) recognize the heterogeneous nature of a group; and (7) use anthropologic strategies when conducting the research (Cohen et al., 2001, p. 194).

Finally, Kirkevold and Bergland (2007) discuss the difficulty of interviewing participants with significant health problems in a traditional interview format lasting from 60 to 90 minutes. They suggest that certain populations such as those with chronic illness may not be able to sustain long, uninterrupted narratives. These authors suggest strategies such as enlarging or varying your sample; maximizing the quality of the interview; repeating the interview over days, weeks, or months; or combining interviews with observation. This may help to build the rich narrative so important in qualitative research.

Choosing the setting and participants appropriately will assist in developing a successful research study. Knowing how to access the site, knowing what to expect from those who are part of a particular group, and knowing how to most effectively develop a trusting relationship with those from whom you intend to learn will support achievement of the research goals.

Achieving Saturation

A feature that is closely related to the topic of sampling is saturation. *Saturation* refers to the repetition of discovered information and confirmation of previously collected data (Morse, 1994). This means that rather than sampling a specific number of individuals to gain significance based on statistical manipulation, the qualitative researcher is looking for repetition and confirmation of previously collected data. For example, Flinck, Astedt-Kurki, and Paavilainen (2008) were interested in describing "intimate partner violence as experienced by men and to formulate the common structure of meanings of experiences of men exposed to intimate partner violence" (p. 322). Their sample included men between 36 and 56 years who were recruited through personal contacts. Flinck et al. stated that saturation was reached when no new themes emerged. Each of the 10 participants was interviewed twice to reach this degree of closure. At the end of the 10 interviews, the researchers were able to recognize the repetition in the data and determined that the new information was surfacing. The repetitive nature of data is the point at which the researcher determines that saturation has been achieved.

Morse (1989), however, warned that saturation may be a myth. She believes that if another group of individuals were observed or interviewed at another time, new data might be revealed. The best that a qualitative researcher can hope for in terms of saturation is to saturate the specific culture or phenomenon at a particular time.

SUMMARY

In this chapter, an explanation of the commonalities of qualitative research have been offered to provide an informed framework for deciding whether qualitative research best suits you as the researcher and the research question you wish to pursue. Introduction to the process is offered to help the reader understand what the similarities and differences are between quantitative and qualitative research paradigms. The intent is to offer the reader an exposure to the processes and terms that are important to qualitative research approaches. It is essential that the reader understands and then embraces the similarities and differences in research paradigms before launching into implementation of a qualitative study. In the next chapter, a description of qualitative data generation and management will be provided to ground the reader in the language and processes of qualitative research. The intent is to offer the reader of this chapter and Chapter 3 a general understanding of qualitative research. In the chapters that follow, a more intensive description of specific approaches will be offered to more completely engage the reader in understanding many of the important qualitative research approaches.

References

Ahern, K. J. (1999). Ten tips for reflexive bracketing. *Qualitative Health Research, 9*(3), 407–412.

Boyd, C. O. (2001). Philosophical foundations of qualitative research. In P. L. Munhall (Ed.), *Nursing research: A qualitative perspective* (pp. 65–89). Sudbury, MA: Jones and Bartlett.

Chuang, Y., & Abbey, J. (2009). The culture of a Taiwanese nursing home. *Journal of Clinical Nursing, 18*(11), 1640–1648.

Cohen, M. Z., Phillips, J. M., & Palos, G. (2001). Qualitative research with diverse populations. *Seminars in Oncology Nursing, 17*(3), 190–196.

Coyne, I. T. (1997). Sampling in qualitative research. Purposeful and theoretical sampling: Merging or clear boundaries? *Journal of Advanced Nursing, 26*, 623–630.

Creswell, J. W. (2003). *Research design: Qualitative, quantitative, and mixed methods approaches* (2nd ed.). Thousand Oaks, CA: Sage.

Denzin, N. K. (2000). Aesthetics and the practice of qualitative inquiry. *Qualitative Inquiry, 6*(2), 253–265.

Field, P. A., & Morse, J. M. (1985). *Nursing research: The application of qualitative approaches*. Rockville, MD: Aspen.

Flinck, A., Astedt-Kurki, P. & Paavilainen, E. (2008). Intimate partner violence as experienced by men. *Journal of Psychiatric and Mental Health Nursing, 15*, 322–327

Glaser, B. G. (1978). *Theoretical sensitivity: Advances in the methodology of grounded theory*. Mill Valley, CA: Sociology Press.

Glaser, B. G., & Strauss, A. (1967). *The discovery of grounded theory*. Chicago: Aldine.

Hayes, P. (2001). Diversity in a global society. *Clinical Nursing Research, 10*(2), 99–101.

Hunter, C.L., Spence, K., McKenna, K., & Iedema, R. (2008). Learning how we learn: An ethnographic study in a neonatal intensive care unit. *Journal of Advanced Nursing 62*(6), 657–664.

Jenks, J. M. (1995). New generation research approaches. In H. J. Streubert & D. R. Carpenter (Eds.), *Qualitative research in nursing* (pp. 242–268). Philadelphia, PA: J. B. Lippincott.

Kirkevold, M., & Bergland, A. (2007). The quality of qualitative data: Issues to consider when interviewing participants who have difficulty providing detailed accounts of their experiences. *International Journal of Qualitative Studies on Health and Wellbeing, 2,* 68–75.

Krasner, D. L. (2001). Qualitative research: A different paradigm—part 1. *Journal of Wound, Ostomy and Continence Nurses Society, 28*(2), 70–72.

Lincoln, Y. S., & Guba, E. G. (1985). *Naturalistic inquiry.* Beverly Hills, CA: Sage.

Maggs-Rapport, F. (2000). Combining methodological approaches in research: Ethnography and interpretive phenomenology. *Journal of Advanced Nursing, 31*(1), 219–225.

McDougall, P. (2000). In-depth interviewing: The key issues of reliability and validity. *Community Practitioner, 73*(8), 722–724.

Morse, J. M. (1989). Strategies for sampling. In J. M. Morse (Ed.), *Qualitative nursing research: A contemporary dialogue* (pp. 117–131). Rockville, MD: Aspen.

Morse, J. M. (1994). Designing funded qualitative research. In N. K. Denzin & Y. S. Lincoln (Eds.), *Handbook of qualitative research* (pp. 220–235). Thousand Oaks, CA: Sage.

Morse, J. M. (1997). Learning to drive from a manual? *Qualitative Health Research, 7*(2), 181–183.

Morse, J.M. (2006). The scope of qualitatively derived clinical interventions. *Qualitative Health Research, 16*(5), 591–593.

Patton, M. Q. (1980). *Qualitative evaluation methods.* Beverly Hills, CA: Sage.

Patton, M. Q. (1990). *Qualitative evaluation and research methods.* Newbury Park, CA: Sage.

Polit, D. F., Beck, C. T., & Hungler, B. P. (2001). *Essentials of nursing research: Methods, appraisal, and utilization* (5th ed.). Philadelphia, PA: Lippincott Williams & Wilkins.

Schutz, A. (1970). *On phenomenology and social relations.* Chicago: University of Chicago Press.

Sixsmith, J., Boneham, M., & Goldring, J. E. (2003). Accessing the community: Gaining insider perspectives from the outside. *Qualitative Health Research, 13*(4), 578–589.

Strauss, A., & Corbin, J. (1990). *Basics of qualitative research: Grounded theory procedures and techniques.* Newbury Park, CA: Sage.

Thompson, C. (1999). Qualitative research into nurse decision making: Factors for consideration in theoretical sampling. *Qualitative Health Research, 9*(6), 815–828.

Topping, A. (2006). Qualitative perspectives. *Nurse Researcher, 13*(4), 4–6.

Volante, M. (2008). Qualitative research. *Nurse Researcher, 16*(1), 4–6.

Woodgate, R. (2000). Part 1: An introduction to conducting qualitative research in children with cancer. *Journal of Pediatric Oncology Nursing, 17*(4), 192–206.

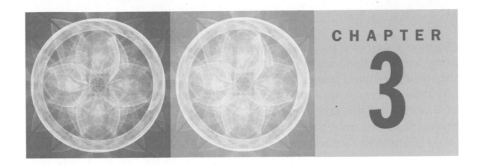

3

Designing Data Generation and Management Strategies

"*I*nquiry is . . . a dialogical process. It is a dialogue with the participants, the data [themselves], the events surrounding the research process, and the investigators as introspective individuals or as interacting team members" (Hall, 2003, p. 494). Therefore, to implement a high-quality qualitative research study, a researcher must make sure that the research question is clear, that the method selected to answer the question is appropriate, and that the people and data sources needed are available. Once this has been achieved, the researcher will then begin collecting data. Once data are collected, they must be analyzed and synthesized; conclusions will need to be drawn and practice implications stated. This chapter explores the strategies for collecting and managing data. General concepts of qualitative research are offered. The specifics of data generation and management to be used for particular qualitative approaches are offered in the chapter that follows.

GENERATING DATA

A variety of strategies can be used to generate qualitative research data: interviews, observations, narrative, and focus groups. "The reconstruction of social phenomena can come in a number of forms: video, photography, film, and text" (Maggs-Rapport, 2000, p. 221). The strategies offered in this chapter are not meant to be exhaustive but rather descriptive of the more common data collection techniques. Each researcher will need to determine, based on the question asked, the research approach selected, the sensitivity of the subject matter, and available resources, which methods of data generation are most appropriate. For example, if the researcher is interested in investigating the experiences of comfort for clients living in a nursing home, those who agree to be interviewed may be more willing to speak in a focus group than face-to-face. As the researcher, you will need to carefully assess the research goals and then match those with the best data collection strategy.

Conducting Interviews

Before entering the field to conduct interviews, researchers have to be open to their influence on the inquiry. An important term to be aware of in discussion of the researcher's role in qualitative inquiry is *reflexivity*. According to Carolan (2003), "reflexivity is a term that is widely used, with a diverse range of connotations, and sometimes with virtually no meaning at all" (p. 8). For the purpose of this chapter, reflexivity is defined as the responsibility of researchers to examine their influence in all aspects of qualitative inquiry—self-reflection. Primeau (2003) states, "reflexivity enhances the quality of research through its ability to extend our understanding of how our positions and interests as researchers affect all stages of the research process" (p. 9). The researcher's position is never fixed, it is an ongoing process of self-critique and self-appraisal (Koch, 2006). "Reflecting on the process of one's research and trying to understand how one's own values and views may influence the findings adds credibility to the research and should be part of any method of qualitative inquiry" (Jootun, McGhee, & Marland, 2009, p. 42). Once researchers are aware of the influence their ideas may have on interpretation of the findings, they can develop a mechanism to maintain a self-reflective stance. This awareness readies them to enter the field and collect data.

One of the most frequently used data collection strategies is the open-ended interview. According to experts in the field, it is the *gold* standard. Ryan, Coughlan, and Cronin (2009) describe three types of interviews; two of these are more appropriate for qualitative research than the third. The standardized interview (or structured) is mostly used in quantitative studies. It contains a preset list of questions that each research subject will be asked. The second is the semistandard (or semistructured) interview that is more flexible. Although there are guide questions, the opportunity for story telling is inherent in the format. The unstandarized (or unstructured) interview uses one or more lead questions. There is limited structure in this type of interview. Robinson (2000) states "the formal qualitative interview is an unstructured conversation with a purpose that usually features audiotape and verbatim transcription of data, and use of an interview guide rather than a rigid schedule of questions" (p. 18). According to Bianco and Carr-Chellman

(2002), "interviews range in type and length and are used for different purposes but are present in virtually all qualitative traditions" (p. 254). It is increasingly popular to conduct qualitative interviews through telephone, discussion boards, or e-mail.

For interviews to be successful, they must be interdependent by nature. Accessing closely held information will only occur if there is mutual trust and respect between researcher and informant (Perry, Thurston, & Green, 2004). When preparing to enter into the interview, the researcher must be cognizant of the fact that the outcome of the interview is an understanding of the meaning of the experience for those who are part of it. Hence, "meaning is not 'just the facts' but rather the understandings one has that are specific to the individual (what was said) yet transcendent of the specific (what is the relationship between what was said, how it was said, what the listener was attempting to ask or hear, what the speaker was attempting to convey or say)" (Dilley, 2004, p. 128). Essential to the interview process is the importance of committing oneself to fully engage in it. Interviews should not be conducted without adequate preparation and understanding of the process, its intent, and the desired outcome. In addition, Lambert and Loiselle (2008) offer some caution with regard to use of interviews, "the assumption that words are accurate indicators of participants' inner experiences' may be problematic" (p. 229). Interviewees may choose only to disclose what they think is socially acceptable. Some of the ways to reduce the effect of obtaining socially acceptable answers is through building trusting relationships, triangulating, and saturating data.

Before entering the field to conduct an interview, it is important for the researcher to consider the social and cultural context in which data will be collected (McDougall, 2000). Interviewers come with histories and cultural value systems; on many levels, the cultural and social expectations of both individuals—interviewer and interviewee—will affect what is said and what is heard. At the extreme, "differences in age, social class, race, and ethnicity between the interviewer and interviewee may inhibit rapport" (p. 722). To facilitate dialogue during data collection, the researcher needs to be aware of cultural differences and work to reduce their impact as much as possible. One of the ways suggested earlier in this text is to use the researcher's journal as a place to chronicle feelings, attitudes, and values relative to the interview process and those who will be interviewed. Another suggestion is to take the time to build rapport with those from whom you will be soliciting information. Whiting (2008) suggests that there are four phases to the interview process: apprehension, exploration, cooperative, and participation phases. Each one being very important to a complete interview. In the process of building a relationship, the researcher can assure the informants that their confidentiality will be protected.

Open-ended interviews provide participants with the opportunity to fully describe their experience. Interviews generally are conducted face-to-face. To facilitate sharing by the research participants, it is a good practice to conduct the interview in a place and at a time that is most comfortable and convenient for the participants. The more comfortable each participant is, the more likely he or she will share important information.

The actual interviews can be brief with a specific objective, such as verifying previously reported information. Or interviewing can cover a longer period, either in one sitting or over a prolonged time. A life history is an example of data collection that may continue for a long time at each sitting and also over weeks, months, or even years.

As stated earlier, the *structured interview* is one in which researchers use a set of preselected questions that they wish to have answered. Structured interviews are more likely to occur in quantitative rather than qualitative research studies. An *unstructured interview* provides the opportunity for greater latitude in the answers provided. In the unstructured interview, the researcher asks open-ended questions, such as "What is it like to care for an abusive client? Can you describe your experience for me?" In this example, there is no defined response. Using these questions, the respondent is able to move about freely in his or her description of caring for an abusive client. The unstructured interview is the preferred technique in a qualitative study.

When engaging in interviews, there are special population-specific concerns that you should be aware of. One in particular that has gained significant attention is age. Robinson (2000) and Docherty and Sandelowski (1999) have addressed interviewing the elderly and children. Robinson found in her work with institutionalized elderly that the interview had six distinct phases. These included (1) introducing; (2) personalizing; (3) reminiscing; (4) contextualizing; (5) closing; and (6) reciprocating. In describing these phases, Robinson clearly states the relevance and importance of allowing the aged individual to lead the conversation. Although interviews may take longer with the elderly, the time for sharing is well worth the richness of the data collected.

Docherty and Sandelowski (1999) offer advice on interviewing children. Based on their review of the literature, researchers should be aware that "developmental age, the target event under investigation, interview structure, multiple interviewers, and research design" (p. 183) are all factors requiring the interviewer's attention. In addition, Docherty and Sandelowski raise the issue of attention span and recall, both of which may not be directly linked to developmental age.

There are also issues around cross-cultural interviewing. This is a complex issue that researchers need to take under consideration when selecting informants. In many cases, the native language of the interviewer and the interviewee may be different thus necessitating an interpreter. The use of interpreters has received little attention in the research literature (Wallin & Ahlstrom, 2006). Those interested in using interpreters for data collection should seek out strong mentors who have experience in this area.

Videoconferencing has also been used to conduct interviews. Sedgwick and Spiers (2009) used this medium to conduct personal interviews for a focused ethnographic study whose informants were dispersed over 640,000 square kilometers in Canada. The researchers found this superior to telephone interviews because it provided the opportunity to pick up visual cues.

Regardless of the data collection strategies used, researchers need to gain access to participants. Access is an extremely important consideration when designing data collection strategies. When interviewing is the major way the researcher will collect data, it is important to determine how he or she will achieve access. The way in which researchers present themselves to prospective study participants will affect the level and type of participation provided. Sixsmith, Boneham, and Goldring (2003) suggest specific strategies for large-scale studies that may assist with access. These include (1) stakeholder analysis; (2) identification of gatekeepers; (3) snowballing; (4) advertising; (5) dispersing questionnaires in public areas that can be used by the subjects to contact researchers for interviews; (6) street interviews; and (7) the ethnographic technique of "being there."

There is a growing body of information regarding the therapeutic nature of qualitative interviews for research participants. The opportunity to give voice to an experience is a validating experience for some. The value of being heard is empowering. However, there are some experiences that are difficult to share and once shared stir up a plethora of feelings. This is particularly true for vulnerable populations. Nurse researchers, because of their education and training, sometimes struggle with when to be the researcher and when to be the nurse. Like many of the topics offered in this section on interviewing, this is yet another area the researcher needs to explore before entering the setting to conduct the interviews. Drury, Francis, and Chapman (2007) suggest that before engaging vulnerable populations, nurses would be well served to be skilled in using an ethical decision-making model to determine when to remain the researcher and when therapeutic intervention is required.

Establishing rapport once on the scene is achieved by conveying a sense of interest and concern for the research informant. The research participant must trust the researcher before he or she will feel comfortable revealing information.

Using Focus Groups

Using focus groups for data collection is another valuable strategy for qualitative researchers. A *focus group* is "a particular form of group interview intended to exploit group dynamics" (Freeman, 2006, p. 491). They are aimed at "promoting self-disclosure among participants, by explicitly capitalizing on group dynamics in discussions" (p. 492). Although focus groups as a method of data collection did not arise from a qualitative tradition, they have been found to be most useful in a number of settings, but most importantly when dealing with sensitive topics. Focus groups are particularly suited to the collection of qualitative data because they have the advantages of being inexpensive, flexible, stimulating, cumulative, elaborative, assistive in information recall, and capable of producing rich data (Fontana & Frey, 1994; MacDougall & Baum, 1997). The major disadvantage of focus groups is *groupthink*, a process that occurs when stronger members of a group or segments of the group have major control or influence over the verbalizations of other group members (Carey & Smith, 1994). Generally, a good group leader can overcome the tendency of *groupthink* if he or she is attentive to its potential throughout data collection. The advantages of a focus group as a data collection strategy outweigh the disadvantages.

Stewart, Shamdasani, and Rook (2007) identify seven common uses of focus groups: collecting background information on a particular topic; generating research hypotheses that can be tested in larger studies; stimulating new ideas and concepts; identifying problems or collecting information about products or services; generating information for instrument development; and assisting with interpretation of previously collected qualitative data. Most of these reflect the use of focus groups in nursing research. What this data collection strategy accomplishes is it provides a forum for members of the group to explore a topic with each other (Redmond & Curtis, 2009). In nursing, focus groups have been used to explore a range of topics in clinical, education, and management areas. They have also been used to collect perspectives on patients and caregivers (Webb & Doman, 2008). Curtis and Redmond (2007) believe that they are not appropriate for use when the purpose of the research is to generalize findings. Further, they are generally not suitable in situations where hierarchical relationships exist (Krueger & Casey, 2007).

Focus groups have been used to collect information on a variety of topics. They are thought to be most useful when the topic of inquiry is considered sensitive. Although the use of focus groups for sensitive topic inquiry is well documented, its overall popularity as a qualitative research data collection strategy is increasing based on many of the advantages cited earlier. Moloney, Dietrich, Strickland, and Myerburg (2003) recommend virtual focus groups, which use computer-mediated communications such as e-mail. Moloney and colleagues differentiate virtual focus groups into two types: discussion boards and chat rooms. Discussion boards refer to "an on-going site where participants are free to log on at any time, read others' postings, and post their own thoughts" (p. 275). Chat rooms refer to "a discussion site that functions in real time, where participants log on at a specific time and converse back and forth . . . instant messenger is a type of a chat room" (p. 275). Researchers should exercise caution, however, when using e-mail as an information exchange medium because anonymity can be compromised. (See Chapter 4 for an expanded discussion of the ethical issues relevant to data collected through the Internet.) If the internet is being considered as the medium for a focus group, the researcher must carefully weigh the complex issues that arise when working in cyberspace.

As stated, there are important considerations before you choose focus group as a data collection strategy. A good focus group session has the potential for learning about both the *focus* and the *group* (Kidd & Parshall, 2000). To do so, the group facilitator must have a solid understanding of group process (Joseph, Griffin, & Sullivan, 2000) and should collect data with at least one other researcher/facilitator (Kidd & Parshall, 2000). Hudson (2003) offers three distinct segments of focus groups: introducing the group, conducting the group, and closing the group. Those planning to use focus groups should be well versed in what each part requires.

In addition, when deciding who should attend a focus group, the researcher must be certain that the people invited to participate "have a shared trait or experience on which the discussion can build" (Lucasey, 2000). Group size should be between 6 and 10 members. Larger group size may preclude everyone from having a chance to speak. Smaller group size may make group members feel as though they cannot speak freely or have to speak when they have nothing to offer.

Recording of focus group data can be problematic and is another area that should be seriously considered before the decision is made to use this strategy for data collection. A number of authors address the complexity of transcribing recorded data when the data are being generated during a focus group. Location of the microphone, intonation, participants talking at the same time, and mechanical difficulties can all preclude complete and accurate data transcription. Fernandez and Griffiths (2007) suggest the use of portable MP3 players to enhance audio recording. The clarity, usability, and storage capabilities surpass conventional tape recorders. Joseph et al. (2000) advocate the use of videotaping as a method of data documentation during focus group activity. Videotaping has proved successful particularly with children's focus groups (Kennedy, Kools, & Krueger, 2001). Videotaping has the advantage of providing a complete recording of an individual's statement, group interaction, and individual behavior; however, it also can be viewed as intrusive and a violation of privacy. Researchers interested in using videotaping will need to consider the positives and negatives of its use.

When videotaping is not possible, Halcomb et al. (2007) recommend two experienced researchers be present at each session. One person who will lead or facilitate the session and a second who will assume the role of notetaker. These authors point out that the note-taker is invaluable in recording nonverbal communication that is lost in audiotaping.

More recently, attention has been directed at the reliability and validity of focus group data. Kidd and Parshall (2000) state that there are three criteria of reliability: stability, equivalence, and internal consistency. *Stability* refers to the consistency of issues over time. Stability becomes an important issue when group membership changes from one meeting of the group to the next.

Equivalence is a term used to describe the consistency of the moderators or coders of the focus group (Kidd & Parshall, 2000). It is essential that, to the extent possible, the same moderator lead the discussion with one group and across groups and that one researcher play a predominant role in analysis. *Internal consistency* of coding relates to the importance of having one team member assume the major responsibility for conducting the analysis, participating in as many groups and debriefings as possible, and communicating regularly with other team members as the analysis proceeds (Kidd & Parshall, 2000, p. 302).

Validity is used by Kidd and Parshall (2000) to describe a form of content validity. In other words, how convinced is the researcher that what the participants have shared is valid information? Paying careful attention to the composition of the group and interviews across groups with similar experiences are two ways to attend to validity of the data when using focus groups.

"The history of focus groups suggests that they were not originally conceived as a stand-alone method" (Kidd & Parshall, 2000). Therefore, to enhance the findings of a study that uses focus groups, the researcher should be prepared to consider using data triangulation. (For a full description of data triangulation, the reader is referred to Chapter 15.) Although not specifically related to validity, Traulsen, Almarsdottir, and Bjornsdottir (2004) have suggested interviewing the focus group moderator as a method to add "a new and valuable dimension to group interview" (p. 714). The purposes of interviewing the moderator include (1) offering information about group interaction and behavior; (2) effectively providing feedback on the research; (3) serving as an additional data point for the final analysis; and (4) adding to the richness of the data specifically about activity/conversation that occurs when the tape or video recorder is not running (Traulsen et al., 2004). The opportunity for other members of the research team to interview the moderator has important potential in adding to the study.

Using Written Narratives

Written responses by qualitative research participants are not new as a data collection strategy. Many researchers prefer written narratives to the spoken word because such narratives permit participants to think about what they wish to share. In addition, written narratives reduce costs by eliminating transcription requirements for audiotape interviews. The disadvantage of written narratives is the lack of spontaneity in responses that may occur. The popularity of the written narrative suggests it has proved an effective means of collecting qualitative research data.

In using written narratives, it becomes extremely important to be clear about what it is that researchers wish the participants to write about. Because the researcher often is not present during the actual writing, it is essential that directions be focused to obtain the desired information. Researchers may need to establish mechanisms to request clarification in the event that the written document provided is unclear.

More recently, the nursing literature includes the term *narrative analysis*. Narrative analysis has been addressed primarily as a research method. Bailey (1996) defines narrative analysis as "the systematic study of stories commonly found in ethnographic interviews" (p. 187). Eaves and Kahn (2000) further share that the "terms narrative and story are used interchangeably and refer to any spoken or written presentation that includes a recounting of events that follow each other in time . . . Narrative explains by clarifying the importance of events that have taken place based on the outcome that has resulted" (p. 29).

The terms *narrative analysis* and *narrative*, as described here, refer to a data collection strategy and are **not** interchangeable concepts. Researchers interested in narrative analysis should read the works of Polkinghorne (1988) and Riessman (1993) to gain a clear understanding of this valuable research methodology. Narrative as referenced here is a data collection strategy used *in place of* or in addition to an interview.

Using Chat Rooms

With the increasing use of computer-mediated communications, the opportunities to collect data online grow daily. Chat rooms on the internet allow interested parties to log on and communicate synchronously. The transmissions and responses occur in real time as opposed to being delayed. A number of chat rooms are available on the Internet. Although their use as a data collection strategy has not been fully developed or completely explored, the opportunities abound. Moloney et al. (2003) point out that narrative data collected in chat rooms have to be copied and pasted when the board is inactive. Also, it is difficult to scroll back to see what has been said. These peculiarities of chat rooms may make them less attractive for use as a data collection strategy. There is also the problem with synchronous communication. It may be easier to engage individuals in electronically mediated data collection when there is not a particular time demand placed on them.

Using Participant Observation

Participant observation is a method of data collection that comes from the anthropologic tradition. Therefore, it is the method of choice in ethnography. Generally, four types of participant observation are discussed in the literature. The first is *complete observer*, in which the researcher is a full observer of participants' activities. There is no interaction between the researcher and participants.

Observer as participant is the second type of participant observation. In this situation, the predominant activity of the researcher is to observe and potentially to interview. The majority of the researcher's time is spent in observation, rather than participation. To "fit" into the setting, the researcher may engage in some activities with the participants.

Participant as observer is the third type of participant observation. In this situation, the researcher acknowledges interest in studying the group; however, the researcher is most interested in doing so by becoming part of the group. A great deal has been written about "going native." This phrase demonstrates the inherent problem in getting too involved. That is, the researcher becomes so engrossed in the groups' activities that he or she loses sight of the real reason for being with the group.

The fourth type of participant observer is called *complete participant*. Complete participation requires that the researcher conceal his or her purpose. The individual becomes a member of the group. The ethical standard accepted by all disciplines makes concealment unacceptable. It is difficult, if not impossible, to justify this method. Because of a real concern for the ethics involved in data collection, individuals should not become complete participants.

Observations can also be structured or unstructured. Structured observations are more commonly found in quantitative research studies where the researcher is looking for something specific during the observation. Unstructured observations are the technique of choice in qualitative research as a way to comprehend the actions and interactions of individuals without a predetermined script. Mulhall (2003) points out that the term *unstructured* is misleading: "Observation within the naturalistic paradigm is not unstructured in the sense that it is unsystematic or sloppy. It does not, however, follow the approach of strictly checking the list of predetermined behaviors such as would occur in a structured observation" (p. 307).

Researchers should explore fully the reasons for selecting the various approaches to participant observation before initiating a study, realizing that, based on the circumstances, they may move among the approaches. There is no requirement to use only one approach. More importantly, the use of only one approach is almost impossible given the nature of fieldwork (Atkinson & Hammersley, 1998). However, it is important for researchers to think carefully about which approach they are interested in using in a given situation.

Using Field Notes

Field notes are the notations ethnographers generally make to document observations. These notes become part of data analysis. When recording field notes, it is important that researchers document what they have heard, seen, thought, or experienced. Chapter 9 offers examples of types of field notes, with detailed descriptions of how to write them.

Qualitative researchers using approaches other than ethnography for their research can use field notes. The field notes or notations made by the researcher may describe observations, assumptions about what is being heard or observed, or personal narrative about what is experienced by the researcher during a particular encounter. These notes can be very important during data collection and analysis. For example, in a phenomenological study conducted by the author (HJS), during the interviews, notes were used to describe the participants' expressions, changes in position, and other observations that would not be captured by voice recordings. These notes were important additions during data analysis because they provided validation for important points made by the participants and facilitated appropriate emphasis on emerging themes.

Little has been written about the use of photos; however, they are commonly used in ethnography as part of the ethnographic record. In addition, photos are included in research presentations to illustrate certain lived experiences. Hansen-Ketchum and Myrick (2008) suggest that photos have a role to play in the conduct of research. The authors offer important considerations of photos as a type of research method. Photograph images have the ability to engage participants in dialogue about particular phenomena, provide a medium for portraying a particular concept or experience or the ability to illustrate a lifeway or personal experience. Photos have the potential to add value to data collection, analysis, and reporting and as such should be considered an important strategy for qualitative researchers.

MANAGING DATA

*H*ow researchers manage data will greatly affect the ease with which they analyze the data. As addressed earlier, researchers may collect data in a number of ways. Storage and retrieval are other important considerations. MacLean, Meyer, and Estable (2004) advise that there is a significant amount of attention needed to improve the accuracy of transcripts. Specifically, they offer that to ensure the quality of transcription, researchers should spot-check the work provided by the transcriptionist. This includes completely checking a subset of all completed interviews. These authors also offer information on the use of voice recognition systems, the potential for inaccurate transcription in highly charged interviews, misinterpretation of content, effect of unfamiliar terminology, language-specific errors, and difficulties in cross-cultural or multilingual transcription. Researchers must be aware of these potential problems and institute measures to minimize them.

Large amounts of qualitative data can be stored on computers using a variety of available computer applications. It is beyond the scope of this book to fully share all the qualitative data collection packages available and their uses. It is important for qualitative researchers interested in using computer software to acquire and preview qualitative data analysis software and work with various software packages to determine which will be the most useful. Working with individuals who have used particular packages offers a significant opportunity to learn about the application without hours of reading and "trial and error." However, it is important to remember that what an "expert" in the program knows and what the program can do may not be the same. Therefore, gaining as much knowledge as possible about computer programs is critical. Also, remember that your purpose and needs relative to data analysis may be different from the "expert" you utilize. In conclusion, the time to review data analysis packages is *before* you begin data collection. It can be very distracting and frustrating to try to develop an understanding of the software during the data collection and analysis phases of your research.

Richards and Richards (1994) note that if data are in text format and are part of a word processing document, computer analysis offers several features. These features include the following:

1. The ability to handle multiple documents on-screen in separate windows, which will facilitate viewing text that is similar throughout the document and will allow "cut and paste" editing.
2. The ability to format files.
3. The ability to include pictures, graphs, or charts to illustrate ideas.
4. The ability to add video or audio data.
5. Good text-searching abilities.
6. Publish and subscribe facility, which allows for text to be changed in one document and automatically updated in a linked document.
7. The ability to link documents using hypertext, which permits readers to easily move from document to document and creates a unique ability to annotate text using hypertext links; these links facilitate memo writing about identified information.

These features are available in computer applications that would not be accessible in the more traditional storage formats such as handwritten files.

Table 3-1 offers an overview of commonly used computer packages. Qualitative researchers will need to practice working with these packages and, in some cases, use computer consultants to navigate the various program features. However, ultimately, the rewards of using a qualitative data analysis package will outweigh the time spent in learning about the various packages.

PERFORMING DATA ANALYSIS

Although data analysis is not always a linear process, analysis usually follows data collection. Neophyte qualitative researchers are faced with the inevitability of a certain ambiguity when beginning data analysis. Qualitative data analysis requires the investigator to use mental processes to draw conclusions. In particular, the researcher will need to use "sensory impressions, intuition, images, experiences, and cognitive comparisons in categorizing the findings and discerning patterns" (Hall, 2003, p. 495). These

Table 3-1 • Computerized Qualitative Data Management Programs	
Computer Program	*Source*
ATLAS/ti 6.0	ATLAS.ti
	http://www.atlasti.com
Ethnograph (Version 6)	Qualis Research Associates
	610 Popes Valley Drive
	Colorado Springs, CO 80914
	(719) 278-0925
	Qualis@Qualisresearch.com
	http://www.qualisresearch.com
Hyper Research 2.8	Research Ware, Inc.
	P.O. Box 1258
	Randolph, MA 02368-1258
	U.S. (888) 497-3737, or Out of US (781) 961-3909
	http://www.researchware.com/
QSR NVivo 8	QSR International (Americas Inc.)
QSR XSight 2	90 Sherman Street
	Cambridge, MA 02140
	USA
	(617) 491-1850
	http://www.qsrinternational.com

LIBRARY UNIVERSITY OF CHESTER

are not skills that the neophyte qualitative researcher is generally comfortable with. The amount of data collected and the style in which data have been stored will either facilitate or impede data analysis. Analysis of qualitative research is a hands-on process. Thorne (2000) states, "unquestionably, data analysis is the most complex and mysterious of all of the phases of a qualitative project" (p. 68). Researchers must become deeply immersed in the data (sometimes referred to as "dwelling" with the data). This process requires researchers to commit fully to a structured analytic process to gain an understanding of what the data convey. It requires a significant degree of dedication to reading, intuiting, analyzing, synthesizing, and reporting the discoveries. It is difficult to fully explain this process because "it is dynamic, intuitive, and creative process of thinking and theorizing" (Basit, 2003, p. 143).

As a neophyte qualitative researcher, interaction with an experienced researcher is the best way to become comfortable with data analysis. In a study reported by Li and Seale (2007), these researchers share how they used observational techniques within a PhD program to develop data analysis skills in their students. In this example, the experts guided the students through a series of exercises within a class to improve data analysis skills. There are times when a mentor may not be available. In these situations, an alternative offered by Walker, Cooke and McAllister (2008) is to use a framework. In this case, the authors share how Morse's cognitive processes were used by a masters student to analyze a research study.

Data analysis in qualitative research actually begins when data collection begins. As researchers conduct interviews or observations, they maintain and constantly review records to discover additional questions they need to ask or to offer descriptions of their findings. Usually these questions or descriptions are embedded in observations and interviews. Qualitative researchers must "listen" carefully to what they have seen, heard, and experienced to discover meaning. The cyclic nature of questioning and verifying is an important aspect of data collection and analysis. In addition to the analysis that occurs throughout the study, an extended period of immersion occurs at the conclusion of data collection. During this period of dwelling, investigators question all prior conclusions in the context of the whole based on what they have discovered. Generally, this period of data analysis consumes a considerable amount of time. Researchers will spend weeks or months with their data based on the amount of information available for analysis.

The actual process of data analysis usually takes the form of clustering similar data. In many qualitative approaches, these clustered ideas are labeled *themes*. Themes are structural meaning units of data. DeSantis and Ugarriza (2000) tell us that themes emerge from the data; they are not superimposed on them. Further, they share that "a theme is an abstract entity that brings meaning identity to a recurrent experience and its variant manifestations. As such, a theme captures and unifies the nature or basis of the experience into a meaningful whole" (p. 400). For example, in a study completed by Clark (2008), participants spoke about faculty incivility. Clark offers the following two statements:

"I played the game and jumped through the hoops. I mean there is hoop jumping and super hoop jumping. Like applying for your license. That's a hoop you've got to go through. But having to do 10 care plans makes you feel like you are back in ninth grade."

"Those old power-hungry women have been demeaning students for too long and it needs to be exposed. They put so much pressure on you and you're constantly under their thumb—being tested and forced to jump through hoops."

Clark (2008) concludes based on these two statements that in the first instance the student is talking about the thoughtless way that students are directed. In the second instance, she interprets this as the student feeling out of control. In her report, she names these *pressuring students to conform to faculty demands* and *anger*, respectively.

Once researchers have explicated all themes relevant to a study, they report them in a way that is meaningful to the intended audience. In a phenomenological study, the researcher will relate the themes to one another to develop an *exhaustive description* of the experience being investigated.

Thorne (2000) shares that in each approach to qualitative data analysis, there is a different purpose for and different process used to draw conclusions. In grounded theory, the process for analyzing data is labeled *constant comparative method*. Using this process, the researcher compares each new piece of data with data previously analyzed. Questions are asked each time relative to the similarities or differences between each compared piece of data. The ultimate goal is the development of a theory about why a particular phenomenon exists as it does. What is the basic social-psychological process that is occurring? For a full description of the process, the reader is directed to Glaser and Strauss (1967).

In phenomenology, the process of interpretation may vary based on the philosophic tradition used. Regardless of the specific tradition, they all support "immersing oneself in data, engaging with data reflectively, and generating a rich description that will enlighten a reader as to the deeper essential structures underlying the human experience" (Thorne, 2000, p. 69).

For ethnographers, the focus of data analysis is to offer a description of a culture based on participant observation, interviews, and artifacts. "Ethnographic analysis uses an iterative process in which cultural ideas that arise during active involvement 'in the field' are transformed, translated or represented in written document" (Thorne, 2000, p. 69). The researcher asks questions, analyzes the answers, develops more questions, and analyzes the answers in a repeating pattern until a full picture of the culture emerges.

Regardless of the methodological approach used, the goal of data analysis is to illuminate the experiences of those who have lived them by sharing the richness of lived experiences and cultures. The researcher has the responsibility of describing and analyzing what is presented in the raw data to bring to life particular phenomena. It is only through rich description that we will come to know the experiences of others. As Krasner (2001) states, "stories illuminate meaning, meaning stimulates interpretation, and interpretation can change outcome" (p. 72).

DEMONSTRATING TRUSTWORTHINESS

Much debate is ongoing regarding rigor or goodness in qualitative research. The debate has mostly moved beyond the positivist convention of reliability and validity. This section of the chapter takes a conservative position regarding the ongoing debate and offers a set of criteria that has been meaningful to qualitative researchers for the past twenty plus years. However, taking the conservative position for the sake of sharing the *fundamentals* of qualitative research does not negate the need for nor the importance of the debate surrounding rigor. It is critical that qualitative researchers clarify "to 'outsiders' what qualitative research is, stressing the utility of qualitative findings, and addressing the quality in qualitative studies [which has] been suggested as means of assessing a place for qualitative research as 'evidence.'" (Nelson, 2008, p. 316). Equally important is the need to constantly question the predominant paradigm's structure and function. Dualist thinking does not advance nursing knowledge, nor does it add substantially to what we know about the people we care for or the lives they lead. Advocacy for being open to alternative ways of knowing is essential. Emden and Sandelowski (1999) offer as an important criterion for addressing rigor in qualitative research a "criterion of uncertainty" (p. 5). This criterion provides for "an open acknowledgement that claims about research outcomes are at best tentative and that there may indeed be no way of showing otherwise" (p. 5).

At the outset, it is important to state that "no one set of criteria can be expected to 'fit the bill' for every research study" (Emden & Sandelowski, 1999, p. 6). Further, it is important to recognize that, ultimately, our decisions regarding the rigor in a research study amount to a judgment call (p. 6). With these two assumptions in mind, rigor in qualitative research is demonstrated through researchers' attention to and confirmation of information discovery. The goal of rigor in qualitative research is to accurately represent study participants' experiences. There are different terms to describe the processes that contribute to rigor in qualitative research. Guba (1981) and Guba and Lincoln (1994) have identified the following terms that describe operational techniques supporting the rigor of the work: *credibility, dependability, confirmability,* and *transferability.*

Credibility includes activities that increase the probability that credible findings will be produced (Lincoln & Guba, 1985). One of the best ways to establish credibility is through prolonged engagement with the subject matter. Another way to confirm the credibility of findings is to see whether the participants recognize the findings of the study to be true to their experiences (Yonge & Stewin, 1988). The act of returning to the informants to see whether they recognize the findings is frequently referred to as *member checking.* Creswell (2003) offers that member checking should be used "to determine the accuracy of the qualitative findings through taking the final report or specific descriptions or themes back to participants and determining whether these participants feel that they are accurate" (p. 196). Important always to the process of assuring credibility using member checks is the importance of weighing a respondent's comments against the larger pool of informants. McBrien (2008) states, "member checking can provide correlating evidence to support the truthfulness and consistency of the findings; however, on the other hand, an over reliance on member checking can potentially compromise the significance of the research findings" (p. 1287).

Another method of improving the credibility of the findings is peer debriefing. Significant debate has arisen around this concept. Peer debriefing has been described by Lincoln and Guba (1985) as "a process of exposing oneself to a disinterested peer in a manner paralleling an analytical sessions . . . for the purpose of exploring aspects of the inquiry that might otherwise remain only implicit within the inquirer's mind" (p. 308). Some authors (Morse, 1994; Cutliffe & McKenna, 1999) contend that an independent colleague has had less contact with the study participants and as such has less ability to judge the adequacy of the interpretation. Despite these objections, "the process may enable the researcher to make reasoned methodological choices and can ensure that emergent themes and patterns can be substantiated in the data" (McBrien, 2008).

Dependability is a criterion met once researchers have demonstrated the credibility of the findings. The question to ask, then, is this: how dependable are these results? Sharts-Hopko (2002) submits that triangulation of methods has the potential to contribute to the dependability of the findings. Similar to validity in quantitative research, in which there can be no validity without reliability, the same holds true for dependability: there can be no dependability without credibility (Lincoln & Guba, 1985).

Confirmability is a process criterion. The way researchers document the confirmability of the findings is to leave an *audit trail*, which is a recording of activities over time that another individual can follow. This process can be compared to a fiscal audit (Lincoln & Guba, 1985). The objective is to illustrate as clearly as possible the evidence and thought processes that led to the conclusions. This particular criterion can be problematic, however, if you subscribe to Morse's (1989) ideas regarding the related matter of saturation. It is the position of Morse that another researcher may not agree with the conclusions developed by the original researcher. Sandelowski (1998a) argues that only the researcher who has collected the data and been immersed in them can confirm the findings.

Transferability refers to the probability that the study findings have meaning to others in similar situations. Transferability has also been labeled "fittingness." The expectation for determining whether the findings fit or are transferable rests with potential users of the findings and not with the researchers (Greene, 1990; Lincoln & Guba, 1985; Sandelowski, 1986). As Lincoln and Guba (1985) have stated,

> It is . . . not the naturalist's task to provide an *index of transferability*; it is his or her responsibility to provide the *database* that makes transferability judgment possible on the part of potential appliers (p. 316).

These four criteria for judging the rigor of qualitative research are important; they define for external audiences the attention qualitative researchers render to their work.

More recently, Pawson et al. (2003) have developed an additional set of criteria to judge the rigor of qualitative research. Although not as widely used as Guba and Lincoln's (1985) criteria, they offer the reader another alternative. Pawson et al.'s model uses the acronym TAPUPAS: transparency, accuracy, purposivity, utility, accessibility, and specificity. The original work provides a full description of each of the criterion.

PRESENTING THE DATA

"There is no one style for reporting the findings of a qualitative research study" (Sandelowski, 1998b, p. 376). Researchers interested in sharing their results must take several things into consideration. First, who is the audience? Second, what is the purpose of the report? Third, for whom am I writing the report? Although presented linearly, the questions offered do not need to be answered linearly. The most important question, which is overarching, is this: how do I most effectively communicate the findings of my study to make them useful for others?

Sandelowski (1998b) offers some important parameters in developing the research report. These include determining focus of the narrative; balancing description, analysis, and interpretation; emphasizing character, scene, or plot; deciding whose voice will be heard; and learning how to effectively use metaphor.

Determining the focus of the study is essential. The researcher must consider carefully what needs to be told. Qualitative research studies create voluminous amounts of data. The researcher needs to decide based on the purpose of his or her study what will be told. For instance, if the purpose of the study is to discover the meaning of health to those who lived in the borderlands, then the purpose is to tell the story of those who experienced living there. The research report should include a rich description of what the meaning of health is for those individuals given the living conditions along the Mexican border.

The way in which one tells the story is guided by the purpose of the study. If the researcher is conducting a descriptive phenomenological study, then the focus is on the description, with less attention to analysis and interpretation. This is not to suggest that the raw data are presented without analysis. Rather, the researcher will have the responsibility of digesting the narrative and distilling it into a meaningful representation of a phenomenon based on those whose experiences are shared.

If, however, the purpose of the research study is to develop a theory about recovery in the aftermath of a major crisis, then the narrative will give rise to analysis and interpretation leading ultimately to the new theory. The descriptions of individuals' recoveries will not be what are highlighted in the report. The descriptions will be the groundwork from which the theory will be derived. The focus will be analysis, interpretation, and reformulation of the data that lead to the creation of the theory.

Sandelowski (1998b) suggests that qualitative researchers also should consider "whether the stories they want to tell are best told by emphasizing, and consciously using devices to showcase, character, scene or plot" (p. 37). For example, if the researcher has studied the history of a college of nursing over 25 years, the researcher can approach the study report in a number of ways. One way is to look at an individual. Let's say the same dean presided over the college for that period of time. The researcher can look at the institution through the eyes of the dean or can analyze the findings within the context of the dean's influence over the college's growth and development. The researcher might also look at the institution in terms of its politics. For instance, if the institution was a publicly funded entity in a state with representation whose primary agenda in the state was improving the health of the populace, then the college can be described based on the effect the politics had in its growth and development. There is no one way to tell the story. The researcher should consider carefully the emphasis of the report.

Deciding whose voice will be heard is a decision that needs careful consideration. Power structures frequently overshadow choice of research topic, data collection, sampling, and analysis. Often, researchers do not even consider how what they share is cloaked in power relationships. Although the researcher needs to stay attuned to the issues of power constantly, it is enormously important when telling the story. Whose voice will be heard and how it will be shared are extremely important. For example, if the researcher has studied the culture of a trauma unit in a major city for the purpose of sharing what life is like for the health professionals and clients who use the unit, the question should be asked, whose voice will be dominant and why? If the researcher tells the story primarily from the health professionals' points of view, is there a slant on the research report that is different than if it is told from the clients' perspectives? Power is an important factor in research. It is a particularly important factor to consider in qualitative research, which has as one of its underlying principles the commitment to convey the experiences of those studied.

Sandelowski (1998b) offers the importance of metaphor and its use in reporting qualitative research. She shares that frequently when metaphor is used in research reports, it is used incorrectly or incompletely. Metaphor is a powerful tool in helping the reader to fully grasp what the researcher is trying to convey. Therefore, it needs to be selected carefully. Those who choose to use it must realize that it is only a tool or device to help the reader understand the data. It is a directional tool and not an outcome.

Finally, graphic medium can be used in data analysis. Hall (2003) speaks about the value of using graphic representations to enhance sharing the richness of data. Similarly, Hansen-Ketchum and Myrick (2008) have offered the value of photography in collection and analysis.

SUMMARY

*D*ata analysis can be described as the heart of qualitative inquiry. It is the point in the research process when researchers have the opportunity to put into words their conceptualizations of the shared experiences. Through the dynamic processes of intuiting, synthesizing, analyzing, and conceptualizing, the researcher distills and then illuminates the experiences or cultures that have been part of the inquiry. Qualitative data analysis requires an openness to possibilities. It necessitates patience with abstraction and a willingness to discover the wholeness of what is shared. Qualitative data analysis entails listening carefully to narrative and sharing description and understanding of what has been said, always maintaining the highest degree of integrity.

The focus of this chapter has been on data collection, management, and analysis. The novice qualitative researcher is advised to pursue a mentor to learn good techniques and to avoid the pitfalls of data collection, management, and analysis. Beck (2003) offers that the most common data analysis problem for neophytes is premature or delayed closure. For the advanced beginner, reading published studies with others and analyzing the data collection methods, data management strategies and reporting of the analysis will be helpful in further developing analysis skills. In this chapter, we have offered information on collecting data using interviews, observation, focus groups, chat rooms, and narratives. This information should be helpful in identifying the most appropriate way to collect data for your study. In the methodological chapters that follow, we offer specific information on data collection strategies that are most appropriate for the specific approach.

In the data management section, the information is focused primarily on computer programs that can help you analyze large amounts of data. There is considerable debate about the usefulness of computer programs given the dynamic nature of the analysis process. It is important, however, that you have the information so that you can make an informed decision based on what you want to achieve. Finally, we offer information on the complexity of data analysis and how very difficult it is to fully describe a process that is creative and dynamic. It is our intention to offer a foundation from which to develop data analysis skills. The integrity of qualitative research findings will be judged on the ability of researchers to tell the story of participants with truthfulness and an attention to context and power.

References

Atkinson, P., & Hammersley, M. (1998). Ethnography and participant observation. In N. K. Denzin, & Y. S. Lincoln (Eds.), *Strategies of qualitative inquiry* (pp. 110–136). Thousand Oaks, CA: Sage.

Bailey, P. H. (1996). Assuring quality in narrative analysis. *Western Journal of Nursing Research, 18*(2), 186–195.

Basit, T. N. (2003). Manual or electronic? The role of coding in qualitative data analysis. *Educational Research, 45*(2), 143–154.

Beck, C. T. (2003). Initiation into qualitative data analysis. *Journal of Nursing Education, 42*(5), 231–234.

Bianco, M. B., & Carr-Chellman, A. A. (2002). Exploring qualitative methodologies in online learning environments. *Quarterly Review of Distance Education, 3*(3), 251–260.

Carey, M. A., & Smith, M. W. (1994). Capturing the group effect in focus groups: A special concern for analysis. *Qualitative Health Research, 4*(1), 123–127.

Carolan, M. (2003). Reflexivity: A personal journey during data collection. *Researcher, 10*(3), 7–14.

Clark, C. M. (2008). Student voices on faculty incivility in nursing education: A conceptual model. *Nursing Education Perspectives, 29*(5), 284–289.

Cutliffe, J. R. & McKenna, H. P. (1999). Establishing the credibility of qualitative research findings: The plot thickens. *Journal of Advanced Nursing, 30*(2), 374–380.

Creswell, J. W. (2003). *Research design: Qualitative, quantitative, and mixed methods/ approaches* (2nd ed.). Thousand Oaks, CA: Sage.

Curtis, E. A. & Redmond, R. (2007). Focus groups in nursing research. *Nurse Researcher, 14*(2), 25–37.

DeSantis, L., & Ugarriza, D. N. (2000). The concept of theme as used in qualitative research. *Western Journal of Nursing Research, 22*(3), 351–377.

Dilley, P. (2004). Interviews and the philosophy of qualitative research. *Journal of Higher Education, 75*(1), 127–132.

Docherty, S., & Sandelowski, M. (1999). Focus on qualitative methods: Interviewing children. *Research in Nursing and Health Care, 22*, 177–185.

Drury, V., Francis, K., & Chapman, Y. (2007). Taming the rescuer: The therapeutic nature of qualitative research interviews. *International Journal of Nursing Practice, 13*, 383–384.

Eaves, Y. D., & Kahn, D. L. (2000). Coming to terms with perceived danger. *Journal of Holistic Nursing, 18*(1), 27–45.

Emden, C., & Sandelowski, M. (1999). The good, the bad and relative, part two: Goodness and the criterion problem in qualitative research. *International Journal of Professional Nursing Practice, 5*(1), 2–7.

Fernandez, R. & Griffiths, R. (2007). Portable MP3 players: Innovative devices for recording qualitative interviews. *Nurse Researcher, 15*(1), 7–15.

Fontana, A., & Frey, J. H. (1994). Interviewing: The art and science. In N. K. Denzin, & Y.S. Lincoln (Eds.), *Handbook of qualitative research* (pp. 361–376). Thousand Oaks, CA: Sage.

Freeman, T. (2006). 'Best practice' in focus group research: Making sense of different views. *Journal of Advanced Research, 56*(5), 491–497.

Glaser, B. G., & Strauss, A. (1967). *The discovery of grounded theory.* Chicago: Aldine.

Greene, J. C. (1990). Three views on nature and role of knowledge in social science. In E. Guba (Ed.), *The paradigm dialogue* (pp. 227–245). Newbury Park, CA: Sage.

Guba, E. G. (1981). Criteria for assessing the trustworthiness of naturalistic inquiries. *Educational Communication and Technology Journal, 29*, 75–92.

Guba, E. G., & Lincoln Y. S. (1994). Competing paradigms in qualitative research. In N. K. Denzin & Y. S. Lincoln (Eds.), *Handbook of qualitative research* (pp. 105–117). Thousand Oaks, CA: Sage.

Halcomb, E. J., Gholizadeh, L., DiGiacomo, M., Phillips, J. & Davidson, P. M. (2007). Literature review: Considerations in undertaking focus group research with culturally and linguistically diverse groups. *Journal of Clinical Nursing, 16*(6), 1000–1011.

Hall, J. M. (2003). Analyzing women's roles through graphic representation of narratives. *Western Journal of Nursing Research, 25*(5), 492–507.

Hansen-Ketchum, P. & Myrick, F. (2008). Photo methods for qualitative research in nursing: An ontological and epistemological perspective. *Nursing Philosophy, 9*, 205–213.

Hudson, P. (2003). Focus group interviews: A guide for palliative care researchers and clinicians. *International Journal of Palliative Nursing, 9*(5), 202–207.

Jootun, D., McGhee, G. & Marland, G. R. (2009). Reflexity: Promoting rigour in qualitative research. *Nursing Standard, 23*(23), 42–46.

Joseph, D. H., Griffin, M., & Sullivan, E. D. (2000). Videotaped focus groups: Transforming a therapeutic strategy into a research tool. *Nursing Forum, 35*(1), 15–20.

Kennedy, C., Kools, S., & Krueger, R. (2001). Methodological considerations in children's focus groups. *Nursing Research, 50*(3), 184–187.

Kidd, P. S., & Parshall, M. B. (2000). Getting the focus and the group: Enhancing analytical rigor in focus group research. *Qualitative Health Research, 10*(3), 293–309.

Koch, T. (2006). Establishing rigour in qualitative research: The decision trail. *Journal of Advanced Nursing, 53*,(1), 91–100.

Krasner, D. L. (2001). Qualitative research: A different paradigm—part 1. *Journal of Wound, Ostomy and Continence Nurses Society, 28*(2), 70–72.

Krueger, R. A. & Casey, M. A. (2007). *Focus groups: A practical guide for applied research* (3rd ed.). London: Sage.

Lambert, S. D. & Loiselle, C. G. (2008). Combining individual interviews and focus groups to enhance data richness. *Journal of Advanced Nursing, 63*(2), 228–237.

Lewins, A. (1996). The CAQDAS Networking Project: Multilevel support for the qualitative research community. *Qualitative Health Research, 6*(2), 298–303.

Li, S. & Seale, C. (2007). Learning to do qualitative data analysis: An observational study of doctoral work. *Qualitative Health Research, 17*(10), 1442–1452.

Lincoln, Y. S., & Guba, E. (1985). *Naturalistic inquiry*. Beverly Hills, CA: Sage.

Lucasey, B. (2000). Qualitative research and focus group methodology. *Orthopedic Nursing, 19*(1), 53–55.

MacLean, L. M., Meyer, M., & Estable, A. (2004). Improving accuracy of transcripts in qualitative research. *Qualitative Health Research, 14*(1), 113–123.

MacDougall, C., & Baum, F. (1997). The devil's advocate: A strategy to avoid group-think and stimulate discussion in focus groups. *Qualitative Health Research, 7*(4), 532–541.

Maggs-Rapport, F. (2000). Combining methodological approaches in research: Ethnography and interpretive phenomenology. *Journal of Advanced Nursing, 31*(1), 219–225.

McBrien, B. (2008). Evidence-based care: Enhancing the rigour of a qualitative study. *British Journal of Nursing, 17*(20), 1286–1289.

McDougall, P. (2000). In-depth interviewing: The key issues of reliability and validity. *Community Practitioner, 73*(8), 722–724.

Moloney, J. F., Dietrich, A. S., Strickland, O. L., & Myerburg, S. (2003). Using Internet discussion boards as virtual focus groups. *Advances in Nursing Science, 26*(4), 274–286.

Morse, J. M. (1989). Strategies for sampling. In J. M. Morse (Ed.), *Qualitative nursing research: A contemporary dialogue* (pp. 117–131). Rockville, MD: Aspen.

Morse, J. M. (1994). Emerging from the data: The cognitive process of analysis in qualitative inquiry. In J.M. Morse (Ed.). *Critical issues in qualitative research methods*. California: Sage.

Mulhall, A. (2003). In the field: Notes on observation in qualitative research. *Journal of Advanced Nursing, 41*(3), 306–313.

Nelson, A. M. (2008). Addressing the threat of evidence-based practice to qualitative inquiry through increasing attention to quality: A discussion paper. *International Journal of Nursing Studies, 45*, 316–322.

Pawson, R., Boaz, A., Grayson, L., Long, A., & Barnes, C. (2003). *Types of quality of knowledge in social care*. London: Social Care Institute for Excellence.

Perry, C., Thurston, M., & Green, K. (2004). Involvement and detachment in researching sexuality: Reflections on the process of semistructured interviewing. *Qualitative Health Research, 14*(1), 135–148.

Polkinghorne, D. E. (1988). *Narrative knowing and the human sciences.* Albany: State University of New York Press.

Primeau, L. A. (2003). Reflections on self in qualitative research: Stories of family. *American Journal of Occupational Therapy, 57*(1), 9–16.

Redmond, R., & Curtis, E. (2009). Focus groups: Principles and practice. *Nurse Researcher, 16*(3), 57–69.

Richards, T. J., & Richards, L. (1994). Using computers in qualitative research. In N. K. Denzin & Y. S. Lincoln (Eds.), *Handbook of qualitative research* (pp. 445–462). Thousand Oaks, CA: Sage.

Riessman, C. K. (1993). *Narrative analysis.* Newbury Park, CA: Sage.

Robinson, J. P. (2000). Phases of the qualitative research interview with institutionalized elderly individuals. *Journal of Gerontological Nursing, 26*(11), 17–23.

Ryan, F., Coughlan, M., & Cronin, P. (2009). Interviewing in qualitative research: The one-to-one interview. *International Journal of Therapy and Rehabilitation, 16*(6), 309–314.

Sandelowski, M. (1986). The problem of rigor in qualitative research. *Advances in Nursing Science, 8*(3), 27–37.

Sandelowski, M. (1998a). The call to experts in qualitative research. *Research in Nursing & Health, 21,* 467–471.

Sandelowski, M. (1998b). Writing a good read: Strategies for re-presenting qualitative data. *Research in Nursing and Health, 21,* 375–382.

Sedgwick, M., & Spiers, J. (2009). The use of videoconferencing as a medium for the qualitative interview. *International Journal of Qualitative Methods, 8*(1), 1–11.

Sharts-Hopko, N. (2002). Assessing rigor in qualitative research. *Journal of the Association of Nurses in AIDS Care, 13*(4), 84–86.

Sixsmith, J., Boneham, M., & Goldring, J. E. (2003). Accessing the community: Gaining insider perspectives from the outside. *Qualitative Health Research, 13*(4), 578–589.

Stewart, D. W., Shamdasani, P. N., & Rook, D. W. (2007). *Focus groups: Theory and practice.* Thousand Oaks, CA: Sage.

Thorne, S. (2000). Data analysis in qualitative research. *Evidence-Based Nursing, 3*(3), 68–70.

Traulsen, J. M., Almarsdottir, A. B., & Bjornsdottir, I. (2004). Interviewing the moderator: An ancillary method to focus groups. *Qualitative Health Research, 14*(5), 714–725.

Walker, R., Cooke, M., & McAllister, M. (2008). A neophyte's journey through qualitative analysis using Morse's cognitive processes of analysis. *International Journal of Qualitative Methods, 7*(1), 81–93.

Wallin, A., & Ahlstrom, G. (2006). Cross-cultural interview studies using interpreters: Systematic literature review. *Journal of Advanced Nursing, 55*(6), 723–735.

Webb, C., & Doman, M. (2008). Conducting focus groups: Experiences from nursing research. *The Journal of Thematic Dialogue, 10,* 51–60.

Whiting, L. S. (2008). Semi-structured interviews: Guidance for novice researchers. *Nursing Standard 22*(23), 35–40.

Yonge, O., & Stewin, L. (1988). Reliability and validity: Misnomers for qualitative research. *Canadian Journal of Nursing, 20*(2), 61–67.

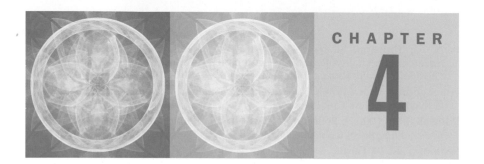

Ethical Considerations in Qualitative Research

*E*thical issues related to professional nursing practice arise daily in the constant struggle to do good for the patient and to avoid harm. All that nurses do in the name of patient care is wrought with tension between these two principles. As science and technology provide avenues to intervene, unanticipated and more complex ethical dilemmas will continue to arise in our practice settings. The ethical dilemmas that emerge are grounded in the fact that direct relationships with human beings are at the heart of nurses' work. Understanding ethical principles in theory, combined with life experience in practice, prepares the nurse to make sound ethical and moral decisions on a daily basis. This knowledge and experience can be transferred to an understanding of ethical issues relevant to the research process.

Ethical issues and standards must be critically considered in both quantitative and qualitative research. Nurse researchers have a professional responsibility to design research that upholds sound ethical principles and protects human rights. Ethical issues related to informed consent, participant–researcher relationships, gaining access, confidentiality, anonymity, sample size, and data analysis are addressed in this chapter. The ethical issues considered are relevant to each of the qualitative research approaches presented in the text and should be considered within the context of the method selected for a particular investigation. The protection of participants must remain at the forefront of all research studies; however, the nature of qualitative methods requires that the researcher remain alert to the possibility of unanticipated ethical dilemmas.

There has been ongoing discussion in the nursing literature regarding the ethical variances that have arisen in qualitative investigations. Clearly, guidelines established for quantitative research investigations require an expanded scope of discussion when applied to qualitative research endeavors (Cutliffe & Ramcharan, 2002; Demi & Warren, 1995; Forbat & Henderson, 2003; Haggman-Laitila, 1999; Karnieli-Miller et al., 2009; Orb, Eisenhauer, & Wynaden, 2001; Robley, 1995). Standards for ethical conduct in the qualitative realm will continue to require in-depth examination. Although qualitative designs have improved guidelines regarding the unique concerns that emerge in this type of research, what has become increasingly clear is that the ethical aspects of the research process will always require ongoing critique and evaluation. Given this understanding, this chapter addresses ethical issues that require critical consideration in any qualitative research endeavor. Table 4-1 provides qualitative researchers with an "ethics checklist" to use as a guide when critiquing the ethical aspects of a research study.

HISTORICAL BACKGROUND

Codes of ethics have been established for the conduct of research in response to human rights violations that have occurred. Sadly, the human atrocities that occurred in the name of research did not happen that long ago. Ethical concerns have high visibility today because of flagrant abuses of subjects that have occurred. As a result of this abuse, some examples of which are highlighted below, varying groups have developed codes of ethics.

- *The Nazi Medical Experiments* (1930s–1940s) implemented by the Third Reich in Europe are one atrocious example of the violation of basic human rights with research participants. Programs of research included sterilization, euthanasia, and medical experiments that were inhumane and generated no useful scientific knowledge. Participants were exposed to permanent physical harm or death and were not allowed to refuse participation (Levine, 1986).

- *The Tuskegee Syphilis Study* (1932–1972) occurred in the United States and was sponsored by the U.S. Public Health Service. The study was conducted to determine the course of syphilis in adult black men. Some participants were unaware that they were participating in a study, and many were uninformed as to the purpose and procedures of the research. Medical treatment for syphilis was deliberately withheld, even after penicillin was determined to be an effective treatment (Levine, 1986).

- *The Jewish Chronic Disease Hospital* (1960s) conducted a study to determine patients' rejection response to live cancer cells. Elderly patients at the Jewish Chronic Disease Hospital in Brooklyn were

Table 4-1 • The "Ethics Checklist": A Guide for Critiquing the Ethical Aspects of a Qualitative Research Study	
Topic	*Guiding Questions*
Phenomenon of interest	1. Is the research study relevant, important, and most appropriately investigated through a qualitative design? Explain. 2. Are there any aspects of the research or phenomenon of interest that appear to be misleading either in terms of the true purpose or misleading to participants? Explain. 3. Is the research primarily being conducted for personal gain on the part of the researcher, or is there evidence that the research will somehow contribute to the greater good? What are the benefits to the participants or society as a whole?
Review of the literature	1. Has all the available literature been reviewed? 2. Are all citations accurate in terms of referencing and quoting? 3. Is the basis for inclusion of the articles referred to explicit?
Research design participants	1. How did the researcher protect the physical and psychological well-being of the participants? 2. Is there evidence that informed or process consent was obtained and freely given? 3. How were vulnerable populations recruited and protected from physical or emotional harm? 4. Did an Institutional Review Board approve the research?
Sampling	1. How was the confidentiality of participants protected? 2. Is there any evidence of coercion or deception?
Data generation	1. If more than one researcher collected data, were they adequately prepared? 2. Is there evidence of falsified or fabricated data? 3. Is there intentional use of data collection methods to obtain biased data? 4. Was data collection covert? If so, does the researcher explain why? 5. Have the participants been misled with regard to the nature of the research? 6. What mechanisms did the researcher employ to ensure authenticity and trustworthiness of data? (e.g., audit trail, reflexive journaling)
Data analysis	1. Was data analysis conducted by more than one person? 2. Is there evidence of data manipulation to achieve intended findings? 3. Is there evidence of missing data that may have been lost or destroyed?
Conclusions and recommen- dations	1. Is there evidence of intentional false or misleading conclusions and recommendations? 2. Is confidentiality violated given the presentation of the findings?

Adapted from Firby, P. (1995). Critiquing the ethical aspects of a study. *Nurse Researcher*, 3(1), 35–41.

injected with live cancer cells. The project was conducted without informed consent and without institutional review (Levine, 1986).

- *The Willowbrook Study* (1950s–1970s) deliberately infected mentally handicapped children with the hepatitis B virus. Admission to the hospital was contingent on parental consent for the children to participate in the study. However, the consent was not informed, and parents were never told of the dangerous consequences of the study (Levine, 1986).

- *The Johns Hopkins Crisis* (2001) is one of the most recent examples leading to concerns regarding research. This study involved the use of healthy volunteers to study the pathophysiology of asthma. The third subject to receive the drug hexamethonium as part of the research protocol died as a result of progressive hypotension and multiorgan failure. The study was criticized because the consent document did not indicate that the inhaled hexamethonium was experimental and did not have U.S. Food and Drug Administration (FDA) approval (Steinbrook, 2002).

Although these examples emerged from quantitative studies that employed a specific intervention, the message is clear. Guidelines are essential, but they do not always answer all the ethical or moral questions that may arise in any research study, whether the design is quantitative or qualitative. It is the responsibility of the researcher to constantly examine and question the ethical components of their work. Participants must be protected, and the researcher must remain sensitive to emerging actual or potential ethical concerns.

Early quantitative investigations paved the way for ethical codes and guidelines. Qualitative researchers are bound by the same codes and must maintain an ongoing dialogue regarding ethical dilemmas encountered during their investigations so that all researchers can benefit from the experience of others. Despite the most vigilant attempts to ensure ethical conduct during a qualitative investigation, new and important considerations are always emerging. Researchers must be willing to share their experiences. For example, Boman and Jevne (2000) report on an experience of being charged with an ethical violation in the conduct of a qualitative investigation. The article centers on a frank discussion of a qualitative research endeavor in which the identity of a study participant was disclosed (Boman & Jevne, 2000). There is much to be learned from this open and honest sharing of the researchers' experience. Similarly, Lawton (2001) discusses ethical concerns related to informed consent and role conflict that emerged during a participant observation study of dying patients. Lawton (2001) and Boman and Jevne (2000) provide relevant examples from personal experience that will serve to enhance the ethical integrity of future studies. Their open and frank discussions leave all researchers in a better position to address ethical issues that present during the conduct of a qualitative investigation.

CODES OF ETHICS

V arious codes of ethics have been developed over the past five decades in response to violations of moral principles and human rights in the conduct of research. The *Nuremberg Code* was developed following the Nazi experiments of the 1930s and 1940s and remains one of the first internationally recognized efforts to establish ethical standards. The code concerns itself with the adequate protection of human subjects, the rights of participants to withdraw from a research study, and the importance of conducting research only by qualified individuals. Other international standards include the *Declaration of Helsinki*, developed in 1964 by the World Medical Association and Finland. This document is similar to the Nuremberg Code but further differentiates between research that has a therapeutic value for participants and that which does not.

In the United States, the National Commission for the Protection of Human Subjects of Biomedical and Behavioral Research, known as the *Belmont Report*, served as a model for many of the guidelines adopted by specific disciplines. The Belmont Report identified three ethical principles relevant to the conduct of research involving human subjects: the principle of respect for persons, beneficence, and justice. The regulations are available online (http://ohsr.od.nih.gov/guidelines/45cfr46.html).

The profession of nursing has developed a *Code of Ethics* that provides guidelines related to practice issues and research (American Nurses Association, 2001). Silva (1995) provides an explicit account of the roles and responsibilities of nurses in the conduct, dissemination, and implementation of nursing research in a document entitled *Ethical Guidelines in the Conduct, Dissemination, and Implementation of Nursing Research*.

ETHICAL ISSUES SPECIFIC TO QUALITATIVE RESEARCH DESIGN

D istinct and conceivably unanticipated ethical issues emanate from the unpredictable nature of qualitative research. As Robley (1995) noted, "ethical considerations relevant to quantitative research impact qualitative investigations in unique and more fragile ways" (p. 45). The ethical dilemmas inherent in issues surrounding informed consent, anonymity and confidentiality, data generation, treatment, publication, and participant–researcher relationships are reviewed in light of the unique issues that emerge in the design and conduct of qualitative investigations. Ethical standards for qualitative investigations must evolve from a sense that the research is dynamic and that the process, by its application, may result in unanticipated ethical concerns. The researcher must remain open to the possibility of new, and, to date, unexamined ethical concerns related to qualitative research. Further, the evolving standards must be grounded in the ethical principles of autonomy, beneficence, and justice.

Researchers must observe certain basic principles when conducting any form of research that involves human subjects. First, participants must not be harmed, thereby supporting the principle of *beneficence*. In any qualitative investigation, if researchers sense that the interview is causing issues to surface that may result in emotional trauma to participants, they must protect the welfare of the participants, perhaps by ending the interview or providing follow-up counseling and referrals. Researchers must obtain informed consent, and informant participation must be voluntary, thereby supporting the principle of *autonomy*. Furthermore, researchers must assure participants that confidentiality and anonymity will be upheld and that participants will be treated with dignity and respect. The principles of *beneficence* and *justice* are upheld in this regard (Beauchamp & Childress, 2001). The three ethical principles of autonomy, beneficence, and justice provide the organizing framework for a meaningful dialogue regarding ethical issues that pertain to qualitative investigations.

INFORMED CONSENT

*I*nformed consent is a topic of regular discussion in health care settings. There is an expectation that, in the clinical setting, when clients sign a consent form, they are fully aware of both the health benefits and the actual or potential risks to their health (hence, the term *informed consent*). Informed consent in research holds similar meaning, with added inherent dimensions.

Informed consent is a prerequisite for all research involving identifiable subjects. Any dialogue referencing informed consent must be grounded in the ethical principle of autonomy that encompasses the notion of being a self-governing person with decision-making capacity. Polit and Beck (2004) defined informed consent as follows: "Informed consent means that participants have adequate information regarding the research; are capable of comprehending the information; and have the power of free choice, enabling them to consent voluntarily to participate in the research or decline participation" (p. 151). The researcher is obligated to provide the participant with relevant and adequate information when obtaining informed consent. At a minimum, participants should have information about the purpose and scope of the study, the types of questions that will potentially be asked, how the results will be used, and how their anonymity will be protected (Richards & Schwartz, 2002). The emergent design of a qualitative investigation, however, presents qualitative researchers with ethical considerations that have the potential to violate the basic premise of informed consent.

Of particular concern is the notion that participants will have adequate information regarding the research study. Although a participant may consent to a study on the life experience of open heart surgery, new issues may emerge within the context of the interview for which the participant and perhaps even the researcher were unprepared. Research with vulnerable populations or topics that deal with sensitive subjects may change the direction of the research or reveal information that is not related to the original purpose of the study.

"As a minimum, it [informed consent] requires that prospective human subjects are given true and sufficient information to help them decide whether they wish to be research participants" (Behi & Nolan, 1995, p. 713). The open, emerging nature of qualitative research methods in most cases makes informed consent impossible because neither researchers nor participants can predict exactly how data will present themselves either through interview or participant observation (Holloway & Wheeler, 1995; Ramos, 1989; Richards & Schwartz, 2002; Robley, 1995). As Robley (1995) pointed out, "Questions of ethics arise within the context of the shifting focus of the study, the unpredictable nature of the research and the trust relationship between the researcher and the participant" (p. 45).

"The inherent unpredictability of the [qualitative] research process undermines the spirit of informed consent and endangers the assurance of confidentiality, two basic ethical safety nets in more quantitative research" (Ramos, 1989, p. 58). For example, in a study on the meaning of quality of life for individuals with type 1 (insulin-dependent) diabetes mellitus, data collection might begin with one open-ended question: "Tell me in as much detail as possible: What does it mean to have quality of life with type 1 insulin-dependent diabetes mellitus?" The researcher's probing questions to elicit a more detailed understanding can open a Pandora's box. Issues surrounding compliance or noncompliance may arise that endanger the client's health, or perhaps the client is depressed and concerned about issues related to loss, death, and dying. What may emerge is impossible to predict, but both researchers and participants must be informed and prepared to address issues that arise as data emerges.

The emergent design of qualitative research demands a different approach to informed consent. *Consensual decision making*, also called *process informed consent*, is more appropriate for the conduct of a qualitative investigation. This approach requires that researchers, at varying points in the research process, re-evaluate participants' consent to participate in the study. According to Munhall (1988), process consent encourages mutual participation: "Because qualitative research is conducted in an ever-changing field, informed consent should be an ongoing process. Over time, consent needs to be renegotiated as unexpected events or consequences occur" (p. 156). Information about how the researcher enters the field, participants' time commitment, and what will become of the findings are all important components to process consent (Munhall, 1988). Participants must know from the beginning of, and be reminded throughout, the investigation that they have the right to withdraw from the research study at any time. A process consent offers the opportunity to change the original consent as the study emerges and change becomes necessary. "Common sense plays a large part in renegotiating informed consent. If our focus should change, we need to ask participants for permission to change the first agreement. Continually informing and asking permission establishes the needed trust to go on further in an ethical manner" (Munhall, 1988, p. 157).

It is essential that researchers and participants discuss and clarify their understanding of the investigation (Alty & Rodham, 1998; Raudonis, 1992). As Alty and Rodham (1998) have emphasized, "At the best of times, it is difficult to know if the person you are talking to really has the same understanding of the topic as you do; indeed, if the researcher has an accurate understanding of what the subject is expressing" (p. 277).

Participant observation is an important approach to data collection in qualitative investigations. This method of data collection is useful in learning about the social practices of participants, the manner in which they relate to each other, and how they interpret their world (Merrell & Williams, 1994; Punch, 1994; Moore & Savage, 2002; Savage, 2000). *Covert participant observation*, which results when participants are unaware they are being observed, presents another ethical concern for qualitative researchers. Covert participant observation is sometimes a necessary component to data generation in some qualitative investigations. The rationale from the researcher's perspective would be to ensure that collected data are true and accurate. This type of data generation is grounded in the idea that, when the participants are aware they are being observed, their behavior will change. For example, Clarke (1996) discussed the use of covert participant observation in a secure forensic unit and the ethical issues that emerged from this method of data generation. Clarke emphasized the need to obtain an "uncontaminated picture of the unit" (p. 37).

A researcher's integrity can become damaged if the researcher uses deception to generate data. Some researchers claim that deception in the form of covert observations—or not completely describing the aims of the study or its procedures—is sometimes necessary to get reliable and valid data (Douglas, 1979; Gans, 1962). Punch (1994) agreed that field-related deception might be necessary, provided the interests of the subjects are protected. Others have argued that the need for covert research is exaggerated (Bulmer, 1982). The use of covert participant observation must be given serious consideration in the conduct of a qualitative investigation. Researchers must consider available alternative solutions for data generation, provided those solutions will maintain the integrity of the study.

Confidentiality and Anonymity

The principle of beneficence, doing good and preventing harm, applies to providing confidentiality and anonymity for research study participants. According to Polit and Beck (2004), "A promise of confidentiality is a pledge that any information participants provide will not be publicly reported in a manner that identifies them and will not be made accessible to others" (p. 150), and "anonymity occurs when even the researcher cannot link a participant to [his/her] data" (p. 149).

The very nature of data collection in a qualitative investigation makes anonymity impossible. The personal, one-to-one interaction during the interview process allows researchers to know the participants in ways that are not possible and unnecessary in quantitative designs. Qualitative research methods such as participant observation and one-to-one interviews make it "impossible to maintain anonymity at all stages; in other words, when using these methods, becoming cognizant of the source of data is unavoidable" (Behi & Nolan, 1995, p. 713).

Small sample size and thick descriptions provided in the presentation of the findings can present problems in maintaining confidentiality (Behi & Nolan, 1995; Boman & Jevne, 2000; Holloway & Wheeler, 1995; Lincoln & Guba, 1987; O'Reilly et al., 2007; Ramos, 1989; Robley, 1995). Davis (1991) discussed thick descriptions as follows: "We learn from our experiences and we need to present the fruits of that learning in a full-bodied way that invites our audience to share that experience with us, and also to judge the legitimacy of our results" (p. 13). Robley (1995) emphasized that thick descriptions are extremely important to the meaning of the research and offered a solution supported by the works of Cowles (1988), Davis (1991), and Lincoln and Guba (1987): "If the narrative requires it, retain it and return to the respondent for permission, verification, and justification" (Robley, 1995, p. 48).

Often, if the research has been conducted close to home and the sample is familiar to others, the details given in the thick slices of data used to support and verify themes may reveal research participants' identities. The researcher must make every effort to ensure that confidentiality is a promise kept. "Guaranteeing confidentiality implies that the research subject's data will be used in such a way that no-one else but the researcher knows the source" (Behi & Nolan, 1995, p. 713). As Robley (1995) has pointed out, "Guarding against disclosure that may create unacceptable risks for the respondents is accomplished in part by respecting the need for withdrawal of revealing material during the interview process, and in part through the process of member checking and negotiated outcomes" (p. 46). In some instances, circulation of the research may need to be restricted to protect participants' identity (Orb et al., 2001).

Orb et al. (2001) note that confidentiality and anonymity can be breached by legal requirements, such as when researchers' data are subpoenaed for legal purposes (p. 95). Audit trails, commonly used to establish the confirmability of research findings, require that other researchers read the raw data. Participants need to know that this may occur within the context of data analysis. Haggerty and Hawkins (2000) discussed the limits of confidentiality within the context of the legal and ethical issues that arose in research they conducted on partner abuse. They emphasize the importance of balancing the rights of participants and furthering knowledge that has the potential to improve health care delivery. Balancing the right to privacy and confidentiality for their participants with legally mandated reporting regarding child abuse, homicidality, and suicidality are addressed.

The process of publication may also result in a breach in confidentiality or anonymity. Permission to use direct quotes must be acquired, and the researcher must be sure that examples of raw data do not reveal the participant's identity. It is imperative that, within the process of gaining consent, the participants know how the results will be used and whether they will be published (Orb et al., 2001). Finally, data may exist in a variety of formats such as written demographic data, taped interviews, videotapes, and photos. All of these formats have the potential to identify participants; they must be stored securely and, at the completion of the study, disposed of properly.

Ethical Considerations Related to the Researcher–Participant Relationship

The principle of justice concerns fair treatment and the right to privacy and anonymity. The data generation strategies associated with a qualitative investigation include such approaches as one-to-one interviews, focus groups, and participant observation. The private and intimate nature of this relationship imposes unique constraints and raises distinct ethical issues for investigators using qualitative methods. The researcher is the tool for data collection and, as such, comes to know participants in a personal way. The boundaries of the relationship may become blurred as the research progresses, and role confusion may lead to ethical concerns for the investigation. As Ramos (1989) explained, "The respondent and the investigator interact verbally, and their relationship can range from one of civil cooperation to camaraderie in problem-solving to the abiding trust and dependency of the therapeutic alliance" (p. 59).

"Nurses are legally, culturally, and historically bound to nurture and protect the health and welfare of their patients" (Ramos, 1989, p. 57). Therefore, when participants confuse the researcher's role with that of a counselor, therapist, or nurse as caregiver and unrelated issues of concern emerge, the protection of the participants' welfare must always take precedence over the research. Researchers must not move from the role of instrument in the investigation to that of counselor or therapist. "Research in nursing constitutes a delicate balance between the principles of rigorous investigation and a nurturing concern for patient welfare" (Ramos, 1989, p. 57). Investigators can attempt to guide the interview and must maintain focus on the topic under investigation. The interview is not a therapeutic intervention, and the researcher should avoid asking questions that might result in participants offering more information than they had originally consented to. Following the closure of the interview, researchers should recap for the participants' issues of concern that emerged during the interview and should also provide follow-up.

Researchers must also consider the selection of participants for a qualitative research study from an ethical standpoint. "An ethical basis for selection would also involve attention to the inclusion of those whose voices need to be heard: women, minorities, children, the illiterate, and those with less personal or professional status. Social responsibility calls for attention to diversity" (Robley, 1995, p. 46).

SENSITIVE ISSUES ARISING IN THE CONDUCT OF QUALITATIVE RESEARCH

*T*he interview may be one of the few opportunities participants have to discuss the issue at hand, and the topic may well be a sensitive one. Alty and Rodham (1998) have given perspective to sensitive issues:

> The ouch! factor is a term that describes certain experiences encountered in the process of conducting qualitative research. These experiences include those ranging from a short sharp shock to the researcher to those situations and experiences that can develop into a chronic ache if not addressed early. (p. 275)

Sensitive issues also may arise in research conducted with vulnerable populations such as dying people (Raudonis, 1992); children and adolescents (Faux, Walsh, & Deatrick, 1988); families (Demi & Warren, 1995); lesbians and gay men (Platzer & James, 1997); those involved in HIV research in poor nations (Mabunda, 2001); and individuals with intellectual disabilities (Llewellyn, 1995). Certain topics such as the "sudden violent death of a loved one, controversial involvement in political activity, a crumbling relationship, legal incarceration, and a life-threatening illness" (Cowles, 1988, p. 163) are extremely sensitive and place participants in a vulnerable situation as the researcher asks the probing questions to elicit the necessary data. Given the intensity of the interaction between researcher and participant, the researcher also may be in a vulnerable position. As Robley (1995) has observed,

> Subjectivity and collaboration makes the researcher vulnerable. Emotionally immersed in the lived experience of others, continually sensitive to the potentially injurious nature of language, and experiencing the rights of passage as an interviewer/observer—all require an inner strength that can be enhanced by self care. The researcher can use the ethics committee as a guide and support throughout the process. [He or she] can use debriefing to explore personal responses and weigh risk/benefits. Personal education in ethics and consultation with experts when it is believed that the nurse researcher is being hurt is advocated. (p. 48)

Similarly, James and Platzer (1999) discuss the risk for harm to both researcher and participant in a qualitative study with lesbians and gay men and their experiences with health care. Their account of the complex emotional and ethical issues that can arise in research with vulnerable groups emphasizes the need for researchers to pay attention to things that cause them discomfort and unease in the process of their research.

Do not stray from the focus of the investigation. Recognize that participants may need to talk, but make clear that the researcher will address the issue after the interview. "All research (particularly that which focuses on sensitive issues) may stir up emotions of such intensity that failure to provide an opportunity for the respondent to talk may be perceived as irresponsible" (Alty & Rodham, 1998, p. 279). Allowing time for feedback and discussion of participants' feelings brings with it the possibility that the researcher will hear too much, but it must be done. After each interview, ask participants if they need follow-up. Provide a contact for additional help (Alty & Rodham, 1998; Dickson-Swift et al., 2008; Holloway & Wheeler, 1995; Richards & Swartz, 2002).

GATHERING, INTERPRETING, AND REPORTING QUALITATIVE DATA

Gathering, interpreting, and reporting qualitative research findings require that researchers spend time planning how data will be collected and then reading and rereading verbatim transcriptions of interviews and field notes. Procedures such as bracketing (defined in Chapter 2) are required if researchers are to have any confidence in the final data analysis. Researchers must keep any presuppositions and personal biases separate or set aside throughout the entire investigation. Having a second researcher review data and verify categories can also serve as a validity check. According to Ramos (1989),

> The investigator, even with the validation of inferences afforded by the relationship with the respondent, imposes his or her logic and values onto the communicated reality of the respondent. He or she imposes his or her subjective reality upon the interpretation of meaning-data from the respondent. The researcher cannot extract correct meanings unilaterally. Without the validation afforded by member checking, a leap in logic could occur, and a serious misinterpretation of sensitive information can occur. (p. 60)

Returning final descriptions to participants so that they may validate that the interpretation of the interview or observation is authentic and true further adds to final data analysis. This procedure can assist researchers in verifying that there were no serious misinterpretations or omissions of critical information. Respondent validation does, however, have limitations. The repeated contact with participants may be impractical and present undue burden on participants (Richards & Schwartz, 2002).

Haggman-Laitila (1999) expands on the discussion of authenticity of data and overcoming the researcher's personal views. Haggman-Laitila bases a discussion of data collection and analysis on the assumption that the researcher cannot detach from his or her own view in phenomenological research. The researcher is able to understand the experiences of an individual only through the researcher's own view. The research process is a balanced cooperative relationship between the subjects and the researcher (p. 13). Given this assumption, Haggman-Laitila offers practical guidelines for the purpose of data gathering and interpretation in a qualitative investigation.

During the process of data gathering, Haggman-Laitila (1999) suggests that researchers plan key interview questions in advance, keep interviews open and discussion-like, verify interpretations by asking more questions and allowing additions and corrections, avoid rhetorical or leading questions, and keep a diary or videotape to facilitate recognition of the researchers' own views during the data analysis process. During data analysis, the researcher must look for additional questions raised in the data, write down questions that emerge during the reading of the data, compare researcher and participant views, re-examine all experiences, and be sure that the presentation of findings is based on the views expressed by the participants. Smith (1999) illustrates the importance of considering the researcher's reflections through the use of a reflexive journal. Smith used the journaling process in his study of the lived experience of suffering among six problem drinkers. The information reported in the reflexive journal added to the contextual richness of the study.

HUMAN SUBJECTS AND INTERNET RESEARCH

*T*he Internet is a comprehensive electronic database of material that represents the opinions and concerns of those individuals who utilize this resource. Qualitative analysis of material communicated on the Internet can describe needs, values, concerns, and preference of consumers and professionals relevant to health and health care. Although the Internet provides innovative access to human interactions, such research raises new issues in research ethics.

Within the context of ethics and Internet research, questions emerge regarding what may be public versus private information, whether informed consent has been obtained, and the extent to which the subjects can be identified. Im and Chee (2002) discuss issues related to the protection of human subjects in Internet research that emerged in a study exploring gender and ethnic diversity in cancer pain experiences. Issues raised in their study include concerns regarding anonymity and confidentiality, security, full disclosure, and fair treatment. The authors focus on mechanisms employed to address ethical concerns that emerged in the study. Similarly, Sixsmith, and Murray, 2001 discussed issues of consent, privacy anonymity and ownership as these concepts relate to internet posts and archives. As more and more research is conducted through the Internet, ethical codes will need to be examined to ensure they address the issues that emerge in this type of research. Traditional tenets of informed consent and public and private information must be questioned when researchers use electronic databases for their research.

SUMMARY

A lthough the ethical principles governing qualitative and quantitative research are similar, the complex, personal, and intense nature of qualitative research requires a fresh perspective regarding the research process. The dynamic nature of qualitative methodologies presents unique concerns regarding informed consent. Treating consent as an ongoing process rather than an isolated event allows participants to re-evaluate their participation in a particular study should the focus change. Qualitative data collection strategies prevent participant anonymity. Maintaining the focus of the research and clarifying the purpose can prevent the development of close, intimate relationships between participants and the researcher from turning into what may be interpreted as therapeutic encounters. Presentation of the findings with thick descriptions and slices of raw data may complicate issues of confidentiality. When writing the analysis, the researcher should take care to prevent the identity of participants from being revealed through the incorporation of examples of raw data. Internet research presents new and emerging concerns regarding anonymity and confidentiality. Additionally, researchers must consider and address the vulnerability of certain populations. These issues are important in the ongoing development and use of qualitative research methods. Finally, it is important to remember that although established ethical guidelines may give some direction, the ethical and moral picture of qualitative research is much more complicated. Even though an ethical review board may have approved a research study, problems may still arise. "We should not simply assume that because research has been accepted by a committee it is morally justifiable in its methods" (Firby, 1995, p. 36). Ethical guidelines for qualitative research will continue to emerge, and researchers must consider those guidelines from a different perspective than those associated with quantitative designs.

References

Alty, A., & Rodham, K. (1998). The ouch! factor: Problems in conducting sensitive research. *Qualitative Health Research, 8*(2), 275–282.

American Nurses Association. (2001). *Code for nurses with interpretive statements.* Kansas City, MO: Author.

Beauchamp, T. L., & Childress, J. F. (2001). *Principles of biomedical ethics* (5th ed.). Oxford, UK: Oxford University Press.

Behi, R., & Nolan, M. (1995). Ethical issues in research. *British Journal of Nursing, 4*(12), 712–716.

Boman, J., & Jevne, R. (2000). Ethical evaluation in qualitative research. *Qualitative Health Research, 10*(4), 547–554.

Bulmer, M. (Ed.). (1982). *Social research ethics.* New York: Macmillan.

Clarke, L. (1996). Covert participant observation in a secure forensic unit. *Nursing Times, 92*(48), 37–40.

Cowles, K. V. (1988). Issues in qualitative research on sensitive topics. *Western Journal of Nursing Research, 10*(2), 163–179.

Cutliffe, J. R., & Ramcharan, P. (2002). Leveling the playing field? Exploring the merits of the ethics-as-process approach for judging qualitative research proposals. *Qualitative Health Research, 12*(7), 1000–1010.

Davis, D. S. (1991). Rich cases: The ethics of thick description. *Hastings Center Report, 21*(4), 12–16.

Demi, A. S., & Warren, N. A. (1995). Issues in conducting research with vulnerable families. *Western Journal of Nursing Research, 17*(2), 188–202.

Dickson-Swift, V., James, E. L., Kippen, S., & Liamputtong, P. (2008). Risk to researchers in qualitative research on sensitive topics: Issues and strategies. *Qualitative Health Research, 18*, 133–144.

Douglas, J. D. (1979). Living morality versus bureaucratic fiat. In C. B. Klockers & F. W. O. Connor (Eds.), *Deviance and decency: The ethics of research with human subjects* (pp. 13–33). Beverly Hills, CA: Sage.

Faux, S. A., Walsh, M., & Deatrick, J. A. (1988). Intensive interviewing with adolescents. *Western Journal of Nursing Research, 10*(2), 180–194.

Firby, P. (1995). Critiquing the ethical aspects of a study. *Nurse Researcher, 3*(1), 35–41.

Forbat, L., & Henderson, J. (2003). "Stuck in the middle with you": The ethics and process of qualitative research with two people in an intimate relationship. *Qualitative Health Research, 13*(10), 1453–1462.

Gans, H. J. (1962). *The urban villagers: Group and class in the life of Italian-Americans.* New York, NY: Free Press.

Haggerty, L. A., & Hawkins, J. (2000). Informed consent and the limits of confidentiality. *Western Journal of Nursing Research, 22*(4), 508–515.

Haggman-Laitila, A. (1999). The authenticity and ethics of phenomenological research: How to overcome the researcher's own views. *Nursing Ethics, 6*(1), 12–22.

Holloway, I., & Wheeler, S. (1995). Ethical issues in qualitative nursing research. *Nursing Ethics, 2*(3), 223–232.

Im, E., & Chee, W. (2002). Issues in protection of human subjects in Internet research. *Nursing Research, 51*(4), 266–269.

James, T., & Platzer, H. (1999). Ethical considerations in qualitative research with vulnerable groups: Exploring lesbians' and gay men's experiences of health care—a personal perspective. *Nursing Ethics, 6*(1), 73–81.

Karnieli-Miller, O., Strier, R., Pessach, L. (2009). Power relations in qualitative research. *Qualitative Health Research, 19*(2), 279–289.

Lawton, J. (2001). Gaining and maintaining consent: Ethical concerns raised in a study of dying patients. *Qualitative Health Research, 11*(5), 693–705.

Levine, R. (Ed.). (1986). *Ethics and regulation of clinical research* (2nd ed.). Baltimore-Munich: Urban & Schwarzenberg.

Lincoln, Y. S., & Guba, E. (1987). Ethics: The failure of positivist science. *Review of Higher Education, 12*, 221–240.

Llewellyn, G. (1995). Qualitative research with people with intellectual disability. *Occupational Therapy International, 2*, 108–127.

Mabunda, G. (2001). Ethical issues in HIV research in poor countries. *Journal of Nursing Scholarship, 33*(2), 111–114.

Merrell, J., & Williams, A. (1994). Participant observation and informed consent: Relationships and tactical decision-making in nursing research. *Nursing Ethics, 1*(3), 163–172.

Moore, L., & Savage, J. (2002). Participant observation, informed consent and ethical approval. *Nurse Researcher, 9*(4), 58–70.

Munhall, P. (1988). Ethical considerations in qualitative research. *Western Journal of Nursing Research, 10*(2), 150–162.

Orb, A., Eisenhauer, L., & Wynaden, D. (2001). Ethics in qualitative research. *Journal of Nursing Scholarship, 33*(1), 93–98.

Platzer, H., & James, T. (1997). Methodological issues conducting sensitive research on lesbian and gay men's experience of nursing care. *Journal of Advanced Nursing, 25*, 626–633.

Polit, D. F., & Beck, C. T. (2004). *Nursing research: Methods, appraisal, and utilization* (7th ed.). Philadelphia, PA: Lippincott Williams & Wilkins.

Punch, M. (1994). Politics and ethics in qualitative research. In N. K. Denzin & Y. S. Lincoln (Eds.), *Handbook of qualitative research* (pp. 86–97). Thousand Oaks, CA: Sage.

Ramos, M. C. (1989). Some ethical implications of qualitative research. *Research in Nursing and Health, 12*, 57–63.

Raudonis, B. A. (1992). Ethical considerations in qualitative research with hospice patients. *Qualitative Health Research, 2*(2), 238–249.

Richards, H. M., & Schwartz, L. J. (2002). Ethics of qualitative research: Are there special issues for health services research? *Family Practice, 19*(2), 135–139.

Robley, L. R. (1995). The ethics of qualitative nursing research. *Journal of Professional Nursing, 11*(1), 45–48.

Savage, J. (2000). Participative observation: Standing in the shoes of others? *Qualitative Health Research, 10*(3), 324–339.

Silva, M. (1995). *Ethical guidelines in the conduct, dissemination, and implementation of nursing research.* Washington, DC: American Nurses Publishing.

Sixsmith, J., & Murray, C. D. (2001). Ethical issues in the documentary data analysis of internet posts and archives. *Qualitative Health Research, 11*(3), 423–432.

Smith, B. A. (1999). Ethical and methodological benefits of using a reflexive journal in hermeneutic-phenomenologic research. *Journal of Nursing Scholarship, 31*(4), 359–363.

Steinbrook, R. (2002). Protecting research subjects: The crisis at John Hopkins. *New England Journal of Medicine, 346*, 716.

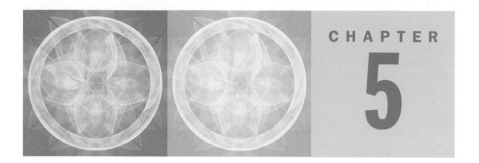

Phenomenology as Method

*P*henomenology has been and continues to be an integral field of inquiry that cuts across philosophic, sociologic, and psychological disciplines. This rigorous, critical, systematic method of investigation is a recognized qualitative research approach applicable to the study of phenomena important to the discipline of nursing. Phenomenological inquiry brings to language perceptions of human experience with all types of phenomena. As several authors have noted, phenomenology, both as philosophy and research approach, allows nursing to explore and describe phenomena important to the discipline (Arrigo & Cody, 2004; Beck, 1994; Caelli, 2000, 2001; McConnell-Henry, Chapman, & Francis, 2009; Ortiz, 2009; Todres & Wheeler, 2001; Van der Zalm & Bergum, 2000). Because professional nursing practice is enmeshed in people's life experiences, phenomenology as a research approach is well suited to the investigation of phenomena important to nursing.

Phenomenological inquiry as a philosophy and developing science continues to undergo interpretation and explication in terms of its pragmatic use as a nursing research method. This chapter addresses the variety of methodological interpretations detailed within the discipline of phenomenological inquiry. Phenomenology as philosophy and as method is discussed, along with fundamental differences between descriptive and interpretive phenomenology. Highlights of specific elements and interpretations of phenomenology as a research approach provide readers with a beginning understanding of common phenomenological language and themes. This chapter also addresses methodological concerns specific to conducting a phenomenological investigation.

Introductory concepts for researchers interested in conducting a phenomenological investigation are presented in the content that follows. The reader should keep in mind that there is no quick step-by-step method to phenomenological inquiry. The methodology is philosophically complex, and the analytic processes required to participate in the method require scientific discipline. Researchers interested in conducting a phenomenological investigation must read original philosophically based work and identify a mentor with expertise in the discipline to acquire an in-depth understanding of phenomenology both as a philosophy and as a research approach.

PHENOMENOLOGY DEFINED

*P*henomenology is a science whose purpose is to describe particular phenomena, or the appearance of things, as lived experience. Cohen (1987) has pointed out that phenomenology was first described as the study of phenomena or things by Immanuel Kant in 1764. Merleau-Ponty (1962), in the preface to his text *Phenomenology of Perception*, asked the question, What is phenomenology? His description reflects the flow of phenomenological thinking, but Merleau-Ponty never offered a definitive answer or step-by-step approach to what phenomenology actually entailed. Essentially, not much has changed. Merleau-Ponty offered the following description:

> Phenomenology is the study of essences; and according to it, all problems amount to finding definitions of essences: the essence of perception, or the essence of consciousness, for example. But phenomenology is also a philosophy, which puts essences back into existence, and does not expect to arrive at an understanding of man and the world from any starting point other than that of their "facticity." It is a transcendental philosophy which places in abeyance the assertions arising out of the natural attitude, the better to understand them: but it is also a philosophy for which the world is always "already there" before reflection begins—as an inalienable presence; and all its efforts are concentrated upon re-achieving a direct and primitive contact with the world, and endowing that contact with a philosophical status. It is the search for a philosophy which shall be a "rigorous science," but it also offers an account of space, time, and the world as we "live" them. It tries to give a direct description of our experience as it is, without taking account of its psychological origin and the causal explanations which the scientist, the historian, or the sociologist may be able to provide. (p. vii)

The historian Herbert Spiegelberg (1975) explained phenomenology as a movement rather than a uniform method or set of doctrines. The account provided by Spiegelberg emphasizes the fluid nature of phenomenology and the fact that a list of steps to the approach would not reflect the philosophic depth of the discipline. Spiegelberg defined phenomenology as "the name for a philosophical movement whose primary objective is the direct investigation and description of phenomena as consciously experienced, without theories about their causal explanation and as free as possible from unexamined preconceptions and presuppositions" (p. 3).

Spiegelberg (1975) and Merleau-Ponty (1962) described phenomenology as both a philosophy and a method. Phenomenology was further explained by Wagner (1983) as a way of viewing ourselves, others, and everything else whom or with which we come in contact in life. "Phenomenology is a system of interpretation that helps us perceive and conceive ourselves, our contacts and interchanges with others, and everything else in the realm of our experiences in a variety of ways, including to describe a method as well as a philosophy or way of thinking" (Wagner, 1983, p. 8).

Omery (1983) addressed the question, What is the phenomenological method? Although researchers have interpreted this question in a variety of ways, the approach is inductive and descriptive in its design. Phenomenological method is "the trick of making things whose meanings seem clear, meaningless, and then, discovering what they mean" (Blumensteil, 1973, p. 189).

Lived experience of the world of everyday life is the central focus of phenomenological inquiry. Schutz (1970) described the world of everyday life as the "total sphere of experiences of an individual which is circumscribed by the objects, persons, and events encountered in the pursuit of the pragmatic objectives of living" (p. 320). In other words, it is the lived experience that presents to the individual what is true or real in his or her life. Furthermore, it is this lived experience that gives meaning to each individual's perception of a particular phenomenon and is influenced by everything internal and external to the individual. Perception is important in phenomenological philosophy and method, as explained by Merleau-Ponty (1956):

> Perception is not a science of the world, nor even an act, a deliberate taking up of a position. It is the basis from which every act issues and it is presupposed by them. The world is not an object the law of whose constitution I possess. It is the natural milieu and the field of all my thoughts and of all my explicit perceptions. Truth does not "dwell" only in the "interior man" for there is no interior man. Man is before himself in the world and it is in the world that he knows himself. When I turn upon myself from the dogmatism of common sense or the dogmatism of science, I find, not the dwelling place of intrinsic truth, but a subject committed to the world. (p. 62)

Phenomenology is as much a way of thinking or perceiving as it is a method. The goal of phenomenology is to describe lived experience. To further clarify both the philosophy and method of phenomenology, it is helpful to gain a sense of how the movement developed historically. An overview of the roots of phenomenology as a philosophy and science follows.

PHENOMENOLOGICAL ROOTS

*T*he phenomenological movement began around the first decade of the 20th century. This philosophic movement consisted of three phases: (1) preparatory; (2) German; and (3) French. The following text describes common themes of phenomenology within the context of these three phases.

Preparatory Phase

The Preparatory phase was dominated by Franz Brentano (1838–1917) and Carl Stumpf (1848–1936). Stumpf was Brentano's first prominent student and, through his work, demonstrated the scientific rigor of phenomenology. Clarification of the concept of intentionality was the primary focus during this time (Spiegelberg, 1965). *Intentionality* means that consciousness is always consciousness of something. Merleau-Ponty (1956) explained "interior perception is impossible without exterior perception, that the world as the connection of phenomena is anticipated in the consciousness of my unity and is the way for me to realize myself in consciousness" (p. 67). Therefore, one does not hear without hearing something or believe without believing something (Cohen, 1987).

German Phase

Edmund Husserl (1857–1938) and Martin Heidegger (1889–1976) were the prominent leaders during the German, or second, phase of the phenomenological movement. Husserl (1931, 1965) believed that philosophy should become a rigorous science that would restore contact with deeper human concerns and that phenomenology should become the foundation for all philosophy and science. According to Spiegelberg (1965), Heidegger followed so closely in the steps of Husserl that his work is probably a direct outcome of Husserl's. The concepts of essences, intuiting, and phenomenological reduction were developed during the German phase (Spiegelberg, 1965).

Essences are elements related to the ideal or true meaning of something, that is, those concepts that give common understanding to the phenomenon under investigation. Essences emerge in both isolation and in relationship to one another. According to Natanson (1973), "Essences are unities of meaning intended by different individuals in the same acts or by the same individuals in different acts" (p. 14). Essences, therefore, represent the basic units of common understanding of any phenomenon. For example, Schwarz (2003) explored how nurses experience and respond to patients' requests for assistance in dying. Schwarz (2003) describes the continuum of interventions provided by the nurses in her phenomenological study that includes "refusal, providing palliative care that might secondarily hasten dying, respecting and not interfering with patients' or families' plans to hasten dying, and providing varying types and degrees of direct AID" (p. 377). In a study examining patient experiences living with rheumatoid arthritis,

Iaquinta and Larrabee (2003) describe the essences of this experience as "grieving while growing, persuading self and others of RA's authenticity, cultivating resilience, confronting negative feelings, navigating the healthcare system, and masterminding new lifeways" (p. 282).

Intuiting is an eidetic comprehension or accurate interpretation of what is meant in the description of the phenomenon under investigation. The intuitive process in phenomenological research results in a common understanding about the phenomenon under investigation. Intuiting in the phenomenological sense requires that researchers imaginatively vary the data until a common understanding about the phenomenon emerges. Through imaginative variation, researchers begin to wonder about the phenomenon under investigation in relationship to the various descriptions generated. To further illustrate, in a study on commitment to nursing (Rinaldi, 1989), the essences of commitment gleaned from the data were varied in as many ways as possible and compared with participants' descriptions. From this imaginative variation, a relationship between the essences of commitment and to whom or what the nurse was committed emerged. For example, the nurse may be committed to clients, colleagues, the employing institution, the profession, or self. To whom or what the nurse is committed is then examined in relationship to the essences of commitment. Researchers might vary the essences of commitment within the descriptions of the person to whom or the thing to which the nurse is committed. Some essences may apply when the issue is commitment to clients, and other essences if the issue is commitment to the institution. In a study on the lived experience of caring for a child with cystic fibrosis, the intuitive process resulted in emergence of phenomena unique to caring for a child with a chronic illness at the time of diagnosis. The essential elements of the experience included Falling Apart, Pulling Together, and Moving Beyond (Carpenter & Narsavage, 2004).

Phenomenological reduction is a return to original awareness regarding the phenomenon under investigation. Husserl specified how to describe, with scientific exactness, the life of consciousness in its original encounter with the world through phenomenological reduction. Husserl (1931, 1965) challenged individuals to go "back to the things themselves" to recover this original awareness. Husserl's reference "to the things" meant "a fresh approach to concretely experienced phenomena, as free as possible from conceptual presuppositions and an attempt to describe them as faithfully as possible" (Spiegelberg, 1975, p. 10).

Phenomenological reduction begins with a suspension of beliefs, assumptions, and biases about the phenomenon under investigation. Isolation of pure phenomenon, versus what is already known about a particular phenomenon, is the goal of the reductive procedure. The only way to really see the world clearly is to remain as free as possible from preconceived ideas or notions. Complete reduction may never be possible because of the intimate relationship individuals have with the world (Merleau-Ponty, 1956).

As part of the reductive process, phenomenological researchers must first identify any preconceived notions or ideas about the phenomenon under investigation. Having identified these ideas, the researchers must bracket or separate out of consciousness what they know or believe about the topic under investigation. *Bracketing* requires researchers to remain neutral with respect to belief or disbelief in the existence of the phenomenon. Bracketing begins the reductive process and, like that process, must continue throughout the investigation. Essentially, researchers set aside previous knowledge or personal beliefs about the phenomenon under investigation to prevent this information from interfering with the recovery of a pure description of the phenomenon. Bracketing must be constant and ongoing if descriptions are to achieve their purest form. Haggman-Laitila (1999) holds the position that the researcher cannot detach from his or her own view and offers practical aspects to help in overcoming the researcher's views during data gathering and analysis. Chapter 4 offers an overview of strategies to address this very issue within the context of ethical standards.

French Phase

Gabriel Marcel (1889–1973), Jean-Paul Sartre (1905–1980), and Maurice Merleau-Ponty (1905–1980) were the predominant leaders of the French, or third phase, of the phenomenological movement. The primary concepts developed during this phase were embodiment and being-in-the-world. These concepts refer to the belief that all acts are constructed on foundations of perception or original awareness of some phenomenon. Lived experience, given in the perceived world, must be described (Merleau-Ponty, 1956). Munhall (1989) explained these key concepts, originally described by Merleau-Ponty, as follows:

> Embodiment explains that through consciousness one is aware of being-in-the-world and it is through the body that one gains access to this world. One feels, thinks, tastes, touches, hears, and is conscious through the opportunities the body offers. There is talk sometimes about expanding the mind or expanding waistlines. The expansion is within the body, within the consciousness. It is important to understand that at any point in time and for each individual a particular perspective and/or consciousness exists. It is based on the individual's history, knowledge of the world, and perhaps openness to the world. Nursing's focus on the individual and the "meaning" events may have for an individual, is this recognition that experience is individually interpreted. (p. 24)

The philosophic underpinnings of phenomenology are complex. Given this understanding, one can appreciate why the methodological applications remain dynamic and evolving. Different philosophers may have different interpretations of phenomenology as both a philosophy and method.

Table 5-1 • (Continued)	
Author(s)	*Procedural Steps*
	4. Eliminate expressions not meeting these two requirements.
	5. Tentatively identify the descriptive constituents; bring together all common relevant constituents in a cluster labeled with the more abstract formula expressing the common theme.
	6. Finally, identify the descriptive constituents by application; this operation consists of checking the tentatively identified constituents against random cases of the sample to see whether they fulfill the following conditions. Each constituent must: a. be expressed explicitly in the description, b. be expressed explicitly or implicitly in some or the large majority of descriptions, c. be compatible with the description in which it is not expressed.
	7. If a description is found incompatible with a constituent, the description must be proved not to be an expression of the experience under study, but of some other experience that intrudes on it.
van Manen (1990)	1. Turn to the nature of lived experience by orienting to the phenomenon, formulating the phenomenological question, and explicating assumptions and preunderstandings.
	2. Engage in existential investigation, which involves exploring the phenomenon: generating data, using personal experience as a starting point, tracing etymologic sources, searching idiomatic phrases, obtaining experiential descriptions from participants, locating experiential descriptions in the literature, and consulting phenomenological literature, art, and so forth.
	3. Engage in phenomenological reflection, which involves conducting thematic analysis, uncovering thematic aspects in life-world descriptions, isolating thematic statements, composing linguistic transformations, and gleaning thematic descriptions from artistic sources.
	4. Engage in phenomenological writing, which includes attending to the speaking of language, varying the examples, writing, and rewriting.
Streubert (1991)	1. Explicate a personal description of the phenomenon of interest.
	2. Bracket the researcher's presuppositions.
	3. Interview participants in unfamiliar settings.
	4. Carefully read the interview transcripts to obtain a general sense of the experience.
	5. Review the transcripts to uncover essences.
	6. Apprehend essential relationships.
	7. Develop formalized descriptions of the phenomenon.
	8. Return to participants to validate descriptions.
	9. Review the relevant literature.
	10. Distribute the findings to the nursing community.

Six Core Steps

Spiegelberg (1965, 1975) identified a core of steps or elements central to phenomenological investigations. These six steps are (1) descriptive phenomenology; (2) phenomenology of essences; (3) phenomenology of appearances; (4) constitutive phenomenology; (5) reductive phenomenology; and (6) hermeneutic phenomenology (Spiegelberg, 1975). A discussion of each of the six elements follows. As Spiegelberg (1965) has explained, the purpose of this discussion is to "present this method as a series of steps, of which the later will usually presuppose the earlier ones, yet not be necessarily entailed by them" (p. 655). As such, phenomenology as a movement is described. A combination of one or more of the elements identified as central to the movement can be found in the plethora of published phenomenological investigations.

DESCRIPTIVE PHENOMENOLOGY

*D*escriptive phenomenology involves "direct exploration, analysis, and description of particular phenomena, as free as possible from unexamined presuppositions, aiming at maximum intuitive presentation" (Spiegelberg, 1975, p. 57). Descriptive phenomenology stimulates our perception of lived experience while emphasizing the richness, breadth, and depth of those experiences (Spiegelberg, 1975, p. 70). Spiegelberg (1965, 1975) identified a three-step process for descriptive phenomenology: (1) intuiting; (2) analyzing; and (3) describing.

Intuiting

The first step, *intuiting*, requires the researcher to become totally immersed in the phenomenon under investigation and is the step in the process whereby the researcher begins to know about the phenomenon as described by the participants. The researcher avoids all criticism, evaluation, or opinion and pays strict attention to the phenomenon under investigation as it is being described (Spiegelberg, 1965, 1975).

The step of intuiting the phenomenon in a study of quality of life would involve the "researcher as instrument" in the interview process. The researcher becomes the tool for data collection and listens to individual descriptions of quality of life through the interview process. The researcher then studies the data as they are transcribed and reviews repeatedly what the participants have described as the meaning of quality of life.

Analyzing

The second step is *phenomenological analyzing*, which involves identifying the essence of the phenomenon under investigation based on data obtained and how the data are presented. As the researcher distinguishes the phenomenon with regard to elements or constituents, he or she explores the relationships and connections with adjacent phenomena (Spiegelberg, 1965, 1975).

As the researcher listens to descriptions of quality of life and dwells with the data, common themes or essences will begin to emerge. Dwelling with the data essentially involves complete immersion in the generated data to fully engage in this analytic process. The researcher must dwell with the data for as long as necessary to ensure a pure and accurate description.

Describing

The third step is *phenomenological describing*. The aim of the describing operation is to communicate and bring to written and verbal description distinct, critical elements of the phenomenon. The description is based on a classification or grouping of the phenomenon. The researcher must avoid attempting to describe a phenomenon prematurely. Premature description is a common methodological error associated with this type of research (Spiegelberg, 1965, 1975). Description is an integral part of intuiting and analyzing. Although addressed separately, intuiting and analyzing are often occurring simultaneously.

In a study on quality of life, phenomenological describing would involve classifying all critical elements or essences that are common to the lived experience of quality of life and describing these essences in detail. Critical elements or essences are described singularly and then within the context of their relationship to one another. A discussion of this relationship follows.

PHENOMENOLOGY OF ESSENCES

*P*henomenology of essences involves probing through the data to search for common themes or essences and establishing patterns of relationships shared by particular phenomena. *Free imaginative variation*, used to apprehend essential relationships between essences, involves careful study of concrete examples supplied by the participants' experiences and systematic variation of these examples in the imagination. In this way, it becomes possible to gain insights into the essential structures and relationships among phenomena. Probing for essences provides a sense for what is essential and what is accidental in the phenomenological description (Spiegelberg, 1975). The researcher follows through with the steps of intuiting, analyzing, and describing in this second core step (Spiegelberg, 1965, 1975). According to Spiegelberg (1975), "Phenomenology in its descriptive stage can stimulate our perceptiveness for the richness of our experience in breadth and in depth" (p. 70).

PHENOMENOLOGY OF APPEARANCES

P *henomenology of appearances* involves giving attention to the ways in which phenomena appear. In watching the ways in which phenomena appear, the researcher pays particular attention to the different ways in which an object presents itself. Phenomenology of appearances focuses attention on the phenomenon as it unfolds through dwelling with the data. Phenomenology of appearances "can heighten the sense for the inexhaustibility of the perspectives through which our world is given" (Spiegelberg, 1975, p. 70).

CONSTITUTIVE PHENOMENOLOGY

C *onstitutive phenomenology* is studying phenomena as they become established or "constituted" in our consciousness. Constitutive phenomenology "means the process in which the phenomena 'take shape' in our consciousness, as we advance from first impressions to a full 'picture' of their structure" (Spiegelberg, 1975, p. 66). According to Spiegelberg (1975), constitutive phenomenology "can develop the sense for the dynamic adventure in our relationship with the world" (p. 70).

REDUCTIVE PHENOMENOLOGY

R *eductive phenomenology*, although addressed as a separate process, occurs concurrently throughout a phenomenological investigation. The researcher continually addresses personal biases, assumptions, and presuppositions or sets aside these beliefs to obtain the purest description of the phenomenon under investigation. Suspending judgment can make us more aware of the precariousness of all our claims to knowledge, "a ground for epistemological humility" (Spiegelberg, 1975, p. 70).

This step is critical for the preservation of objectivity in the phenomenological method. For example, in a study investigating the meaning of quality of life for individuals with type 1 (insulin-dependent) diabetes mellitus, the investigator begins the study with the reductive process. The researcher identifies all presuppositions, biases, or assumptions he or she holds about what quality of life means or what it is like to have diabetes. This process involves a critical self-examination of personal beliefs and an acknowledgment of understandings that the researcher has gained from experience. The researcher takes all he or she knows about the phenomenon and brackets it or sets it aside in an effort to keep what is already known separate from the lived experience as described by the participants.

Phenomenological reduction is critical if the researcher is to achieve pure description. The reductive process is also the basis for postponing any review of the literature until the researcher has analyzed the data. The researcher must always keep separate from the participants' descriptions what he or she knows or believes about the phenomenon under investigation. Therefore, postponing the literature review until data analysis is complete facilitates phenomenological reduction.

INTERPRETIVE NURSING RESEARCH AND HERMENEUTIC PHILOSOPHY

Interpretive frameworks within phenomenology are used to search out the relationships and meanings that knowledge and context have for each other (Lincoln & Guba, 1985). Increasingly, published nursing research is grounded in the philosophic theory of hermeneutics, and several authors have discussed the philosophic underpinnings of this particular research approach, offering clarity and direction for others (Crist & Tanner, 2003; Geanellos, 2000; Todres & Wheeler, 2001; Van der Zalm & Bergum, 2000). A phenomenological-hermeneutic approach is essentially a philosophy of the nature of understanding a particular phenomenon and the scientific interpretation of phenomena appearing in text or written word. Hermeneutics as an interpretive approach is based on the work of Ricoeur (1976), Heidegger (1962), and Gadamer (1976). The methodology allows for increasingly sensitive awareness of humans and their ways of being-in-the-world (Dreyfus, 1991). Allen and Jenson (1990) emphasized that

> The value of knowledge in nursing is, in part, determined by its relevance to and significance for an understanding of the human experience. In order to obtain that understanding, nursing requires modes of inquiry that offer the freedom to explore the richness of this experience. Hermeneutics offers such a mode of inquiry. With this interpretive strategy, a means is provided for arriving at a deeper understanding of human existence through attention to the nature of language and meaning. (p. 241)

Hermeneutic phenomenology is a "special kind of phenomenological interpretation, designed to unveil otherwise concealed meanings in the phenomena" (Spiegelberg, 1975, p. 57). Gadamer (1976) elaborated by noting that hermeneutics bridges the gap between what is familiar in our worlds and what is unfamiliar: "Its field of application is comprised of all those situations in which we encounter meanings that are not immediately understandable but require interpretive effort" (p. xii). As in all research, congruence between the philosophic foundations of the study and the methodological processes of the research are critical. The basic elements of hermeneutic philosophy and interpretive inquiry are addressed in the following narrative within the context of the work of Ricoeur (1976), Heidegger (1927/1962), and Gadamer (1976).

Paul Ricoeur's interpretive approach is one way in which nurse researchers can apply hermeneutic philosophy to a qualitative investigation. Ricoeur (1976) describes the interpretive process as a series of analytic steps and acknowledged the "interrelationship between epistemology (interpretation) and ontology (interpreter)" (Geanellos, 2000, p. 112). Crist and Tanner (2003) also describe the interpretive process of hermeneutic phenomenology. They note that although it is not required, having a team of researchers that can debate, brainstorm, and discuss interpretations adds depth and insight to the content area of the inquiry (Crist & Tanner, 2003). A major difference between hermeneutic phenomenology and other interpretations of phenomenological research methods is the fact that the method does not require researchers to bracket their own preconceptions or theories during the process (Lowes & Prowse, 2001). Analysis is essentially the hermeneutic circle, which proceeds from a naïve understanding to an explicit understanding that emerges from explanation of data interpretation. As described by Allen and Jenson (1990),

> The hermeneutical circle of interpretation moves forward and backward, starting at the present. It is never closed or final. Through rigorous interaction and understanding, the phenomenon is uncovered. The interpretive process that underlies meaning arises out of interactions, working outward and back from self to event and event to self. (p. 245)

There are three main steps to the process of hermeneutic phenomenology:

1. First, during the *naïve reading*, the researcher reads the text as a whole to become familiar with the text and begins to formulate thoughts about its meaning for further analysis. Lindholm, Uden, and Rastam (1999) in a study on nursing management note that during this particular component of data analysis, they "read all the interviews individually to gain a sense of the whole text. Their impressions of the text were then documented and discussed. The naïve reading directed attention to the phenomenon of power" (p. 103).

2. *Structural analysis* follows as the second step and involves identifying patterns of meaningful connection. This step is often referred to as an *interpretive reading*. To illustrate, Lindholm et al. (1999) noted that the researchers met to compare and discuss the texts. They describe this step in the following manner: "The text was divided into meaning units, which were transformed with the contents intact. Arising from every transformed meaning unit a number of labels were created, to discover common themes. During the analysis, there was continuous movement between the whole and the parts of the text" (p. 103).

3. Third, *interpretation of the whole* follows and involves reflecting on the initial reading along with the interpretive reading to ensure a comprehensive understanding of the findings. Several readings are usually required. Lindholm et al. (1999) performed a separate interpretation of their data during this step and described themes and subthemes within the data.

important to nursing requires that researchers study lived experience as it is presented in the everyday world of nursing practice, education, and administration. Human experience is the central tenet, and how human beings experience phenomena important to nursing practice directs phenomenological investigations.

A holistic perspective and the study of experience as lived serve as the foundation for phenomenological inquiry. A positive response to the following questions will help researchers clarify whether phenomenological method is the most appropriate approach for the investigation. First, researchers should ask, Is there a need for further clarity on the chosen phenomenon? Evidence leading researchers to conclude that phenomena need further clarity may be that there is little if anything published on a subject, or perhaps what is published needs to be described in more depth. Second, researchers should consider the question, Will the shared lived experience be the best data source for the phenomenon under investigation? Because the primary method of data collection is the voice of the people experiencing a particular phenomenon, researchers must determine that this approach will provide the richest and most descriptive data. Third, as in all research, investigators should ask, What are the available resources, the time frame for the completion of the research, the audience to which the research will be presented, and my own personal style and ability to engage in the method in a rigorous manner while accepting the inherent ambiguity?

Topics appropriate to phenomenological research method include those central to humans' life experiences. Examples include happiness, fear, being there, commitment, being a chairperson, being a head nurse, or the meaning of stress for nursing students in the clinical setting. Health-related topics suitable for phenomenological investigation might include a myriad of topics such as the meaning of pain, living with chronic illness, and end-of-life issues. Chapter 6 offers readers a selective sample of published research using phenomenological research methodology in the areas of practice, education, and administration.

ELEMENTS AND INTERPRETATIONS OF THE METHOD

Researcher's Role

As lived experience becomes the description of a particular phenomenon, the investigator takes on specific responsibilities in transforming the information. Reinharz (1983) articulated five steps that occur in phenomenological transformation as the investigator makes public what essentially was private knowledge. The first transformation occurs as people's experiences are transformed into language. During this step, the researcher, through verbal interaction, creates an opportunity for the lived experience to be shared (Reinharz, 1983). In the example of research on quality of life for individuals with type 1 diabetes mellitus, the researcher would create an opportunity for individuals living with this chronic illness to share their experiences related to the meaning of quality of life.

The second transformation occurs as the researcher transforms what is seen and heard into an understanding of the original experience. Because one person can never experience what another person has experienced in exactly the same manner, researchers must rely on the data participants have shared about a particular experience and from those develop their own transformation (Reinharz, 1983). In this instance, the researcher studying quality of life takes what participants have said and produces a description that lends understanding to the participants' original experiences.

Third, the researcher transforms what is understood about the phenomenon under investigation into conceptual categories that are the essences of the original experience (Reinharz, 1983). Data analysis of interviews addressing the meaning of quality of life would involve clarifying the essences of the phenomenon. For example, the data may reveal that quality of life for an individual with type 1 diabetes mellitus may center on freedom from restrictions in daily activities, independence, and prevention of long-term complications.

Fourth, the researcher transforms those essences into a written document that captures what the researcher has thought about the experience and reflects the participants' descriptions or actions. In all transformations, information may be lost or gained; therefore, it is important to have participants review the final description to ensure that the material is correctly stated and nothing has been added or deleted (Reinharz, 1983).

Fifth, the researcher transforms the written document into an understanding that can function to clarify all preceding steps (Reinharz, 1983). The intent of this written document, often referred to as the exhaustive description, is to synthesize and capture the meaning of the experience into written form without distorting or losing the richness of the data. In other words, the exhaustive description of quality of life would reveal the richness of the experience identified from the very beginning of the investigation as perceived by individuals with type 1 diabetes mellitus.

In addition to the five transformational steps outlined by Reinharz (1983), the investigator must possess certain qualities that will permit access to data that participants possess. The abilities to communicate clearly and to help participants feel comfortable expressing their experiences are essential qualities in a phenomenological researcher. The researcher is the instrument for data collection and must function effectively to facilitate data collection. The researcher must recognize that personal characteristics such as manner of speaking, gender, age, and other personality traits may interfere with data retrieval. For this reason, researchers must ask whether they are the appropriate people to access a given person's or group's experiences (Reinharz, 1983).

Data Generation

Purposive sampling is used most commonly in phenomenological inquiry. This method of sampling selects individuals for study participation based on their particular knowledge of a phenomenon for the purpose of sharing that knowledge. "The logic and power of purposeful sampling lies in selecting information-rich cases for study in depth. Information-rich cases are those from which one can learn a great deal about issues of central importance to the purpose of the research, thus the term purposeful sampling" (Patton, 1990, p. 169).

Sample selection provides the participants for the investigation. Researchers should contact participants, once they have agreed to participate, before the interview to prepare them for the actual meeting and to answer any preliminary questions. At the time of the first interview, the researcher may obtain informed consent and permission to tape-record, if using this data-gathering instrument. Piloting interview skills and having a more experienced phenomenological researcher listen to the tape of an interview can assist in the development of interviewing skills. According to Benoliel (1988), an "effective observer-interviewer needs to bring knowledge, sensitivity, and flexibility into a situation. Interviewing is not an interpersonal exchange controlled by the interviewer but rather a transaction that is reciprocal in nature and involves an exchange of social rewards" (p. 211).

Researchers should help participants describe lived experience without leading the discussion. Open-ended, clarifying questions such as the following facilitate this process: What comes to mind when you hear the word *commitment*? What comes to mind when you think about quality of life? Open-ended interviewing allows researchers to follow participants' lead, to ask clarifying questions, and to facilitate the expression of the participants' lived experience. Interviews usually end when participants believe they have exhausted their descriptions. If interviews are not feasible, researchers may ask participants to write an extensive description of some phenomenon by responding to a pre-established question or questions. The concern with written responses versus tape-recorded interviews is that descriptions may not reveal the depth and detail that can be achieved through interviews. During the interview, researchers can help participants explain things in more detail by asking questions. This valuable opportunity is eliminated when participants write their descriptions.

The interview allows entrance into another person's world and is an excellent source of data. Complete concentration and rigorous participation in the interview process improve the accuracy, trustworthiness, and authenticity of the data. However, researchers must remember to remain centered on the data, listen attentively, avoid interrogating participants, and treat participants with respect and sincere interest in the shared experience.

Data generation or collection continues until the researcher believes saturation has been achieved, that is, when no new themes or essences have emerged from the participants and the data are repeating. Therefore, predetermination of the number of participants for a given study is impossible. Data collection must continue until the researcher is assured saturation has been achieved.

Morse (1989) stated that saturation is a myth. She proposed that, given another group of informants on the same subject at another time, new data may be revealed. Therefore, investigators will be able to reach saturation only with a particular group of informants and only during specific times. "The long term challenge for the phenomenologist interested in generating theory is to interview several samples from a variety of backgrounds, age ranges and cultural environments to maximize the likelihood of discovering the essences of phenomena across groups" (Streubert, 1991, p. 121).

Ethical Considerations

The personal nature of phenomenological research results in several ethical considerations for researchers. Informed consent differs in a qualitative study as opposed to a quantitative investigation. There is no way to know exactly what might transpire during an interview. Researchers must consider issues of privacy. When preparing a final manuscript, researchers must determine how to present the data so that they are accurate yet do not reveal participants' identities. For an in-depth discussion of ethical issues in qualitative research, see Chapter 4.

Data Treatment

Researchers may handle treatment of the data in a variety of ways. Use of open-ended interviewing techniques, tape recordings, and verbatim transcriptions will increase the accuracy of data collection. High-quality tape-recording equipment is essential. Researchers will make handwritten notes. Adding handwritten notes to verbally transcribed accounts helps to achieve the most comprehensive and accurate description. A second interview may be needed, giving researchers an opportunity to expand, verify, and add descriptions of the phenomenon under investigation and assist participants in clarifying and expounding on inadequate descriptions. In addition, often participants will have additional thoughts about the phenomenon under study after the initial interview. Following an interview, researchers should immediately listen to the tape, checking that the interview made sense and verifying the need for a follow-up interview. Also, researchers should make extensive, detailed notes immediately after the interview in case the tape recording has failed.

When data collection begins, so, too, does data analysis. From the moment researchers begin listening to descriptions of a particular phenomenon, analysis is occurring. These processes are inseparable. Therefore, the importance of the reductive process cannot be overemphasized. Separating one's beliefs and assumptions from the raw data occurs throughout the investigation. Journaling helps in continuing the reductive process. Researchers' use of a journal can facilitate phenomenological reduction. Writing down any ideas, feelings, or responses that emerge during data collection supports reductive phenomenology. Drew (1989) has offered the added perspective that journaling that addresses a researcher's own experience can be "considered data and examined within the context of the study for the part it has played in the study's results" (p. 431).

Following data collection and verbatim transcription, researchers should listen to the tapes while reading the transcriptions for accuracy. This step will help to familiarize them with the data and begin immersing them in the phenomenon under investigation.

Data Analysis

Data analysis requires that researchers dwell with or become immersed in the data. The purpose of data analysis, according to Banonis (1989), is to preserve the uniqueness of each participant's lived experience while permitting an understanding of the phenomenon under investigation. This begins with listening to participants' verbal descriptions and is followed by reading and rereading the verbatim transcriptions or written responses. As researchers become immersed in the data, they may identify and extract significant statements. They can then transcribe these statements onto index cards or record them in a data management file for ease of ordering later in the process. Apprehending or capturing the essential relationships among the statements and preparing an exhaustive description of the phenomenon constitute the final phase. Through free imaginative variation, researchers make connections between statements obtained in the interview process. It is critical to identify how statements or central themes emerged and are connected to one another if the final description is to be comprehensive and exhaustive.

Microcomputers and word processing software can make data storage and retrieval more efficient. Examining available software packages for qualitative data analysis may be an appropriate option, depending on researchers' personal preferences. See Chapter 3 for an in-depth discussion of data generation and management strategies including available software for data storage, retrieval, and analysis.

Review of the Literature

The review of the literature generally follows data analysis. The rationale for postponing the literature review is related to the goal of achieving a pure description of the phenomenon under investigation. The fewer ideas or preconceived notions researchers have about the phenomenon under investigation, the less likely their biases will influence the research. A cursory review of the literature may be done to ensure the necessity of the study and the appropriateness of method selection. Once data analysis is complete, researchers review the literature to place the findings within the context of what is already known about the topic.

Trustworthiness and Authenticity of Data

The issue of trustworthiness in qualitative research has been a concern for researchers engaging in these methods and is discussed at length in the literature (Beck, 1993; Krefting, 1991; Yonge & Stewin, 1988). The issue of rigor in qualitative research is important to the practice of good science.

The trustworthiness of the questions put to study participants depends on the extent to which they tap the participants' experiences apart from the participants' theoretical knowledge of the topic (Colaizzi, 1978). Consistent use of the method and of bracketing prior knowledge helps to ensure pure description of data. To ensure trustworthiness of data analysis, researchers return to each participant and ask if the exhaustive description reflects the participant's experiences. When the findings are recognized to be true by the participants, the trustworthiness of the data is further established. If elements are noted to be unclear or misinterpreted, the researchers must return to the analysis and revise the description.

Requesting negative descriptions of the phenomenon under investigation is helpful in establishing authenticity and trustworthiness of the data. For example, in the study investigating the meaning of quality of life in individuals with type 1 diabetes mellitus, the researcher may ask, "Can you describe a situation in which you would feel that you did not have quality of life?" This question gives an opportunity to compare and contrast data.

Finally, the audit trail is critical to establishing authenticity and trustworthiness of the data. This process allows the reader to clearly follow the line of thinking that the researcher used during data analysis. Clear connections between how the research moved from raw data to interpreted meanings are made through detailed examples. Rigor in qualitative research is a critical component to the process. Data analysis occurs through complex mental processes, critical thinking, and analysis. Researchers must prepare their final descriptions in such a way that the line of thinking and interpretation that occurred is clear to the reader and true to the data.

SUMMARY

*P*henomenology is an integral field of inquiry to nursing, as well as philosophy, sociology, and psychology. As a research method, phenomenology is a rigorous scientific process whose purpose is to bring to language human experiences. The phenomenological movement has been influenced by the works of Husserl, Brentano, Stumpf, Merleau-Ponty, and others. Hermeneutic phenomenology offers a different approach to qualitative understanding through the interpretive process of the written and spoken word. Concepts central to the method include intentionality, essences, intuiting, reduction, bracketing, embodiment, and being-in-the-world.

Phenomenology as a method of research offers nursing an opportunity to describe and clarify phenomena important to practice, education, and research. Researchers selecting this approach for the investigation of phenomena should base their decision on suitability and a need for further clarification of the selected phenomenon. Specific consideration must be given to the issues of researcher as instrument, data generation, data treatment and authenticity, and trustworthiness of data. Investigations that use this approach contribute to nursing's knowledge base and can provide direction for future investigations.

The relevance of phenomenology as a research method for nursing is clear. Within the qualitative paradigm, this method supports "new initiatives for nursing care where the subject matter is often not amenable to other investigative and experimental methods" (Jasper, 1994, p. 313). Nursing maintains a unique appreciation for caring, commitment, and holism. Phenomena related to nursing can be explored and analyzed by phenomenological methods that have as their goal the description of lived experience.

References

Allen, M. N., & Jenson, L. (1990). Hermeneutical inquiry, meaning and scope. *Western Journal of Nursing Research, 12*(2), 241–253.

Arrigo, B., & Cody, W. K. (2004). A dialogue on existential-phenomenological thought in psychology and in nursing. *Nursing Science Quarterly, 17*(1), 6–11.

Banonis, B. C. (1989). The lived experience of recovering from addiction: A phenomenological investigation. *Nursing Science Quarterly, 2*(1), 37–42.

Beck, C. T. (1993). Qualitative research: The evaluation of its credibility, fittingness, and auditability. *Western Journal of Nursing Research, 15*(2), 263–265.

Beck, C. T. (1994). Phenomenology: Its use in nursing research. *International Journal of Nursing Studies, 31*(6), 499–510.

Benoliel, J. Q. (1988). Commentaries on special issue. *Western Journal of Nursing Research, 10*(2), 210–213.

Blumensteil, A. (1973). A sociology of good times. In G. Psathas (Ed.), *Phenomenological sociology: Issues and applications.* New York, NY: Wiley.

Caelli, K. (2000). The changing face of phenomenological research: Traditional and American phenomenology in nursing. *Qualitative Health Research, 10*(3), 366–377.

Caelli, K. (2001). Engaging with phenomenology: Is it more of a challenge than it needs to be? *Qualitative Health Research, 11*(2), 273–281.

Carpenter, D. R., & Narsavage, G. (2004). One breath at a time: Living with cystic fibrosis. *Journal of Pediatric Nursing, 19*(1), 25–31.

Cohen, M. Z. (1987). A historical overview of the phenomenological movement. *Image, 19*(1), 31–34.

Cohen, M. Z., Ley, C., & Tarzian, A. J. (2001). Isolation in blood and marrow transplantation. *Journal of Nursing Scholarship, 23*(6), 592–609.

Colaizzi, P. F. (1978). Psychological research as the phenomenologist views it. In R. Valle & M. King (Eds.), *Existential phenomenological alternative for psychology* (pp. 48–71). New York, NY: Oxford University Press.

Crist, J. D., & Tanner, C. A. (2003). Interpretation/analysis methods in hermeneutic phenomenology. *Nursing Research, 52*(3), 202–205.

Diekelmann, N. (2001). Narrative pedagogy: Heideggerian hermeneutical analysis of lived experiences of students, teachers, and clinicians. *Advances in Nursing Science, 23*(3), 53–71.

Drew, N. (1989). The interviewer's experience as data in phenomenological research. *Western Journal of Nursing Research, 11*(4), 431–439.

Dreyfus, H. L. (1991). *Being-in-the-world: A commentary on Heidegger's being and time.* Division I. Cambridge, MA: MIT Press.

Gadamer, H. G. (1976). *Philosophical hermeneutics* (D. E. Linge, Trans. & Ed.). Los Angeles, LA: University of California Press.

Geanellos, R. (2000). Exploring Ricoeur's hermeneutic theory of interpretation as a method of analyzing research texts. *Nursing Inquiry, 7*(2), 112–119.

Giorgi, A. (1985). *Phenomenology and psychological research.* Pittsburgh, PA: Duquesne University Press.

Haggman-Laitila, A. (1999). The authenticity and ethics of phenomenological research: How to overcome the researcher's own views. *Nursing Ethics, 6*(1), 12–22.

Heidegger, M. (1962). *Being and time.* New York: Harper & Row. (Original work published 1927.)

Husserl, E. (1931). *Ideas: General introduction to pure phenomenology* (W. R. Boyce Gibson, Trans.). New York, NY: Collier.

Husserl, E. (1965). *Phenomenology and the crisis of philosophy* (Q. Laver, Trans.). New York, NY: Harper & Row.

Iaquinta, M. L., & Larrabee, J. H. (2003). Phenomenological lived experience of patients with rheumatoid arthritis. *Journal of Nursing Care Quality, 19*(3), 280–289.

Jasper, M. A. (1994). Issues in phenomenology for researchers of nursing. *Journal of Advanced Nursing, 19*, 309–314.

Krefting, L. (1991). Rigor in qualitative research: The assessment of trustworthiness. *American Journal of Occupational Therapy, 45*(3), 214–222.

Lincoln, Y. S., & Guba, E. G. (1985). *Naturalistic inquiry.* Beverly Hills, CA: Sage.

Lindholm, M., Uden, G., & Rastam, R. (1999). Management from four different perspectives. *Journal of Nursing Management, 7*, 101–111.

Lowes, L., & Prowse, M. A. (2001). Standing outside the interview process? The illusions of objectivity in phenomenological data generation. *International Journal of Advanced Nursing, 31*, 219–255.

McConnell-Henry, T., Chapman, Y., & Francis, K. (2009). Unpacking Heideggerian phenomenology. *Southern Online Journal of Nursing Research, 9*, 6.

Merleau-Ponty, M. (1956). What is phenomenology? *Cross Currents, 6*, 59–70.

Merleau-Ponty, M. (1962). *Phenomenology of perception* (C. Smith, Trans.). New York, NY: Humanities Press.

Morse, J. M. (1989). *Qualitative nursing research: A contemporary dialogue.* Rockville, MD: Aspen.

Munhall, P. (1989). Philosophical ponderings on qualitative research. *Nursing Science Quarterly, 2*(1), 20–28.

Natanson, M. (1973). *Edmund Husserl: Philosopher of infinite tasks.* Evanston, IL: Northwestern University Press.

Omery, A. (1983). Phenomenology: A method for nursing research. *Advances in Nursing Science, 5*(2), 49–63.

Ortiz, M. R. (2009). Hermeneutics and nursing research: History, processes, and exemplar. *Southern Online Journal of Nursing Research, 9*, 6.

Paley, J. (1997). Husserl, phenomenology and nursing. *Journal of Advanced Nursing, 26*, 187–193.

Paterson, G. J., & Zderad, L. T. (1976). *Humanistic nursing.* New York, NY: Wiley.

Patton, M. Q. (1990). *Qualitative evaluation and research methods* (2nd ed.). Newbury Park, CA: Sage.

Reinharz, S. (1983). Phenomenology as a dynamic process. *Phenomenology and Pedagogy, 1*(1), 77–79.

Ricoeur, P. (1976). *Interpretation theory: Discourse and the surplus of meaning.* Fort Worth, TX: Texas Christian University Press.

Ricoeur, P. (1981). *Hermeneutics and the social sciences* (J. Thompson, Trans. & Ed.). New York, NY: Cambridge University Press.

Rinaldi, D. M. (1989). The lived experience of commitment to nursing. Dissertation Abstracts International (University Microfilms No. 1707).

Rose, P., Beeby, J., & Parker, D. (1995). Academic rigour in the lived experience of researchers using phenomenological methods in nursing. *Journal of Advanced Nursing, 21*, 1123–1129.

Schutz, A. (1970). *On phenomenology and social relations.* Chicago: University of Chicago Press.

Schwarz, J. K. (2003). Understanding and responding to patients' requests for assistance in dying. *Journal of Nursing Scholarship, 35*(4), 377–384.

Spiegelberg, H. (1965). *The phenomenological movement: A historical introduction* (2nd ed., Vol. 1–2). Dordrecht, The Netherlands: Martinus Nijhoff.

Spiegelberg, H. (1975). *Doing phenomenology.* Dordrecht, The Netherlands: Martinus Nijhoff.

Streubert, H. J. (1991). Phenomenological research as a theoretic initiative in community health nursing. *Public Health Nursing, 8*(2), 119–123.

Tarzian, A. J. (2000). Caring for dying patients who have air hunger. *Journal of Nursing Scholarship, 32*(2), 137–143.

Todres, L., & Wheeler, S. (2001). The complexity of phenomenology, hermeneutics and existentialism as a philosophical perspective for nursing research. *International Journal of Nursing Studies, 38*, 1–8.

Van der Zalm, J. E., & Bergum, V. (2000). Hermeneutic phenomenology: Providing living knowledge for nursing practice. *Journal of Advanced Nursing, 31*(1), 211–218.

van Kaam, A. (1984). *Existential foundation of psychology.* New York, NY: Doubleday.

van Manen, M. (1990). *Researching the lived experience.* Buffalo: State University of New York.

Wagner, H. R. (1983). *Phenomenology of consciousness and sociology of the life and world: An introductory study.* Edmonton, Alberta: University of Alberta Press.

Yonge, O., & Stewin, L. (1988). Reliability and validity: Misnomers for qualitative research. *Canadian Journal of Nursing Research, 20*(2), 61–67.

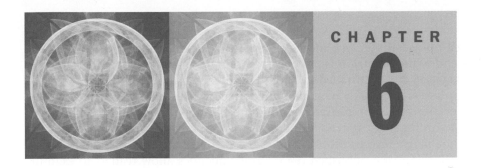

Phenomenology in Practice, Education, and Administration

*T*he acceptance of qualitative methods as legitimate approaches to the discovery of knowledge continues to grow as an increasing number of nurse researchers apply these methods to investigations that have as their phenomena of interest people's life experiences. Very often in nursing, we are faced with practice, education, and administrative experiences that seem to present patterns that are familiar to us. To validate our perceptions, research must be conducted to explore and describe phenomena fully and accurately. This process, in turn, leads to improved understanding and ultimately better outcomes in all domains of nursing. Hudacek's (2000) book, *Making a Difference: Stories from the Point of Care,* uses phenomenological principles to analyze nurse stories. Her work has implications for nursing practice, education, and administration. As evidenced by published works, phenomenology as one approach to qualitative investigations has made a significant contribution to the substantive body of nursing knowledge. Qualitative methods allow exploration of the life experiences of human beings in ways that respect and acknowledge the importance of all knowledge to be gained through subjective experiences and the importance of accepting different ways of knowing.

This chapter provides an overview and critique of three phenomenological investigations, published as journal articles, in the areas of nursing practice, education, and administration. An article by Doumit and colleagues (2010)

"Coping with Breast Cancer: A Phenomenological Study" is reprinted at the end of the chapter. It is provided as a sample of a phenomenological investigation and is critiqued to offer the reader an example of the process used to assess the quality of a phenomenological investigation. The practice, education, and administrative studies presented in this chapter were reviewed according to the criteria found in Box 6-1. These guidelines offer readers of qualitative investigations a guide to recognizing the essential methodological points of a published report. The guidelines allow readers to examine how the research has contributed to the scientific base of nursing knowledge. This chapter also provides readers with selected examples of published research using the phenomenological method. These examples are presented in Table 6-1.

Box 6-1

Qualitative Critique Criteria

Focus/Topic

1. What is the focus or the topic of the study? What is it that the researcher is studying? Is the topic researchable? Is it focused enough to be meaningful but not too limited so as to be trivial?

2. Why is the researcher using a qualitative design? Would the study be more appropriately conducted in the quantitative paradigm?

3. What is the philosophical tradition or qualitative paradigm upon which the study is based?

Purpose

1. What is the purpose of the study? Is it clear?

Significance

1. What is the relevance of the study to what is already known about the topic?

2. How will the results be useful to nursing and/or health care?

Method

1. Given the topic of the study and the researcher's stated purpose, how does the selected research method help to achieve the stated purpose?

2. What methodological components/strategies has the researcher identified to conduct the study?

3. Based on the material presented, how does the researcher demonstrate that he or she has followed the method?

4. If the researcher used any form of triangulation, explain how he or she maintained the integrity of the study.

Sampling

1. How were participants selected?

2. Explain how the selection process supports a qualitative sampling paradigm.

3. Are the participants in the study the appropriate people to inform the research? Explain.

Box 6-1 *(Continued)*

Data Collection

1. How does the data collection method reported support discovery, description, or understanding?
2. What data collection strategies do the researcher use?
3. Does the researcher clearly state how human subjects were protected?
4. How was data saturation achieved?
5. Are the data collection strategies appropriate to achieve the purpose of the study? Explain.

Data Analysis

1. How were data analyzed?
2. Based on the analysis reported, can the reader follow the researcher's stated processes?

Findings/Trustworthiness

1. How do the reported findings demonstrate the participants' realities?
2. How does the researcher relate the findings of the study to what is already known?
3. How does the researcher demonstrate that the findings are meaningful to the participants?

Conclusions/Implications/Recommendations

1. How does the researcher provide a context for use of the findings?
2. Are the conclusions drawn from the study appropriate? Explain.
3. What are the recommendations for future research?
4. Are the recommendations, conclusions, and implications clearly related to the findings? Explain.

APPLICATION TO PRACTICE

*M*any nursing interventions performed in clinical settings lend themselves to quantitative measurement. Examples include measurement of blood pressure, central venous pressure, or urine-specific gravity. However, nurses enmeshed in practice settings are well aware that much of what is done for patients is subjective and based on how nurses come to know their patients and the patients' life experiences. For example, caring, reassurance, and quality of life are phenomena central to nursing practice, but they do not necessarily lend themselves to quantitative measurement. Even areas of practice that are studied primarily from a quantitative perspective can be enriched when examined from a qualitative lens. Therefore, phenomena unique to the practice of professional nursing need investigative approaches suitable to their unique nature. Phenomenology as a qualitative research method has been used to explore a variety of practice-related experiences and facilitates understanding of subjective interactive experiences (Crist, 2005; Ennis & Gregory, 2007; McNeill, 2004; Merrill & Grassley, 2008; Rosedale, 2009; Thomas-MacLean, 2004). Examples of published research related to the practice domain can be found in Table 6-1.

Table 6-1 • *(Continued)*

Author(s)	Date	Domain	Phenomenon of Interest	Sample	Data Generation	Findings
Ruddock & Turner	2007	Education	To explore if having an international learning experience as part of a nursing education program promoted cultural sensitivity in nursing students	Six females and one male Danish nursing students enrolled in a diploma or BSN school of nursing who took part in an international exchange program to Jamaica, Malta, Greenland, or Australia	In-depth conversational interviews, transcribed verbatim, the initial question "What was it like to live and learn in another country?" was followed by probing questions to clarify meanings attached to the experience	Findings captured three fused horizons: experiencing transition from one culture to another, adjusting to cultural differences, and developing cultural sensitivity and growing personally. Findings indicate that RNs find it hard to include cultural dimensions of care at the top of their working agenda
Ennis & Gregory	2007	Practice	Nurses perceptions of caring while working on surgical wards	Ten female registered nurses working on surgical units	Semistructured interviews, tape-recorded, and transcribed verbatim	Lamentation and loss was the significant theme identified and the essential structures supporting the theme included lack of time, lack of caring support, tasking, increased acuity, lack of continuity of care, emotional divestment, and not caring for each other. The nurses in the study mourned the loss of caring in modern practice

Illingworth	2006	Education	To further understanding of the concept of role models among third-year nursing students	A purposive sample of 10 third-year nursing students, 5 males and 5 females, enrolled in a mental-health nursing course	One focus group, tape-recorded and transcribed, discussion led by researcher	Central characteristics of the phenomenon of role models included having an enabling attitude, respect toward others, sharing practitioner, functional role, and humanism
Carpenter & Narsavage	2004	Practice	The lived experience of parents caring for a child newly diagnosed with cystic fibrosis	Eleven families caring for children newly diagnosed with cystic fibrosis	One focus group, tape-recorded and transcribed verbatim. Detailed written narratives from study participants	Three major themes emerged that were fluid in nature. They included falling apart, pulling together, and moving beyond. Subthemes were evident within each of the major themes described. Families reported moving back and forth among the three main areas of adjustment depending on the health of the child or other life events that occurred
McNeill	2004	Practice	Experiences of fathers who have a child with juvenile rheumatoid arthritis (JRA)	22 fathers	Semistructured interviews, tape-recorded and transcribed verbatim	A substantive theory of a father's experience of caring for a child with JRA. Fathers were profoundly affected. JRA served as a catalyst for meaningful involvement, and a multitude of emotions were expressed. Efforts to remain strong for others created high levels of stress

exclusively. The educational domain of nursing also lends itself to qualitative investigation in areas such as educational experiences, developing cultural sensitivity, or the effect of evaluation on student performance in the clinical setting.

Nursing education is an important area of research that can be studied using qualitative approaches. An overview and critique of the study "Developing cultural sensitivity: Nursing students' experiences of a study abroad programme" by Ruddock and Turner (2007) is provided for this example of the phenomenological method applied to the educational domain of nursing.

The phenomenon of interest for this study is relevant to nursing education and had as its purpose to understand if "having an international learning experience as part of a nursing education programme promoted cultural sensitivity in nursing students" (Ruddock & Turner, 2007, p. 361). The authors discussed the relevance of their study through a literature review on topics related to the lack of cultural sensitivity among health care personnel, the development of cultural sensitivity through self-awareness and international experiences, and the need for cultural sensitivity in a multicultural society. The authors support their study with the following statement: "To meet the needs of all members of multicultural societies, nurses need to develop cultural sensitivity and incorporate this into caregiving" (p. 361).

The method chosen by Ruddock and Turner (2007) is a Gadamerian hermeneutic phenomenological approach. This research method is consistent with this branch of phenomenological research. Gadamer (1989) describes a fusion of horizons which is never closed and may be continuously refined and extended. This fusion occurs when one's own preunderstanding meets a new strange horizon resulting in a new understanding. By using a reflexive approach, Ruddock and Turner (2007) improved their "understanding of the literature, how cultural sensitivity develops, and participants' understanding, to enable different vantage points to come together through language, text, and conversation" (p. 364). Participant selection also was described in great detail. The selection of participants supported a qualitative framework in that it was purposeful, and subjects had experience with the phenomenon under investigation. Participants were recruited by asking the international exchange coordinator to mail a description of the study to undergraduate nursing students enrolled in either a diploma or bachelor of nursing course who took part in an international exchange. Students were invited to contact the researcher directly if they were interested. Six females and one male took part in the study. Ruddock and Turner (2007) also address protection of human subjects and note that ethical principles were honored:

> The study was approved by the university and hospital Ethics
> Committee where the study was undertaken. After an initial meeting to answer questions related to the study, students who expressed

definite interest in being involved were asked to sign a consent form and an interview was arranged. To protect confidentiality, we have used pseudonyms to designate the students (p. 363).

The data collection strategies used by Ruddock and Turner (2007) support phenomenological approaches to discovery, description, and understanding. The strategies used by the researchers are detailed and appropriate to achieve the purposes of the study. Data were analyzed using a method described by Turner (2003), which embraced Gadamer's philosophy of understanding as well as the language associated with Gadamerian hermeneutics. Ruddock and Turner (2007) provide an in-depth description of the analysis process and relevant findings. Discussion of the findings demonstrates how the data reflected participants' realities and how the researcher related findings of the study to what is already known. Ruddock and Turner (2007) identified three fused horizons from analysis: experiencing transition from one culture to another, adjusting to cultural differences, and developing cultural sensitivity and growing personally. Examples of raw data related to each fused horizon are provided, allowing the reader to follow the line of thinking of the researcher and adding credibility to the study. The conclusions drawn from the study are appropriate, and recommendations for future research are made. The article makes an important contribution to the literature on cultural diversity and nursing education.

APPLICATION TO ADMINISTRATION

The qualitative research literature addressing issues uniquely related to nursing administration is limited, possibly because many of the issues that lend themselves to qualitative education in nursing administration overlap with the practice arena. For example, studies related to professional nurse behavior and work satisfaction, successful leadership strategies, and perspectives on nurse empowerment would cross over between administration and practice. An example of this overlap is the study by Duchscher (2001), "Out in the real world: Newly graduated nurses in acute-care speak out." This article describes the perceptions of five nurses regarding their work environment. Although the implications from the study relate directly to nursing practice, they can also be applied to nursing administration in that the result provides "insight into, and enhances understanding of, recruitment and retention issues for nursing administrators who serve as gatekeepers to the practice orientations and ongoing workplace environments of new nursing graduates" (p. 426). This study, reported as a phenomenological investigation, provides an example of how this particular methodology can be applied to nursing administration.

For purposes of the critique, the following study, which is purely administrative, is reviewed. The study "Management from four different perspectives" by Lindholm, Uden, and Rastam (1999) is presented as one example of the application of qualitative research in the area of nursing administration. The phenomenon of interest, clearly identified in the study, focused on gaining an understanding of the process of nursing management in a developing organization. The specific rationale for using a qualitative format, as well as the philosophic underpinnings of the approach, was clearly described. Despite the fact that the Swedish health care system has a variety of management positions to which nurses have legal access, nurses have traditionally held middle management positions. Ongoing decentralization has moved nurses into senior management positions. Therefore, "Elucidating the significance of nursing management increases the possibility of developing the management area of the nursing profession and of using recently acquired knowledge to influence the development of the nursing profession" (Lindholm et al., 1999, p. 102).

The purpose of the study was to "illuminate nursing management in a developing organization from the perspectives of nurse managers, chief physicians, hospital directors and politicians, respectively" (Lindholm et al., 1999, p. 102). The authors make explicit their purpose and support it with a review of the literature.

The sample included 15 nurse managers, 11 chief physicians, and 3 politicians who were chairmen of the local health boards. "The nurse managers were all women, except for one. In the other groups all the participants were men"(Lindholm et al., 1999, p. 102).

The method used to collect data was compatible with the research purpose and adequately addressed the phenomenon of interest. Lindholm et al. (1999) interviewed their participants individually. All interviews were tape-recorded and transcribed verbatim. The authors used Ricoeur's process of phenomenological hermeneutics. Detailed examples of the steps of the hermeneutic circle are provided, demonstrating for the reader how the researchers followed the stated method. Although the researchers do not make an explicit statement regarding data saturation, they do comment that the interviews were comprehensive and "provided good coverage of the issues leaving no need to increase the number of informants" (Lindholm et al., 1999, p. 102).

Data analysis followed the phenomenological hermeneutic approach inspired by Ricoeur. The author provides clear examples of the data analysis process in relationship to each step of the hermeneutic circle.

> The first step was the naïve reading of each interview to acquire a sense of the whole of the text, to gain an impression and to formulate ideas for further analysis. The second step was a structural analysis to identify meaning units, to explain, through revealing the structure and the internal dependent relations, what constitutes the static state of the text. The third step was the understanding of the interpreted whole, from reflection on the naïve reading and the structural analysis (Lindholm et al., 1999, p. 103).

The findings demonstrate the participants' realities, and the researchers relate the findings of the study to what is already known. Through the discussion of the findings, the researchers provide a context for their use and conclusions are drawn. Recommendations for future research are made and the conclusions and implications are clearly related to the findings. This work makes an important contribution to the nursing administration knowledge base.

SUMMARY

*T*he body of published phenomenological research has grown considerably since the first publication of this book. Clearly, the body of practice-related research is expanding, with considerable development of research in the area of education and administration. Examples of phenomenological research applied to the areas of nursing practice, education, and administration emphasize the important contribution that phenomenological research has made to nursing's substantive body of knowledge. The critiquing guidelines provide the reader with a guide to evaluating phenomenological research. Examples of phenomenological research using the method interpretations described in Chapter 5 have been highlighted to facilitate method comprehension and application.

Phenomenology as a research approach provides an avenue for investigation that allows description of lived experiences. The voice of professional nurses in practice, education, and administration can be a tremendous source of data that have yet to be fully explored. Identifying subjective phenomena unique to the domains of nursing education, practice, and administration is important to the ever-expanding body of nursing knowledge.

References

Barritt, L., Beekman, T., Bleeker, H., Mulderij, K. (1984) *Analyzing phenomenological descriptions. Phenomenology Pedagogy, 41*(2), 1–17.

Carpenter, D. R., & Narsavage, G. (2004). One breath at a time: Living with cystic fibrosis. *Journal of Pediatric Nursing, 19*(1), 25–31.

Crist, J. D. (2005). The meaning for elders of receiving family care. *Journal of Advanced Nursing, 49*, 485–493.

Diekelmann, N., Ironside, P. (1998). Hermeneutics. In Fitzpatrick J, ed. Encyclopedia of Nursing Research. New York, NY: Springer; 1998: 50–68.

Doumit, M.A.A., Huijer, H. A., Kelly, J. H., Saghir, N. E., Nassar, N. (2010). *Coping with Breast Cancer, A Phenomenological Study. Cancer Nursing, 33*(2), 33–39.

Duchscher, B. J. (2001). Out in the real world: Newly graduated nurses in acute-care speak out. *Journal of Nursing Administration, 31*(9), 426–439.

Ennis, C. & Gregory, D. (2007). Lamentation and loss: Expressions of caring by contemporary surgical nurses. *Journal of Advanced Nursing, 58*, 339–347.

Gadamer, H. G. (1989). Hermeneutics. In J. Weinsheimer, & D. Marshall (Eds.), *Truth and method* (2nd rev. ed., pp. 306–309). New York: Crossroad.

Giorgi, A. (1985). *Phenomenology and Psychological Research*. Pittsburgh, PA: Duquesne University Press.

Hudacek, S. (2000). *Making a difference: Stories from the point of care*. Indianapolis, IN: Sigma Theta Tau Press.

Hudacek, S. (2008). Dimensions of caring: A qualitative analysis of nurses' stories. *Journal of Nursing Education, 47* (3), 124–129.

Illingworth, P. (2006). Exploring mental health students' perceptions of role models. *British Journal of Nursing, 18*, 812–815.

Lindholm M., Uden, G., & Rastam, L. (1999). Management from four different perspectives. *Journal of Nursing Management, 7*, 101–111.

Linton J. & Farrell M. J. (2009). Nurses' perceptions of leadership in an adult intensive care unit: A phenomenology study. *Intensive & Critical Care Nursing, 25* (2), 64–71.

McNeill, T. (2004). Fathers' experience of parenting a child with juvenile rheumatoid arthritis. *Qualitative Health Research, 14*(4), 526–545.

Megginson, L. A. (2008). RN-BSN education: 21st century barriers and incentives. *Journal of Nursing Management, 16*, 47–55.

Merrill, E. & Grassley, J. (2008). Women's stories of their experiences as overweight patients. *Journal of Advanced Nursing, 64*, 139–146.

Rosedale, M. (2009). Survivor loneliness of women following breast cancer. *Oncology Nursing Forum, 36*, 175–183.

Ruddock, H. C. & Turner, DS. (2007). Developing cultural sensitivity: Nursing students' experiences of a study abroad programme. *Journal of Advanced Nursing, 59*, 361–369.

Ruth-Sahd, L. A. & Tisdell, E. J. (2007). The meaning and use of intuition in novice nurses: A phenomenological study. *Adult Education Quarterly, 57*, 115–140.

Schwarz, J. K. (2003). Understanding and responding to patients' requests for assistance in dying. *Journal of Nursing Scholarship, 35*(4), 377–384.

Thomas-MacLean, R. (2004). Memories of treatment: The immediacy of breast cancer. *Qualitative Health Research, 14*(5), 628–643.

Turner, DS. (2003). Horizons revealed: From methodology to method. *International Journal of Qualitative Methods, 2*, 1–17.

Research Article

Coping with Breast Cancer: A Phenomenological Study

Myrna A. A. Doumit, PhD, RN; Huda Abu-Saad Huijer, RN, PhD, FEANS; Jane H. Kelley, PhD, RN; Nagi El Saghir, MD; Nada Nassar, RN, MSN

Background: *Breast cancer is the most common malignancy affecting women worldwide. In Lebanon, a country of 4 million people, breast cancer is also the most prevalent type of cancer among Lebanese women.*

Objective: *The purpose of this study was to gain a more in-depth understanding of the coping strategies espoused by Lebanese women with breast cancer.*

Methods: *The study followed purposeful sampling and saturation principles in which 10 female participants diagnosed as having breast cancer were interviewed. Data were analyzed following a hermeneutical process as described by Diekelmann and Ironside (Encyclopedia of Nursing Research. 1998:50–68).*

Results: *Seven main themes and 1 constitutive pattern emerged from the study describing the Lebanese women's coping strategies with breast cancer. The negative stigma of cancer in the Lebanese culture, the role of women in the Lebanese families, and the embedded role of religion in Lebanese society are bases of the differences in the coping strategies of Lebanese women with breast cancer as compared to women with breast cancer from other cultures.*

Conclusion: *These findings cannot be directly generalized, but they could act as a basis for further research on which to base a development of a framework for an approach to care that promotes coping processes in Lebanese women living with breast cancer.*

Implications for Practice: *Nursing and medical staff need to have a better understanding of the individual coping strategies of each woman and its impact on the woman's well being; the creation of informal support group is indispensable in helping these women cope with their conditions.*

Keywords: Breast cancer, Coping, Culture, Qualitative, Women's issues

Authors' Affiliations: School of Nursing, American University of Beirut, Beirut, Lebanon (Drs Doumit and Huijer); University of Mississippi, Medical Center, Jackson (Dr Kelley); and School of Medicine, American University of Beirut (Dr El Saghir), and American University of Beirut Medical Center (Ms Nassar), Beirut, Lebanon.

This research was supported by a grant from the Medical Practice Plan at the American University of Beirut.

Corresponding author: Myrna A. A. Doumit, PhD, RN, School of Nursing, American University of Beirut, Beirut, Lebanon (ma12@aub.edu.lb).

Accepted for publication October 12, 2009.

From Doumit MAA, Huijer HA-S, Kelley JH, et al. *Cancer Nursing.* vol. 33, issue 2, pp. E33–E39. Copyright © 2010 by Lippincott Williams & Wilkins. Reprinted with permission.

*B*reast cancer is the most frequent malignancy affecting women worldwide. In Lebanon, a country of 4 million people, breast cancer is also the most prevalent type of cancer among Lebanese women. It corresponds to 42% of all female cancers (Lebanese Ministry of Public Health, World Health Organization, and National Non-communicable Diseases Programme).[1] It is noted that at least half of the women with breast cancer will survive 5 years, as has been found for those living in developing countries.[2] Therefore, as the survival rates of breast cancer increase, the number of women living with long-term consequences of breast cancer treatment will also augment. Women's responses to and coping with the diagnosis of breast cancer have become an area of growing concern to many researchers.[3–5] However, most research on women's coping with breast cancer has been conducted in western countries. So far, no documented research study is found on the experience of coping in Lebanese women with breast cancer. Consequently, the intention of this study was to gain more in-depth insights into how Lebanese women cope with breast cancer so that culturally sensitive care can be provided.

Background

Breast cancer diagnosis, and its subsequent treatment, is a traumatic experience with intense impact on all facets of human life.[4,6] Several studies have investigated coping strategies and their effect on cancer. According to Taleghani et al,[7] Iranian women used a religious approach for coping. They used positive suggestions, hope, and intentional forgetfulness as coping mechanisms. Coping strategies as described by African American women included relying on prayer, avoiding negative people, developing a positive attitude, having a will to live, and receiving support from family, friends, and support groups.[8] In a study on 100 newly diagnosed women with breast cancer in China, Li and Lambert[9] reported that planning, positive reframing, and self-distraction were the most commonly used coping strategies. Manual et al,[10] in a study on coping in young women diagnosed as having breast cancer, reported that the most frequently used coping strategies were positive cognitive restructuring, wishful thinking, making changes, social support engaging in physical activity, using medications, and resting. This study also highlighted that different coping strategies were considered best in response to different stressful aspects of dealing with cancer. Comparable results were also highlighted by Stanton et al.[11] In a study on coping following breast cancer and psychological adjustments, Hack and Degner[12] reported that women who respond to their breast cancer diagnosis with passive acceptance and resignation are at a significant risk for poor long-term psychological adjustment. Butow et al[13] reported that women with metastatic breast cancer who minimized the effect of cancer as a disease on their lives survived longer. Those who used minimization as a coping strategy revealed that the cancer did not influence social, work, or family life, nor was it an important cause of anxiety or depression. These women, who accepted their illness and its life-threatening potential, showed a better social adjustment, an ability to shift between appropriate mourning for their loss of health and approaching death, and a tendency to concentrate on ongoing positive aspects of their lives. These results imply that adequate support, active coping, and finding positive meaning in life can lead to a diminution of cancer's effect.

Although research has indicated that coping strategies have a great impact on women's adaptation and response to breast cancer, nothing is known about how Lebanese breast cancer women cope with breast cancer. Therefore, the intent of the present study was to gain a more in-depth understanding of the coping strategies followed by breast cancer Lebanese women so that culturally sensitive healthcare and culturally relevant coping strategies could be encouraged by healthcare providers.

Methods

Design

Our reflections on the concept of coping with breast cancer emerged while conducting a qualitative study about the lived experience of Lebanese women with breast cancer[14] following a phenomenological approach as described by Barritt et al.[15] This approach was chosen because it allows descriptions of phenomena as experienced in life and aims to offer an understanding of the internal meaning of a person's experience in the world.[16] Thus, a comprehensive, culturally competent understanding of the phenomenon was obtained.

The idea of coping with breast cancer emerged from the participants' interviews as an important feature for living with the diagnosis of breast cancer. A second analysis of textual data (narratives) from the initial study was done following a 7-stage hermeneutical process as described by Diekelmann and Ironside.[17] The previous interviews became the narratives that constituted the text for the present analysis. The second analysis was conducted immediately at the end of data collection when the researchers realized that coping was an important element of the women's lived experience. The focus of the second analysis was the coping process. To maintain scientific rigor in the second analysis, researchers' biases were reduced by careful attention to the text, use of team approach for analysis, and verification of the findings with the participants. In addition, findings were supported in the text by participants' excerpts.

Participants

Ten participants were chosen based on purposive sampling, saturation principles, and according to the following inclusion criteria: (1) Lebanese Arabic speaking; (2) living in Lebanon; (3) age of 25 years or older; (4) diagnosed as having breast cancer, stages (I-III); (5) without distant metastases, previous history of mental disorders, or the existence of other forms of cancer or other chronic diseases; and (6) agreed to be interviewed without the presence of a third person to ensure liberty for the participant to express her feelings.

Recruitment Strategies and Techniques

After securing the approval of the institutional review board of the American University of Beirut, the primary researcher talked about the study with community intermediaries (nurses, housewives, friends) and oncologists. After the community intermediaries identified the participant, the primary researcher phoned each potential participant and presented a request to join the study. Then, the researcher arranged for an interview date, time, and place with each participant according to her preferences. All participants read and signed a consent form.

Setting

All interviews were conducted at the participants' homes in rural and urban areas of Lebanon.

Data Collection

Data were collected between December 2007 and May 2008. Interviews were conducted in Arabic by the researcher. Each interview was translated to English by a translator and back translated to Arabic by a research assistant to check for accuracy of translation. In each interview, the participant was the main speaker, and the researcher was mostly a listener and a facilitator. The participants were reminded that their participation is voluntary and that at any time they could decline or withdraw from the study without any obligation. At the end of the second interview, each woman received a "mug" as a token of appreciation for her participation in the study.

The interviews were audio taped, and field notes were recorded. Each interview was coded so that only the researcher has a knowledge of the persons who participated. Participants were guaranteed confidentiality, and pseudonyms were used. The code list and the original tapes were placed in a locked file cabinet in the researcher's office for a period of 3 years, at which time the notes will be destroyed and the tapes erased.

The interval between the first and second interviews was 2 weeks. The first interview took 50 to 60 minutes, and the second interview took 30 to 40 minutes. The objective of the second interview was to validate the preliminary analysis with the participant. It is worth noting that the consensus between the researcher's interpretation and the participants was almost more than 95% in all interviews.

The first set of interviews was based on the following broad or grand tour question: "What has it been like for you since you were diagnosed with breast cancer?" Moreover, during the second interview, each participant was asked to validate if the statements, ideas, and words reported by the researcher illustrate her experience of coping with breast cancer.

Analysis

The second data analysis started at the end of the first study. Narratives (texts) were interpreted following a 7-stage hermeneutical process as described by Diekelmann and Ironside.[17] The objective of this process is to portray shared practices and common meanings. The analysis team included the principal investigator and an experienced graduate assistant in qualitative analysis. Each text was examined as a whole to gain an overall understanding. Possible common meanings were identified from the texts with excerpts to support the interpretation. The researchers compared their interpretations for similarities and differences at biweekly meetings, reaching further clarification and consensus by returning to the original text. All texts were reread to uncover themes that linked them. Researchers described a constitutive pattern that showed the relationship across themes among all texts. According to Diekelmann and Ironside,[17] the discovery of a constitutive pattern forms the highest level of hermeneutical analysis. A situation is constitutive when it gives actual content to a person's self-understanding or to a person's way of being in the world. Furthermore, themes were validated by the participants of the study. At the end, the principal investigator produced the final summary, including verbatim quotes that allow for validation by the reader. This multistage process permitted clarification and validation, which helped in eliminating unconfirmed meanings. The hermeneutic circle involves constant checking of the whole and the parts of the text. It is worth noting that the continuous reference to the text guaranteed that interpretations were grounded and focused.[17]

Results

Sample Description

The sample consisted of 10 women; their ages ranged between 36 and 63 years, with a mean age of 51.3 years. Participants' experience with breast cancer ranged between 4 months and 9 years. Three women underwent total mastectomy of 1 breast, 1 participant endured partial mastectomy of 1 breast, and 6 participants had lumpectomy also on 1 side. Eight participants were still married at the time of the interview, and 2 were widowed. Three participants were living in rural areas and 7 in urban areas. All participants had children. The participants' educational background varied between intermediate (n = 3), secondary (n = 2), and university (n = 5).

Findings

All participants described their journey with the disease process as a nonstop fight against cancer. They also described cancer as a cut in their lives that they had to deal with. Despite the differences in the time since diagnosis, most participants spoke about similar facilitating and hindering factors for coping. Seven main themes and 1 constitutive pattern emerged from the study. Four themes described the participants' facilitating coping factors with the diagnosis of breast cancer, and 3 themes were considered as hindering factors to coping.

Facilitating Coping Factors

Cancer is Something from God All participants regardless of their religious background dealt with cancer as something coming from God that they had to accept because they had no power to change the situation.

Sirine, a 63-year-old lady, said:

Nothing happens to us except what God wishes for us. I had it so I have to accept it but I wish it had not happened. I am relying on God. . .

Sonia, a 55-year-old lady, talked about the issue and said:

I told them (my friend), let it be God's will. I did not feel anything, it did not affect me. I felt let it be God's will; it is ok. I felt that faith, true faith penetrated me; truly. Just yesterday I was telling my friends thank God that so far until now I have not felt that something has happened to me, I feel normal. Normal like if I have a simple flu. Thank God, this is God's will. I do not know. I told him my God let it be your will. If God wants this, what can you do? You have to tolerate it.

Cancer is Similar to Any Other Disease, Mainly Diabetes All participants, while describing their experience with cancer, repeated that cancer is not different or more dangerous than other diseases, and they specifically named diabetes. They all compared cancer to diabetes in terms of chronicity and complications.

Hala, a 36-year-old mother, said:

The cancer patient is much better than the diabetic patient. At least you do not have to worry about your food and medication every day. And the consequences of diabetes sometimes are much worse than cancer. . .

Kathy, a 44-year-old mother, also had similar ideas about cancer; she stated:

I consider cancer like any other disease. It does not mean death to me, it does not scare me, I consider it like diabetes. . .

Positive Support from Work, Family, and Husband Positive support from work environment, family, and husband helped the women diagnosed as having breast cancer to cope with their diagnosis and disease. By positive support, the women meant no differentiation in the conduct of others toward them.

Tina, a 48-year-old woman, mentioned:

It means a lot to be treated like a normal person. The normal treatment that I received from the school where I teach helped me a lot. The director refused to decrease my teaching hours saying that I could make it, and in fact, his trust in me made me feel strong inside. At home we did not change our way of living. My husband insisted that we go out as usual; he did not allow me to stay in bed. I think all this helped me to move ahead from after a "cut" (cancer considered as a cut in her life), a cut that passed in my life. When my children and friend were present, I used to forget that I was sick. I used to stop thinking of my disease. You know I used to think that I have people that I love and that they love me too; this idea used to relieve me. My husband had a big role in all this. . .

Irene, a 59-year-old lady, added:

The support that my relatives and friends gave me boosted my morale; it helped me a lot. My daughter played a big role. At school, the director refused to change the class that I teach because I am teaching a graduating class, and I felt that it was not fair for them (students), but to tell you the truth, the director's decision made me feel stronger and it helped me to fight. . .

Sharing the Experience with People Who Know Sharing information with other people who lived the same experience was considered as a helping factor. Benefiting from others' experiences and also sharing one's own experience were considered as important factors for coping with breast cancer.

Luma, a 62-year-old lady, stated:

If we were living in a normal country, there should have been a center where you could meet with people who had had the same experience. It helps a lot to ask them how they behaved. What did they do? I like to speak with a person who has lived the experience because people who have lived the experience understand you better and can help you. . . . I do not like to speak to people whom I know, like friends and family. . .

Sabine, a 48-year-old lady, revealed in this regard:

My sister's friend had gone through the same experience, and she helped me a lot when I talked to her. I felt more relaxed because I stopped feeling that I was going to the unknown. After my talks with her, I started to accept the issue better, and I felt as if I was preparing myself psychologically for what I was going to go through. There is a big difference between expecting things or to be suddenly shocked by things. . . later, I was called by a lady who was newly diagnosed with breast cancer and she started asking me questions. I felt very happy to be able to provide her with answers; this action gave me satisfaction. . .

Hindering Factors for Coping

Changed Body Image The hair loss was the main aspect that disturbed the participants of this study. They all reported that the hair loss was very detrimental to their coping and self-esteem.

Lamis, a 50-year-old lady, said:

I cried because I was losing my hair, losing my hair. When my hair started to fall, I was prepared for it; however, one day I was doing sports, and suddenly under the shower, I lost all my hair. I started crying, I called my husband and I felt crashed from inside. . .

Fear of Reoccurrence The idea that cancer might hit again was always present in the participants' mind. This idea was preventing them from coping with their current situation. It was disturbing them from inside.

Sirine, the 62-year-old lady, said:

I am always afraid to have it in another place. They say it can hit again, it can hit in different places. This is why I am always afraid. This idea is bothering me a lot, it is disturbing me, and it is preventing me from continuing my life normally . . . . This idea that cancer might hit again is haunting me day and night. . . .

Being Pitied by Others Being pitied by others was reported as very disturbing. Participants reported that they were obliged to hide their disease and their suffering for others not to pity them. This idea of being pitied by others prevented them from coping with their condition; on the contrary, it pushed them to hide their proper feelings and physical sufferings.

Sandra, a 48-year-old lady, said in this regard:

I do not like others to pity me to say "YA HARAM" [meaning more or less "what" in English]. The person with diabetes suffers more than I do, and they do not pity him.

Constitutive Pattern

Cancer is a Cut in Our Lives that We have to Fight The constitutive pattern linked the related themes across text. Overall, the participants of this study described their journey with breast cancer as a continuous battle. Participants were trying to gain this battle by using positive coping strategies; however, through their journey, they were faced by hindering factors that at times prevented them from coping with breast cancer. The pattern, "Cancer is a cut in our lives that we have to fight," was present across all interviews and across all themes. This fight against breast cancer made the participants more aware of their needs and rights as patients. This pattern runs across all interviews and across all identified themes.

Discussion

This is the first qualitative study that has portrayed how Lebanese women cope with breast cancer. This study sheds light on an important aspect of this group of women's coping strategies. According to the results of this study, Lebanese women viewed cancer as a major cut in their lives (which might be expressed as an intrusion), and they described their journey with cancer as a continuous battle. The major positive coping strategy noticed was their reliance on God. It is worth noting that Lebanon is known for its religious diversity. The 2 main prevailing religions in the Lebanese culture are Christianity and Islam.[17] However, there are as many as 18 diverse sects. The term *God* is recurrently used in the Lebanese language. Most Lebanese, regardless of religion, consider God as powerful, capable, and the source of miracles. This positive relationship with God and full reliance on Him gave all participants hope that God is in control. Participants coped with disease, having in mind that it is something from *Him*. It is worth noting that God was perceived as powerful, compassionate, and fair. Results suggested that this belief in God helped participants to accept their diagnosis, cope with their disease, and to bear willingly the consequences. This belief in relating to God evoked in the participants the feeling of hope and the need to cope. Studies conducted in different parts of the world reported that religion offers hope to those with cancer; it plays a big role in facilitating the disease acceptance process, and it has been found to have a positive effect on the quality of life of cancer patients.[7,18–20] However, as noted by Hack and Degner,[12] women who respond to their breast cancer diagnosis with passive acceptance and resignation are at a significant risk for poor long-term psychological adjustment. The use of belief and relationship with God to foster hope and strength to cope with the disease is the positive coping aspect that must be contrasted with the passive acceptance leading to resignation and a sense of helplessness, which was not expressed by the participants of this study.

The second emerging theme related to comparing cancer to an acceptable chronic disease in the Lebanese culture, diabetes, which was not highlighted in any of the reviewed research articles. All participants defended their need to communicate and speak about their breast cancer by comparing cancer to diabetes. It is worth noting that diabetes as a disease is better accepted than cancer within the Lebanese culture, especially when it comes to matters of stigma and marriage. Breast cancer is known for its familial inheritance. So mothers with breast cancer were living with guilt feelings, thinking that their daughters may not be chosen for marriage if it is known that their mothers have breast cancer. This issue does not exist for diabetes. Assessing the perception of people toward cancer and comparing it to other chronic diseases within the Lebanese culture needs further investigation.

The third theme is related to the impact of positive support from work, family, and husband on the coping process. Participants of this study stressed the important and pivotal role that family members, and especially husbands if available, can play on the morale and coping strategies of the women diagnosed as having breast cancer. The positive support received from the family and husbands of the participants helped them to accept their conditions and gave them the support needed to engage in their fight against cancer. These findings coincide with those of other studies[8,21] that highlighted the important role that the family plays in terms of support and coping. All the participants of the study wanted to survive for the sake of their children; for the sake of seeing them growing and enjoying life with them. This attitude is well explained within the Lebanese culture, where the mother plays an important and central role in the family. These results are in line with other studies conducted by Henderson et al[8] and Ashing et al,[22] in which the primary concern of women was to survive and combat the disease for the sake of their children. In addition to the previous 2 factors, work environment also had an influence but in a different way. Working women reported that they maintained their work and work pace as before because they were afraid from being labeled as "cancer patients," which means being pitied by others, a condition that they do not like. They forced themselves to cope with their disease and succeed in their battle. The success was translated by keeping their jobs without any change in the job description and by hiding their diagnosis from colleagues. Participants described this situation as successful, but nevertheless, it was achieved through "selfcoercion." They all reported an obligation to do that in order not to be pitied by others. This condition led all participants to complain about the negative cancer stigma within the Lebanese culture. This attachment to work, as experienced by Lebanese women, contradicts the results of studies[23–25] that reported a voluntary stop or reduction in working hours after breast cancer, along with a changing attitude among cancer survivors, who began attaching less importance to work than prior to their diagnosis and valuing a more balanced approach to life. On the other hand, Steiner et al[26] and Nachreiner et al[27] reported that returning to work enhances the patients' quality of life and could be perceived as a sign of recovery.

Sharing the experience with people who know, with people who went through similar experiences, was a request and a need. All participants who shared their experiences with survivors of breast cancer reported better coping mechanisms because they knew what to expect. Also, discussing their own experience with other patients who were newly diagnosed as having breast cancer boosted the participants' morale and gave them the feeling that they were still useful and strong. This feeling helped them to develop positive coping strategies. This sort of interaction and mutual communication were reported to be very beneficial and useful by the participants. These findings advocate the necessity to create patient support groups. Actually, participants themselves raised the need for such a group. These results match the results of a study conducted by Landmark et al,[21] in which women stressed the importance of fellowship with others who are in the same situation. Recognizing that one is not alone and that others share comparable thoughts and feelings seems to offer support. For the participants of this study, information sharing was viewed as a resource that enhanced coping.

The change in the physical appearance, specifically hair loss, was conceived by the participants of this study as a hindering factor for coping. The hair loss could be linked to the concept of loss of control. It is worth noting that control is a principal concept in the psychological theories of emotional well-being, adjustment, and coping.[28] Similar results were found by Frith et al[29] and Perreault and Bourbonnais,[4] in which losses impacted not only the physical dimension but also the psychological, social, and spiritual dimensions of the individual. In Lebanon, a woman's hair loss has perhaps even deeper meaning for her sense of being a woman. The major cultural roles of Lebanese women are still to gain a husband, have his sons, and keep him interested in her. Even though many Lebanese women now have a higher education and work in professions, the cultural norms of the male-dominated society are intact. This sense of losing her feminine attractiveness would be expected to have a greatly negative effect on her coping. The participants in this study did not reveal negative coping elements based on the loss of attractiveness, which would have been expected. Participants were afraid that, despite wearing a wig, people might know that they have cancer, and they might start pitying them.

The fear of being pitied by others was another factor that was perceived as a hindering feature for coping by the participants of this study. This factor of being pitied was not found in any of the reviewed articles, and it needs further clarification within the Lebanese culture. In speculation, we could say that this fear might be due to the nature of the reciprocal relationship within the Lebanese culture. If a person cannot reciprocate, he/she is perceived as weak or vulnerable. According to Lam and Fielding,[30] people want to keep away from being perceived as different and stigmatized in the society. This sense of being pitied also reduces perceived status relative to the others who are doing the pitying. Status is an important and pervasive aspect of Lebanese and Middle Eastern culture in general. Loss of perceived status increases the sense of vulnerability and would be perceived as hindering the ability to cope.

The fear of the recurrence of breast cancer was perceived as a threat by the participants. They all reported that this idea haunted them day and night and prevented them from coping. Similar results were reported by Bottorf et al[31] and Browall et al.[32]

Conclusion

Our findings provide increased in-depth understanding of Lebanese women's coping strategies for dealing with breast cancer. The constitutive pattern, "Cancer is a cut in our lives that we have to fight," represents the tie between all themes. This pattern, in addition to all emerging themes, reverberated in all interviews regardless of the time since diagnoses and the age of the woman interviewed. All participants reported a precipitous change in their lives and difficulties at times in coping with those sudden changes accompanying breast cancer. Different coping strategies were found to have different impacts on the participants' lives and morale. Healthcare workers need to be conscious of a multitude of factors including the motivational and hindering factors for coping with breast cancer. The findings of this study highlight the importance of identifying the motivational factors for coping in women living with breast cancer. Therefore, a specific assessment of coping strategies as an initial approach to patient care is highly suggested, and the creation of informal support group is needed to help these women cope with their conditions. Moreover, the results of this study can serve as a framework for further studies leading to the development of an approach to care that promotes coping processes in Lebanese women living with breast cancer. Furthermore, nursing and medical curricula need to sensitize students to the concept of coping in relation to breast cancer and its impact on the women's well-being.

Acknowledgments

The authors thank all the women who shared their experiences with them. They also thank Ms Samar Nassif, RN, MSN, for her remarkable contributions.

References

1. Ministry of Public Health, WHO. *National Non-Communicable Diseases Programme. Lebanon:* National Cancer Registry; 2002.
2. WHO. Stewart BW, Kleihues P, eds. *World Cancer Report.* Lyon. IARC Press; 2003.

3. Vachon MLS. Meaning, spirituality, and wellness in cancer survivors. *Semin Oncol Nurs.* 2008;24(3):218–225.

4. Perreault A, Bourbonnais FF. The experience of suffering as lived by women with breast cancer. *Int J Palliat Nurs.* 2005;11(10):510–519.

5. Bertero C, Chamberlain Wilmoth M. Breast cancer diagnosis and its treatment affecting the self: a meta synthesis. *Cancer Nurs.* 2007;30(2):194–202.

6. Fenlon DR, Rogers AE. The experience of hot flushes after breast cancer. *Cancer Nurs.* 2007;30(2):E19–E26.

7. Taleghani F, Yekta Z, Nasrabadi AN. Coping with breast cancer in newly diagnosed Iranian women. *J Adv Nurs.* 2006;54(3):265–272.

8. Henderson PD, Gore SV, Davis B, Condon EH. African American women coping with breast cancer: a qualitative analysis. *Oncol Nurs Forum.* 2003;30(4):641–648.

9. Li J, Lambert VA. Coping strategies and predictors of general well-being in women with breast cancer in the People's Republic of China. *Nurs Health Sci.* 2007;9(3):199–204.

10. Manual J, Burwell S, Crawford S, et al. Younger women's perceptions of coping with breast cancer. *Cancer Nurs.* 2007;30(2):85–94.

11. Stanton A, Danoff-Burg S, Huggins M. The first year after breast cancer diagnosis: hope and coping strategies as predictors of adjustments. *Psychooncology.* 2002;11(2): 93–102.

12. Hack TF, Degner LF. Coping responses following breast cancer diagnosis predict psychological adjustment three years later. *Psychooncology.* 2004;13(4):235–247.

13. Butow PN, Coates AS, Dunn SM. Psychological predictors of survival: metastatic breast cancer. *Ann Oncol.* 2000;11(4):469–474.

14. Doumit M, El Saghir N, Abu-Saad Huijer H, Kelley J, Nassar N. Living with breast cancer, a lebanese experience. *Eur J Oncol Nurs.* 2009. doi.10.1016/j.ejon.

15. Barritt L, Beekman T, Bleeker H, Mulderij K. Analyzing phenomenological descriptions. *Phenomenol Pedagogy.* 1984;2:1–17.

16. Van Manen M. *Researching Lived Experience.* New York, NY: State University of New York Press; 1990.

17. Diekelmann N, Ironside P. Hermeneutics. In: Fitzpatrick J, ed. *Encyclopedia of Nursing Research.* New York, NY: Springer; 1998:50–68.

18. Ryan P. Approaching death: a phenomenologic study of five older adults with advanced cancer. *Oncol Nurs Forum.* 2005;32:1101–1108.

19. Weaver AJ, Flannelly KJ. The role of religion/spirituality for cancer patients and their caregivers. *South Med J.* 2004;97(12):1210–1214.

20. Livneh H. Psychological adaptation to cancer: the role of coping strategies. *J Rehabil.* 2000;66(2):40–49.

21. Landmark BT, Bohler A, Loberg K, Wahl AK. Women with newly diagnosed breast cancer and their perceptions needs in a health-care context. *J Nurs Health Care Chronic Illn.* 2008;17(3):192–200.

22. Ashing TK, PadillaG, Tejero J, Kagawa-Singer M. Understanding the breast cancer experience of Asian American women. *Psychooncology.* 2003;12(1): 38–58.

23. Maunsell E, Brisson C, Dubois L, Lauzier S, Fraser A. Work problems after breast cancer: an exploratory qualitative study. *Psychooncology.* 1999; 8(6):467–473.

24. Maunsell E, Drolet M, Brisson J, Brisson C, Masse B, Deschenes L. Work situation after breast cancer: results from a population-based study. *J Natl Cancer Inst.* 2004;96(24): 1813–1822.

25. Main DS, Nowels CT, Cavender TA, Etschmaier M, Steiner F. A qualitative study of work and work return in cancer survivors. *Psychooncology.* 2005;14(11):992–1004.

26. Steiner JF, Cavender TA, Main DS, Bradley CJ. Assessing the impact of cancer on work outcomes: what are the research needs? *Cancer.* 2004; 101(8):1703–1711.

27. Nachreiner NM, Dagher R, McGovern PM, Baker BA, Alexander BH, Gerberich SG. Successful return to work for cancer survivors. *AAOHN J.* 2007;55(7):290–295.

28. Walker J. *Control and the Psychology of Health.* Buckingham, UK: Open University Press; 2001.

29. Frith H, Harcourt D, Fussell A. Anticipating an altered appearance: women undergoing chemotherapy treatment for breast cancer. *Eur J Oncol Nurs.* 2007;11(5):385–391.

30. Lam WT, Fielding R. The evolving experience of illness for Chinese women with breast cancer: a qualitative study. *Psychooncology.* 2003;12(2): 127–140.

31. Bottorf JL, Grewal SK, Balneaves LG, Naidu PM, Johnson JL, Sawhney R. Punjabi women's stories of breast cancer symptoms: gulti (lumps), bumps, and darad (pain). *Cancer Nurs.* 2007;30(4):E36–E45.

32. Browall M, Gaston-Johansson F, Danielson E. Postmenopausal women with breast cancer: their experiences of the chemotherapy treatment period. *Cancer Nurs.* 2006;29(1):34–42.

Grounded Theory as Method

Grounded theory is a research method used to discover new dimensions of the social processes at play in people's lives. Grounded theory method is rooted in the precepts of Symbolic Interactionism and was developed by two sociologists (Glaser & Strauss, 1967) as an alternative to theory verification. In contrast to research methods that were designed to describe phenomenon, the primary purpose of grounded theory research is to develop a theory. The concepts, and ultimately, the theories discovered through grounded theory research are derived directly from the data, which means that the theory is "grounded" in the experiences of the participants. Once key concepts, or dimensions, are identified, the researcher must also develop theoretical connections among the concepts, explaining what is going on in the area being studied.

Grounded theory is an inductive process used to generate theory from the individual level, which could then be generalized and applied to nursing practice. Grounded theories can help nurses understand how individuals and their families move through major life events, such as cardiac surgery or facing death. Grounded theory studies of nursing practice issues are especially important to nurses. For example, a grounded theory study on "Moral Reckoning" explained how nurses face and work through moral distress in the workplace (Nathaniel, 2006). Using grounded theory method enables researchers to develop explanations about concepts that are derived from empirical data (Hutchinson, 2001).

Glaser and Strauss (1967) first developed and published the method in: *The Discovery of Grounded Theory*. Nurse researchers used grounded theory to study phenomena important to professional nursing as early as the 1960s but it has been used more extensively in the last decade (cf., Beck, 1993, 2002; Benoliel, 1967; D'Abundo & Chally, 2004; Johnson & Delaney, 2006; Wiitavaara, Barnekow-Bergkvist, & Brulin, 2007). Benoliel (1996) noted that grounded theory began to influence nursing knowledge development in the early 1960s. In her manuscript, "Grounded Theory and Nursing Knowledge," she examined how the method has contributed to nursing's body of substantive knowledge from the 1960s through the 1990s. Benoliel (1967) suggested that the major focus of the contributions to nursing knowledge over these decades was on "adaptations to illness, infertility, nurse adaptation and interventions, and status passages of vulnerable persons and groups" (p. 406).

Since the publication of Glaser and Strauss' text, grounded theory research has expanded significantly. The method has continued to evolve and has become an extensively applied research approach. The methodology makes important contributions to nursing's development of a substantive body of knowledge, primarily because of its ability to develop middle-range theory, which can be tested empirically and readily applied to clinical practice, policy development, and public awareness campaigns.

This chapter reviews fundamental characteristics of grounded theory and addresses methodological issues specific to engaging in this research approach. The chapter also reviews the systematic techniques and procedures of analysis essential to grounded theory investigations. Additional reading of primary sources and mentoring by a grounded theory expert is necessary to grasp the nuances of the method in a comprehensive manner, although novices are encouraged to conduct grounded theory research (Glaser, 2009a).

GROUNDED THEORY ROOTS

Grounded theory method was discovered by two sociologists in 1967. Dr. Barney Glaser earned a PhD in sociology from Columbia University, and Dr. Anselm Strauss earned a PhD in sociology from the University of Chicago. The authors commented that the paradigms that guided their doctoral educations were philosophically opposed, but allowed a blending of two schools of thought to form a new way of developing theory, which is grounded in the experiences of the participants. The grounded theory perspective values the experience of the individual, and posits that theoretical processes are always at play, but are elusive to the untrained eye. Grounded theory method, then, is a way to discover these unseen processes.

Grounded theory method is heavily indebted to the discipline of sociology and draws on the "field research" approach to the discovery of new knowledge. Field research is conducted in naturalistic settings such as hospitals, outpatient clinics, and nursing homes. The basic assumption is that theories about people's actions or experience can be discovered by observing and interacting with the social group, rather than theorizing from the outside.

Through keen observation and data gathering, the grounded theory researcher explores the basic psychosocial processes at play in the area of interest. A basic psychosocial process is characterized by stages or phases that might or might not have fixed time frames. Additionally, basic social processes are pervasive, variable, and account for change over a period of time (Glaser, 1978). A basic psychosocial process is believed to transcend time and place, and thus occurs without regard to culture, race, or place.

This broad view of human processes is largely a product of the philosophical underpinnings of the grounded theory perspective. The development of grounded theory method was ideologically influenced by Symbolic Interactionism focused on the individual within a society. Glaser and Strauss (1967) agreed that a sociologist's focus should be on the individual within a society, but opposed the application of grand theories to "field work" because they believed that "armchair theories" (p. 14), which were not derived from the experiences of the individuals who had lived it, could not be effectively applied in "the field," or in the discipline of nursing, to practice.

Nurse researchers have widely recognized the significance of grounded theory as a valuable method to investigate phenomena important to nursing and have used this approach extensively. Benoliel (1996), a pioneer in the use of grounded theory method for nursing research, examined the roots of grounded theory in nursing and its development over the past several decades. She identified the knowledge generation that occurred during this period as the Decade of Discovery, 1960–1970; followed by the Decade of Development, 1970–1980; the Decade of Diffusion, 1980–1990; and the Decade of Diversification, the 1990s.

During the Decade of Discovery (1960–1970), grounded theory emerged as a major research method within the field of sociology. As the method entered the Decade of Development (1970–1980), seminars for the continued development of grounded theorists emerged, as well as funding for postdoctoral research training programs (Benoliel, 1996). The Decade of Diffusion (1980–1990) resulted in even further expansion of the research method, and nursing became visible as a group of researchers who could explain and implement grounded theory method. Nursing journals gave more attention to grounded theory, and university centers evolved that focused on grounded theory research in nursing (Benoliel, 1996). The Decade of Diversification (the 1990s) resulted in the dissemination of the knowledge gained through grounded theory research.

Today, several methodological issues have been raised by attempts to refine, or as Glaser (2009a) called it "remodel" grounded theory (Cutliffe, 2000; Kelle, 2005). In the 1990s, Baker, Wuest, and Stern (1992) discussed method slurring between grounded theory and phenomenology, which mixed steps from both methods, and addressed the importance of being specific about method. But, recently, O'Connor, Netting, and Thomas (2008) addressed the additional slurring of approaches to grounded theory.

To illustrate the shifts occurring in grounded theory discussions, Annells (1996) suggested that grounded theory had been traditionally understood within a postpositivist paradigm, but believed it is increasingly viewed within a postmodern context. Clarke (2003) also envisioned a postmodern approach to grounded theory and proposed using situational analyses to supplement traditional data analysis. Charmaz (2006) put forth the notion of constructivist grounded theory, and later (2008) described grounded theory as an "emergent method," meaning that it is "inductive, indeterminate, and open-ended" (p. 155). Although Corbin (Corbin & Strauss, 2008) expressed her admiration for these interpretations, Glaser (2002) conveyed his disdain. He stated that such interpretations of grounded theory method are merely others' attempts to remodel grounded theory method, while using its terminology to gain legitimacy (Glaser, 2002, 2009b).

Grounded theory, in all of its variations allows researchers to discover new dimensions of phenomena, empowering them to become theorists in their own right. Accordingly, grounded theory research does not begin with an existing theory, or preconceived ideas. Rather, the goal is to generate theory in a specific substantive area. The primary purpose of grounded theory research is the discovery of theory from methodical data collection and analysis (Glaser & Strauss, 1967; Glaser, 1978). But, if a researcher chooses to interpret data through a particular framework, it should be declared (Corbin & Strauss, 2008).

FUNDAMENTAL CHARACTERISTICS OF GROUNDED THEORY METHOD

Although grounded theory method was originally developed by both Glaser and Strauss (1967), a split occurred with the publication of *Strategies in Qualitative Research* by Strauss and Corbin (1990). The authors stated that the text offered practical advice to novices on the implementation of grounded theory research. But, Glaser reacted strongly to its publication, demanding that Strauss and Corbin "withdraw the book pending a rewriting of it" (Glaser, 1992, p. 1). The book was not withdrawn, and a schism began, dividing grounded theory researchers into two camps, those who follow Glaser's approach (which is also called Glaserian or Classic Grounded Theory), and those who follow Strauss and Corbin's approach (which is also called Straussian Grounded Theory).

The exact differences between Classic and Straussian approaches to research have been thoroughly discussed (Heath & Cowley, 2004; Hernandez, 2008) in the literature, and major differences will be highlighted in this chapter. Table 7-1 also provides the reader with a concise comparison between the two approaches. Both approaches share the same basic terminology, and the jargon is commonly used in other forms of qualitative studies (Glaser, 2009b)

Table 7-1 • Comparison of Classic and Straussian Grounded Theory

	Glaser & Strauss/Glaser	Strauss & Corbin/ Corbin & Strauss
Epistemology	No preconceived ideas about the area of study. No literature review is to be conducted. The researcher begins from a position of naiveté and learns from the experts (those who lived it).	Researchers can gain insights into data through literature review. Theories are considered a lens through which the researcher approaches the data and should be named, if used.
Research question/ research problem	The researcher studies an area of interest; a specific research question is not needed. A life-cycle interest, such as mothering is best. The researcher trusts that the participants will reveal their main concern.	A research question is stated. An example given by Corbin & Strauss (2008) is "How do women with a pregnancy complicated by a chronic illness manage their pregnancy and life in a way to secure a positive pregnancy outcome?" (p. 25)
Ethical considerations	Grounded theory is about concepts, not people. Transcription of interviews is not necessary, but information about specific individuals should be confidential.	Interviews can be transcribed, and this is recommended for novices. Data should be stored securely. Confidentiality should be ensured.
Data gathering	No interview guide is needed because these are based on preconceptions. The participants are considered the experts and will reveal their main concern. Field notes can be used, as well as photos, news articles, historical documents, and other information that clarifies the concepts. "All is data."	Unstructured interviews are recommended. Observations of the participants are also part of the data, but are subject to interpretation and should be clarified with the participants. Themes are identified and supported with data.
Data analysis	The researcher sorts and resorts memos until the major concepts become clear. Then, the theoretical connections among the concepts should be stated.	Computer programs can be used to aid data analysis.
Results	The results of the study should be "written up" from the memos. The study will result in a substantive theory that explains what is going on in the area of interest. Numerous theories can be discovered from one study.	Data analysis, at a minimum, results in themes and concepts. Theories can also be developed from the data, but this is not the necessary outcome.
Evaluation	Fit, Work, Relevance, and Modifiability.	Fit, applicability, concepts, contextualization of concepts, logic, depth, variation, creativity, sensitivity, and evidence of memos.

where no original verbiage existed. Key terms will be reviewed to help the reader understand the terminology used when discussing grounded theory. Only succinct definitions are offered here; the reader is referred to Glaser (1978, 1992, 1998) for complete explanations of the terms.

> *Memoing:* Informal notes taken by the researcher to capture ideas about the data, emerging theoretical codes, and relationships among the codes. Memos are free-form and private. They should not be shared or evaluated by others (Glaser, 1998).
>
> *Theoretical Sampling:* A process by which the researcher decides what data to collect next (Glaser & Strauss, 1967). Theoretical sampling is a conscious decision to find new data sources that can clarify the researcher's understanding about the concepts that have been discovered, or how the concepts are related (Glaser, 1998).
>
> *Saturation:* "Saturation means that no additional data are being found whereby the [researcher] can develop properties of the category" (Glaser & Strauss, 1967, p. 61).
>
> *Theoretical completeness:* all of the categories in the substantive theory are saturated, and the theory explains how the main concern is continually resolved (Glaser, 1998).
>
> *Coding:* A way of fracturing the data and then grouping it according to the concepts each incident represents. These codes will eventually explain what is happening in the data (Glaser, 1978).
>
> *Substantive Codes:* The names assigned to similar groups of raw data (Glaser, 1978).
>
> *Theoretical Codes:* The names given to codes that explain how the substantive codes are related to each other (Glaser, 1978).
>
> *Core Category:* The main concern of the participants. The core category explains most of what is going on in the data, and will emerge from the data (Glaser, 1978).
>
> *Selective Coding:* A way of limiting data collection through theoretical sampling by coding for a core category only (Glaser, 1978).
>
> *Constant Comparison:* Comparing "incident to incident, and then when incidents emerge, incident to concept (Glaser, 1992, p. 39).

SELECTION OF GROUNDED THEORY AS A METHOD

Grounded theory research entails the identification of the theoretical connections among the concepts. By clarifying the connections among concepts, the researcher develops a theory that is grounded in the data, and relevant to the substantive area. Glaser and Strauss (1967) referred to this type of theory as a *substantive theory*. Examples pertinent to nursing might include taking care of oneself in a high-risk environment (Rew, 2003) or concerns of intimate partners or patients experiencing sudden cardiac arrest after implantation of an internal defibrillator (Dougherty, Pyper, & Benoliel, 2004). Theories that are broader in scope, and are usually developed through comparative analysis, are referred to as *formal theories*. A formal theory differs from a substantive theory in that it is applicable to more than one substantive area (Glaser & Strauss, 1967).

The goal of grounded theory is not specifically to empirically test the theories that are developed. However, some researchers (Hogan & Schmidt, 2002) have tested theories that were empirically derived through grounded theory research. Such empirically derived and tested theories are particularly important to health professionals because "evidence based practice must be rooted in evidence based theories" (Wright & Hogan, 2008, p. 350). The need for more middle-range theories in nursing that can be empirically tested is one reason for using grounded theory to conduct scientific investigations of phenomena important to nursing. But, it is important to stress that theories discovered through grounded theory analysis do not need to be empirically tested to be considered valid.

Corbin and Strauss (2008), however, noted that "not everyone wants to develop theory, in fact, theory development these days seems to have fallen out of fashion, being replaced by descriptions of "lived experience" and "narrative stories" (p. 55). Although they consider theory development a worthwhile effort, they do not necessarily see it as the main goal of grounded theory research. Rather, they noted the importance of discovering concepts and themes from the data, and stated that grounded theory researchers must learn how to "keep a balance between conceptualization and description" (p. 51).

Novice grounded theory researchers should carefully consider their goals when choosing a research approach, and be sure to work with an experienced mentor. Most importantly, the researcher should study the differences between Classical and Straussian methods and state which approach was used. Clearly delineating the type of study being conducted will help to curtail confusion between the approaches.

ELEMENTS AND INTERPRETATION OF THE METHOD

When individuals choose to conduct a grounded theory investigation, usually they have decided there is some observed social process requiring description and explanation. Corbin (Corbin & Strauss, 2008) believes that there is not "one reality out there waiting to be discovered" (p. 10), and views qualitative research as a way to view events from the perspective of the other. Corbin suggested that qualitative researchers choose a problem area in one of four ways: (1) the suggestion of an advisor or mentor; (2) based on the review of literature; (3) personal or professional experience; or (4) from doing the research. Corbin and Strauss (2008) questioned whether the choice of a research method is purely analytical, or whether qualitative researchers are predisposed to frame questions in a way that demands qualitative inquiry. Haverkamp and Young (2007) suggested that qualitative researchers typically approach inquiry with the goal of understanding, rather than verification.

When a researcher wishes to gain deeper understanding of psychosocial processes and build a theory to explain what is going on in the area of interest, grounded theory method is appropriate. Application of grounded theory research techniques to the investigation of an observed social process important to nursing education, practice, or administration involves the application of several nonlinear steps. Grounded theory techniques are described in the following narrative as they relate to the methodological steps familiar to the research process. Development and refinement of the research question, sample selection, researcher's role, and ethical considerations in grounded theory investigations are described along with procedures for data generation, treatment, and analysis.

Research Question

The main purpose of using grounded theory method is to explore social processes with the goal of developing theory (Glaser & Strauss, 1967). According to Glaser (1992), the grounded theory researcher does not need to specify a problem prior to beginning a research study. The researcher chooses an area of interest and discovers "what is going on that is an issue and how it is handled" (p. 22). Christiansen (2008) explained that the classic grounded theory approach entails choosing a "general and loosely formulated research topic" (p. 30). To do otherwise indicates that the researcher has preconceived ideas about what the issues or problems are in the substantive area, and violates the method. Notably, a review of the literature is not conducted prior to beginning the study. Glaser (1992) stated clearly, "There is a need not to review any of the literature in the substantive area under study. This dictum is brought about by the concern to not contaminate, be constrained by, inhibit, stifle, or otherwise impede the researcher's effort . . ." (p. 31).

The lack of a thorough review of literature and explications of gaps in understanding that support the proposed study can be problematic for those crafting thesis or dissertation proposals within guidelines specified by academic departments or universities. Xie (2009) discussed the potential problems with presenting a proposal for a grounded theory study to a doctoral committee, and offered advice on striking a balance between doctoral program requirements and the principles of classic grounded theory. Although it can be challenging, Xie stated, "the persuasions [presented in the article] . . . convinced my committee that grounded theory was not just the best methodology for this study, but was in fact the only appropriate choice" (p. 32). O'Connor et al. (2008) addressed the need to be clear about the choice of research methods when trying to meet the concerns of positivistic Institutional Review Boards. The authors offered guidelines for researchers and those who serve on review panels which help differentiate grounded theory approaches. They explained, "Strauss moved his original methodology with Glaser toward interpretism when he joined with Corbin and integrated symbolic interactionism and a more postpositivistic stance into the method" (p. 39), and thus, different review criteria should apply.

According to Corbin and Strauss (2008), the research question in a grounded theory investigation identifies the phenomenon to be studied. Once a problem is identified for study, the research question is framed to delimit the scope of the study. Specifically, the question lends focus and clarity about what the phenomenon of interest is (Strauss & Corbin, 1990, 1998; Corbin & Strauss, 2008). Furthermore, researchers need a research question or questions that will give them the flexibility and freedom to explore a phenomenon in depth. Also underlying this research approach is the assumption that all of the concepts pertaining to a given phenomenon have not yet been identified, at least not in this population or place; or if so, then the relationships between the concepts are poorly understood or conceptually undeveloped (Strauss & Corbin, 1990, 1998; Corbin & Strauss, 2008).

An example of a research question appropriate for guiding a Straussian Grounded Theory study is "How do women with a pregnancy complicated by a chronic illness manage their pregnancy and life in a way to secure a positive pregnancy outcome?" (Corbin & Strauss, 2008, p. 25). The authors explained that a question such as this would be considered too vague and nondirectional for quantitative studies, but is appropriate for gaining the perspectives of the participants. Corbin and Strauss (2008) further emphasized that qualitative research need not be limited to individuals, but can focus on groups as well. The research question then specifies the group to be studied, or the area of interest, and allows the researcher to consider where to gather data.

Sampling

Glaser's (1992) approach to data gathering is to take a broad perspective, and enter the area of interest with an open mind. Once the problems begin to emerge, the researcher will determine where to go next for data; this is called theoretical sampling. As an example, if a researcher chose to study pregnancy, she would begin her study by talking with women who have been or are pregnant. She might find that the women's main concern is "managing physical change," in which case, she may then choose to further explore this concept with older adults. Theoretical sampling limits the collection of data, but it is not possible to predetermine how many participants will be "needed" for the study. Data collection should continue until the theoretical completeness is achieved, meaning that the discovered theory explains the action in the substantive area (Glaser, 1992, 1998).

For researchers using Straussian Grounded Theory, participants should be chosen based on their experience with the social process under investigation. The sample size is determined by the data generated and their analysis.

Data collection should continue until saturation is reached. Corbin and Strauss (2008) explained that saturation "is the point in the research when all the concepts are well defined and explained" (p. 145). The researcher can gain closure by constant questioning and re-examination of the data (Hutchinson, 2001), and some (Guest, Bunce, & Johnson, 2006) have suggested that saturation can occur after as few as 12 interviews.

Researcher's Role

Glaser (1992, 1998) advised grounded theory researchers to reduce their preconceptions to the greatest extent possible. This means that the researcher must enter the field as one who is naïve, willing to learn from those who are the experts. The experts are the individuals or groups who can give the researcher insights into the substantive area. The main concern of the participants cannot be predetermined, and the researcher must trust that it will be evident through the grounded theory approach. This type of openness comes naturally to novices (Glaser, 2009). The researcher does not need to demonstrate competence in particular skills but does need to be open to what is going in the focus area.

Strauss and Corbin (1990, 1998) identified several skills needed for doing qualitative research: the ability "to step back and critically analyze situations, to recognize and avoid bias, to obtain valid and reliable data, and to think abstractly" (p. 18). Furthermore, "a qualitative researcher requires theoretical and social sensitivity, the ability to maintain analytical distance while at the same time drawing upon past experience and theoretical knowledge to interpret what is seen, astute powers of observation, and good interactional skills" (p. 18). To conduct a grounded theory investigation, researchers must possess excellent interpersonal and observational skills, compelling analytical abilities, and writing skills that facilitate communication in written word, with a high degree of accuracy, regarding what they have learned.

Corbin and Strauss (2008) also discussed the role of interpretation in the collection and analysis of data. They believe researchers enter the field from cultural, professional, or gender-specific perspectives. Thus, although they believe it is best to not begin a study using a theoretical framework, they recommend that if one is used it be identified. For example, Van and Meleis (2003) specified that they used an integrated theoretical perspective in their Grounded Theory study of African American women's grief after involuntary pregnancy loss. Stating one's theoretical perspective helps readers understand how the researcher approached data analysis and interpreted the findings.

Ethical Considerations

Researchers must also consider the ethical implications of conducting a grounded theory investigation or, for that matter, any qualitative investigation. Obtaining informed consent, maintaining confidentiality, and handling sensitive information are a few examples of ethical considerations re-searchers must address. Because it is impossible to anticipate what sensitive issues might emerge during data collection in a grounded theory investiga-tion, researchers must be prepared for unexpected concerns. Chapter 4 provides an extensive discussion of ethical considerations pertinent to qual-itative investigations.

Steps in the Research Process

Grounded theory research requires that data collection and analysis take place concurrently (Glaser & Strauss, 1967). However, if data is collected and analysis is not simultaneously undertaken, such as when data are col-lected by another person, grounded theory method, and theoretical sam-pling can still take place (Corbin & Strauss, 2008). For the purposes of clarity, each of the steps in the research process will be discussed individu-ally in the following sections, despite the fact that the steps actually overlap in practice.

DATA GENERATION

Researchers may collect grounded theory data from interviews, observa-tions, documents, or from a combination of these sources (Glaser & Strauss, 1967). Daily journals, participant observation, formal or semi-structured interviews, and informal interviews are valid means of generating data. As concepts and categories emerge during data analysis, the required sampling of particular data sources continues until theoretical saturation is reached. No limits are set on the number of participants, interviewees, or data sources because it is not possible to know beforehand where the data will lead (Glaser, 1978).

Individual interviews can also be conducted, but Glaser (1998) opposes recording and transcribing interviews. Rather, the researcher is advised to jot down theoretical notes during interviews. Memos are used to capture the re-searcher's ideas about the concepts and to ask questions about the data as it is being collected and analyzed. Additionally, Glaser cautions against the use of interview guides because they are based on perceived ideas about what will emerge. Rather, Glaser recommends "adjusted conversational in-terviewing" (p. 173).

Corbin and Strauss (2008) agreed that multiple data sources can be used to inform one's understanding of concepts, but they are not specifically opposed to interview guides as long as the questions are open-ended and allow the participants to discuss their concerns. They recommend unstruc-tured interviews, and caution novice researchers to be aware that their ques-tions may change based on the concepts that are found during the study. Corbin and Strauss are also not opposed to the recording of interviews, but advise researchers to ask permission to jot down notes about important concepts that are discussed after the recorder is turned off.

DATA ANALYSIS

As the researcher collects data through interviews, participant observation, field notes, and so forth, coding begins. Coding entails line by line examination of the data to identify concepts, and conceptualize underlying patterns. This type of close analysis of the data is called open coding, and results in many theoretical codes. The code can be a word or phrase taken directly from the data, which is called an "in vivo" code (Glaser, 1978).

As the researcher continues to review data, she compares it to other data, and to the codes that have already been developed. Through this process, data that represent similar facets of the same concept are grouped together by the technique called constant comparison. Constant comparison is a general method that can be used in other types of qualitative inquiry. It allows the researcher to group data into similar categories, and develop themes or concepts. But, to generate hypotheses about how concepts are related, the researcher must ask questions about the data and continually capture her thoughts about the emerging concepts. Memoing is recommended to aid conceptualization and theory building (Glaser, 1978, 1992).

Glaser (1998) recommended that memos be free-form, and hand written. He does not recommend the use of computer programs, and stated, "it hinders and cops out on the skill of doing grounded theory" (p. 185). Table 7-2 presents a sample of a field note with codes and memos. The memos are intentionally incomplete, and informal to show development over time. Glaser noted that memos become more precise over time, as the researcher gains experience and becomes more theoretically sensitive.

In contrast to Glaser's recommendations regarding memos, Strauss and Corbin (1990, 1998) laid out specific features of memos and diagrams, advising that memos should be dated, contain a heading, include short quotes, and references. Additionally, they advised researchers to remain conceptual (not get caught up in details), stay flexible, and keep multiple copies of memos (p. 203). Recently (2008), Corbin and Strauss discussed the use of qualitative computer programs as an aid in organizing, storing, and analyzing data.

Memos help the researcher to discover the core category, which occurs over and over in the data. Glaser (1978) explained, "the researcher undertakes the quest for this essential element of the theory, which illuminates the main theme of the actors in the setting, and explicates what is going on in the data" (p. 94). The core variable serves as the foundational concept for theory generation, and "the integration and density of the theory are dependent on the discovery of a significant core variable" (Hutchinson, 2001, p. 222). The core category "accounts for most of the variation in a pattern of behavior [and] has several important functions for generating grounded theory: integration, density, saturation, completeness, and delimiting focus (Glaser, 1992, p. 75)." Similarly, Strauss (1987) explained that the core category recurs frequently in the data, links various data, is central, and

Table 7-2 • Example of a Field Note With Codes and Memos		
Field Note	*Code*	*Memo*
Senior level nursing student completed first home visit. In postconference, the student discussed feeling confident in her skills and reflected on how far she has come since sophomore year.	Looking back	Taking pride in accomplishments by reflecting on a time when you did not know how to do something.
		Energized reviewing
Sophomore level nursing student worked with a client this morning and engaged in life review. The student shared what the client said about her childhood in Poland. The student then discussed her own childhood.	Looking back	Happy times—maybe there were unhappy times, too. Looking back isn't always good.
		Emotive reviewing
Formal Interview with nursing student: "Whenever I feel like I want to change my major, I just look back at all the work I've put into this"	Looking back	Her expression conveyed pride in her work. Handling changes by looking back. What kinds of changes? Moving forward? Growing up? Retrospective . . . (?)
Informal interview with staff nurse/discussing the students. She began to talk about her experiences as a student, including working night shift, and wearing a cape over her uniform. She also mentioned that gloves were not worn during patient care.	Looking back	Looking back can be a way of earning respect by reflecting on how things were harder then. Is this still a way of dealing with change? What process is this a part of?
		Retrospective appraisal

explains much of the variation in all the data, has implications for a more general or formal theory, moves theory forward, and permits maximum variation and analyses.

When the core variable becomes clear, the researcher can begin selective coding, which means limiting coding to only those data that pertain to the core variable. As the theoretical codes saturate, the researcher must begin the process of sorting memos, which Glaser explained in detail (1998). Sorting enables the investigator to develop hypotheses about the concepts and helps to ensure parsimony of the substantive theory (Glaser, 1992, 1998). When theoretical saturation is reached, meaning that the main concern of the participants is clear, and the theory explains how that concern is continually resolved, the researcher can write up the research findings.

Production of the Research Report

The research report for a grounded theory investigation presents the theory, which is substantiated by supporting data from field notes. The report should give readers an idea of the sources of the data, how the data were rendered, and how the concepts were integrated. A good report reflects the theory in ways that allow an outsider to grasp its meaning and apply its concepts.

EVALUATION OF GROUNDED THEORIES

According to Glaser and Strauss (1967), when a grounded theory is generated from data obtained from those who have lived an experience, the researcher can feel confident "in his bones" that the results are credible (p. 225). The theory that is developed in the study should meet five criteria, as defined by Glaser and Strauss (1967): (a) to predict and explain behavior, (b) to further advance theory in a field, (c) to be useful in practice, (d) to provide perspective, and (e) to guide future research. The researcher bears the burden of conveying credibility to the reader by supporting each theoretical assertion with data (Glaser, 1978; Glaser & Strauss, 1967). The reader must be provided with enough supportive evidence to easily make the connections among the theoretical suppositions.

Readers with experience in the area of study are expected to judge the applicability of the substantive theory in various structures or settings. As Glaser and Strauss stated:

> [I]t is important to note that when a theory is deemed inapplicable to a social world or social structure, then it cannot be invalid for that situation. . . . The invalidation or adjustment of a theory is only legitimate for those social worlds or structures to which it is applicable. (Glaser & Strauss, 1967, p. 232)

This statement indicates that the researcher must delimit clearly the boundaries of the theory and to which situations the theory is or is not applicable and support each assertion with data.

Glaser and Strauss developed systematic criteria for judging the veracity of a grounded theory, which included four criteria: fit, work, relevance, and modifiability (Glaser, 1978, 1992, 1998; Glaser & Strauss, 1967). Strauss and Corbin (1990) identified four criteria for judging the applicability of theory to a phenomenon: (1) fit; (2) understanding; (3) generality; and

(4) control. If theory is faithful to the everyday reality of the substantive area and is carefully induced from diverse data, then it should fit that substantive area. Corbin and Strauss (2008) also explained that these criteria were developed for research that resulted in a theory. Although "the criteria also have significance for more descriptive forms of research" (p. 300), they offered a means of judging the quality of descriptive findings that result from qualitative inquiry. These include: (1) fit, (2) applicability, (3) concepts, (4) contextualization of concepts, (5) logic, (6) depth, (7) variation, (8) creativity, (9) sensitivity, and (10) evidence of memos.

SUMMARY

Grounded theory is a research method that provides a means to theory development from data (Glaser & Strauss, 1967; Glaser, 1978, 1992, 1998), and can also result in description (Corbin & Strauss, 2008). The fundamental characteristics and application of the approach include determining an area of interest, data collection and analysis, and evaluation. When used by nurses, grounded theory can increase middle-range substantive theories and help explain theoretical gaps among theory, research, and practice. Grounded theory has continued to evolve and has become an extensively applied research approach. The methodology makes important contributions to nursing's development of a substantive body of knowledge, primarily due to its ability to develop middle-range theory, which can be tested empirically. Chapter 8 addresses grounded theory method as it has been applied in nursing education, practice, and administration.

References

Annells, M. (1996). Grounded theory method: Philosophical perspectives, paradigm of inquiry, and postmodernism. *Qualitative Health Research, 6,* 379–393.

Baker, C., Wuest, J., & Stern, P. N. (1992). Method slurring: The grounded theory/ phenomenology example. *Journal of Advanced Nursing, 17,* 1255–1360.

Beck, C. T. (1993). Teetering on the edge: A substantive theory of postpartum depression. *Nursing Research, 42*(1), 42–48.

Beck, C. T. (2002). Releasing the pause button: Mothering twins during the first years of life. *Qualitative Health Research, 12*(5), 593–608.

Benoliel, J. Q. (1967). *The nurse and the dying patient.* New York, NY: Macmillan.

Benoliel, J. Q. (1996). Grounded theory and nursing knowledge. *Qualitative Health Research, 6*(3), 406–428.

Charmaz, K. (2006). *Constructing grounded theory.* Thousand Oaks, CA: Sage.

Charmaz, K. (2008). Grounded theory as an emergent method. In S. N. Hesse-Biber, & P. Levy, (Eds.). *Handbook of emergent methods* (pp. 155–170). New York, NY: The Guilford Press.

Christiansen, Ó. (2008). The rationale for the use of Classic GT. *The Grounded Theory Review, 7,* 19–37.

Clarke, A. E. (2003). Situational analysis: Grounded theory mapping after the postmodern turn. *Symbolic Interaction, 26,* 553–576.

Corbin, J., & Strauss, A. (2008). *Basics of qualitative research* (3rd ed.). Los Angeles, CA: Sage Publications.

Cutliffe, J. R. (2000). Methodological issues in grounded theory. *Journal of Advanced Nursing, 31*(6), 1476–1484.

D'Abundo, M., & Chally, P. (2004). Struggling with recovery: Participant perspectives on battling an eating disorder. *Qualitative Health Research, 14*(8), 1094–1106.

Dougherty, C. M., Pyper, G. P., & Benoliel, J. Q. (2004). Domains of concern of intimate partners of sudden cardiac arrest survivors after ICD implantation. *Journal of Cardiovascular Nursing, 19*(1), 21–31.

Glaser, B. (1978). *Theoretical sensitivity*. Mill Valley, CA: Sociology Press.

Glaser, B. G., & Strauss, A. (1967). *The discovery of grounded theory: Strategies for qualitative research*. New York, NY: Aldine.

Glaser, B. G. (1992). *Emergence vs. forcing: Basics of grounded theory analysis*. Mill Valley, CA: Sociology Press.

Glaser, B. (1998). *Doing grounded theory: Issues and discussions*. Mill Valley, CA: Sociology Press.

Glaser, B. (2002). Constructivist grounded theory? *Forum: Qualitative Social Research. 3*, 1–13. Retrieved from http://www.qualitative-research.net/index.php/fqs/article/viewArticle/ 825/17 92. Accessed on October 2009.

Glaser, B. (2009a). The novice GT researcher. *The Grounded Theory Review: An International Journal, 8*, 1–21.

Glaser, B. (2009b). *Jargonizing: Using the grounded theory vocabulary*. Mill Valley, CA: Sociology Press.

Guest, G., Bunce, A., & Johnson, L. (2006). How many interviews are enough? An experiment with data saturation and variability. *Field Methods, 18*, 59–82.

Haverkamp, B. E., & Young, R. A. (2007). Paradigms, purpose, and the role of the literature: Formulating a rationale for qualitative investigators. *The Counseling Psychologist, 35*, 265–294.

Heath, H., & Cowley, S. (2004). Developing a grounded theory approach: A comparison of Glaser and Strauss. *International Journal of Nursing Studies, 41*, 141–150.

Hernandez, C. A. (2008). Are there two methods of grounded theory? Demystifying the methodological debate. *The Grounded Theory Review, 7*, 39–54.

Hogan, N. S., & Schmidt, L. A. (2002). Testing the grief to personal growth model using structural equation modeling. *Death Studies, 26*, 615–634.

Hutchinson, S. (2001). Grounded theory: The method. In P. L. Munhall (Ed.), *Nursing research: A qualitative perspective* (pp. 209–243). Sudbury, MA: Jones and Bartlett.

Johnson, M. E., & Delaney, K. R. (2006). Keeping the unit safe: A grounded theory study. *American Psychiatric Nurses Association. 12*, 13–21.

Kelle, U. (2005). Emergence vs. forcing of empirical data? A crucial problem of grounded theory reconsidered. Retrieved September 27, 2009, from http://www.qualitative-research.net/index.php/fqs/article/viewArticle/467/1000

Nathaniel, A. K. (2006). Moral reckoning in nursing. *Western Journal of Nursing Research, 28*, 419–438.

O'Connor, M. K., Netting, F. E., & Thomas, M. L. (2008). Grounded theory: Managing the challenge for those facing institutional review board oversight. *Qualitative Inquiry, 14*, 28–45.

Rew, L. (2003). A theory of taking care of oneself grounded in experiences of homeless youth. *Nursing Research, 52*(4), 234–241. Retrieved from www.nursingresearchonline.com. Accessed on October 2009.

Strauss, A. (1987). *Qualitative analysis for social scientists*. New York, NY: Cambridge University Press.

Strauss, A., & Corbin, J. (1990). *Basics of qualitative research: Grounded theory procedures and techniques*. Newbury Park, CA: Sage.

Strauss, A., & Corbin, J. (1998). *Basics of qualitative research: Grounded theory procedures and techniques*. Newbury Park, CA: Sage.

Van, P. & Meleis, A. I. (2003). Coping with grief after involuntary pregnancy loss: Perspectives of African American women. *Journal of Obstetric, Gynecologic & Neonatal Nursing, 32*, 28–39.

Wiitavaara, B., Barnekow-Bergkvist, M. & Brulin, C. (2007). Striving for balance: A grounded theory study of health experiences of nurses with musculoskeletal problems. *International Journal of Nursing Studies, 44*, 1379–1390.

Wright, P. M. & Hogan, N. S. (2008). Grief theories and models: Applications to hospice nursing practice. *Journal of Hospice & Palliative Nursing, 10*, 350–356.

Xie, S. L. (2009). Striking a balance between program requirements and GT principles: Writing a compromised GT proposal. *The Grounded Theory Review, 8*, 35–47.

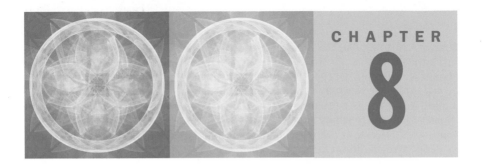

Grounded Theory in Practice, Education, and Administration

Grounded theory research creates opportunities for nurses to develop substantive theories regarding phenomena important for nursing practice as well as the administrative and educative processes that are inherent to the discipline.

In Chapter 7, methodological issues related to grounded theory investigations were described. This chapter examines published grounded theory studies in the areas of nursing practice, education, and administration. Two important questions guided the direction of this chapter: *When should grounded theory be used?* and *How has the method been used to study issues in nursing education, administration, and practice?* Three research studies will be reviewed using the guidelines for evaluating grounded theory research presented in Box 8-1. A reprint of Bach, Ploeg, and Black's (2009) article is provided at the end of this chapter to assist readers in understanding the critiquing process. The chapter also provides readers with an overview of selected studies that highlight how nurse researchers have used grounded theory research in the investigation of phenomena important to nursing (Table 8-1).

CRITIQUE GUIDELINES

Glaser and Strauss (1967) and Corbin and Strauss (2008) offered guidelines for judging Classic or Straussian Grounded Theory studies, which were discussed in Chapter 7. Researchers conducting grounded theory

Box 8-1

Guidelines for Critiquing Research Using Grounded Theory Method

Focus/Topic

1. What is the focus or the topic of the study? What is it that the researcher is studying? Is the topic researchable? Is it focused enough to be meaningful but not too limited so as to be trivial?

2. Has the researcher identified why the phenomenon requires a qualitative format? What is the rationale for selecting the grounded theory approach as the qualitative approach for the investigation?

Purpose

1. Has the researcher made explicit the purpose for conducting the research?

Significance

1. Does the researcher describe the projected significance of the work to nursing?

2. What is the relevance of the study to what is already known about the topic?

Method

1. Given the topic of the study and the researcher's stated purpose, how does grounded theory methodology help to achieve the stated purpose?

2. Is the method adequate to address the research topic?

3. What approach is used to guide the inquiry? Does the researcher complete the study according to the processes described?

Sampling

1. Does the researcher describe the selection of participants and protection of human subjects?

2. What major categories emerged?

3. What were some of the events, incidents, or actions that pointed to some of these major categories?

4. What were the categories that led to theoretical sampling?

5. Did the research specify how and why participants were selected for the study?

Data Generation

1. Does the researcher describe data collection strategies?

2. Have participants been allowed to guide the direction of the inquiry?

3. How did theoretical formulations guide data collection?

Data Analysis

1. Does the researcher describe the strategies used to analyze the data?
   a. Has the theoretical construction been checked against the participants' meanings of the phenomenon?
   b. Are the researcher's views and insights about the phenomenon articulated?
   c. Has the literature been related to each category that emerged in the theory?

2. Does the researcher address the credibility, auditability, and fittingness of the data?

3. Does the researcher clearly describe how and why the core category was selected?

Box 8-1 *(Continued)*

Empirical Grounding of the Study: Findings

1. Are concepts grounded in the data?
2. Are the concepts systematically related?
3. Are conceptual linkages described, and are the categories well developed? Do they have conceptual density?
4. Are the theoretical findings significant? If yes, to what extent?
5. Were data collection strategies comprehensive and analytical interpretations conceptual and broad?
6. Is there sufficient variation to allow for applicability in a variety of contexts related to the phenomenon investigated?

Conclusions, Implications, and Recommendations

1. How does the researcher provide a context for use of the findings?
2. Are the conclusions drawn from the study appropriate? Explain.
3. What are the recommendations for future research?
4. Are the recommendations, conclusions, and implications clearly related to the findings?

Adapted from Chiovitti, R., & Prian, N. (2003). Rigour and grounded theory research. *Journal of Advanced Nursing Practice, 44*(4), 427–435, and Strauss, A., & Corbin, J. (1990). *Basics of qualitative research: Grounded theory procedures and techniques.* Newbury Park, CA: Sage.

studies should evaluate their studies according to those recommendations. But, general guidelines can be challenging to apply, especially for novices who critique research to gain a deeper understanding of the method as well as the subject.

Therefore, specific criteria for evaluating grounded theory investigations are provided to help reviewers focus on critical elements of the method (see Box 8-1). When reviewers are critiquing any published investigation, it is important to recognize that journal restrictions, page limitations, or other external forces beyond the author's control may have necessitated deletion of certain material, resulting in a limited critique of the research. Readers interested in more detailed discussion of method in a published study should contact the author.

APPLICATION TO PRACTICE

Grounded theory method offers an important opportunity for nurses interested in examining clinical practice issues and developing substantive theory. An example of grounded theory research related to the practice arena is the study "Nursing Roles in End-of-Life Decision Making in Critical Care Settings" by Bach et al. (2009); this is the reference for critique in this section. This study provides an example of grounded theory research in the investigation of phenomena important to nursing practice.

Table 8-1 • Selective Sampling of Grounded Theory Research Studies

Author(s)	Date	Domain	Phenomenon of Interest	Sample	Data Generation	Findings
Crowe, V.L.H. & Bitterman, J.E.	2009	Practice	Depression	25 individuals who had a history of depression, but were not acutely depressed at the time of the interview. Other data sources included online information, autobiographical literature, and instruments developed by the researchers.	Interviews, review of online information, and quantitative data.	A theory of "Unprivitizing" was developed from the data, which involved start talking, help-finding, and self-knowing. A transition period followed, which led to "Integrating". Integrating involved self-discovery, self-caretaking, and meaning making.
Chiovitti, R.F.	2008	Practice	Caring	17 Registered Nurses licensed with the College Of Nurses of Ontario	Individual interviews which led to theoretical sampling.	A theory of "Protective empowering" was discovered, and involves six main categories: respecting the patient, not taking the patient's behavior personally, keeping the patient safe, encouraging health, authentic relating, and interactive teaching.

Table 8-1 • *(Continued)*

Author(s)	Date	Domain	Phenomenon of Interest	Sample	Data Generation	Findings
Wells, J.N., Cagle, C.S., Bradley, P., & Barnes, D. M.	2008	Practice	Caregiving experiences of Mexican American Women.	34 female Mexican American family caregivers of cancer patients.	Two interviews by bilingual and bi-cultural students research assistants.	The process of caring for a family member with cancer involved becoming stronger. Subprocesses included: life restructuring, strategizing, and struggling.
Hanson, K. & Stenvig, T.E.	2008	Education	Neophyte baccalaureate-prepared nurses' views of educators' attributes.	6 RNs who completed a baccalaureate program within the 6–18 months of the interview.	Individual interviews which were guided by open-ended questions.	Categories of positive clinical educator attributes were discovered: educator knowledge, interpersonal presentation, and teaching strategies.
Mills, J, Francis, K. & Bonner, A.	2008	Education	Nurses' experiences of mentoring	Nine rural nurses who had experience with mentoring others.	Eleven individual interviews, email dialogue, and situational mapping.	The overall study resulted in a theory of "cultivating and growing" rural nurses which was found to be a two part process involving getting to know a stranger and walking with another. In this paper, the researchers described the process of getting to know a stranger. It entailed "looking after each other, the importance of a name, and building a foundation."

Author	Year	Area	Topic	Sample	Method	Findings
Luhanga, F., Yonge, O. & Myrick, F.	2008	Education	Preceptorship	Twenty-two nurses who precepted students in their final clinical practicum.	One to one interviews with preceptors lasting 20–50 minutes.	Several student behaviors caused preceptors to deem their practice unsafe: inability to demonstrate knowledge and skills, attitude problems, unprofessional behavior, and poor communication skills.
Reid-Searl, K, Moxham, L., Walker, S. & Happell, B.	2008	Education	Medication administration errors by nursing students	Interviews with 28 undergraduate nursing students, using open-ended questions.	Recorded and transcribed interviews were analyzed using constant comparison to generate categories.	The core category was "supervision." The central problem was "shifting levels of supervision" and involved a shift from close supervision to no supervision. These levels were named: being with, being over, being near, and being absent.
Sherman, R.O., Bishop, M., Eggenberger, T., & Karden, R.	2007	Administration	Leadership skills and competency.	Ninety-eight experienced nurse managers and 22 inexperienced nurse managers ($n = 120$).	One-hour transcribed interviews which were guided by interview questions.	The nursing leadership competency model was developed, which included six categories: personal mastery, interpersonal effectiveness, financial management, human resource management, caring, and systems thinking.

Table 8-1 • (Continued)

Author(s)	Date	Domain	Phenomenon of Interest	Sample	Data Generation	Findings
Bondas, T.	2009	Administration	Nursing leadership	Sixty-five first line nurse managers	Nurse managers were asked to write narrative responses to open-ended questions that were coded using line by line analysis.	The core category was "Preparing the air for Nursing Care" and included two major categories "Creating the direction and content of nursing care" and "Concerned about nursing care."
McGilton, K.S., Bowers, B., McKenzie-Green, B., Boscart, V., & Brown, M.	2009	Administration	Long Term Care nurses' understanding of the charge nurse's role.	Individual interviews with 16 charge nurses employed at 8 facilities.	Interviews were transcribed and analyzed using line by line dimensional analysis.	The data analysis resulted in the discovery of three dimensions of the supervisor role in long-term care: (1) Against all odds getting through the day, (2) stepping in work, (3) leading and supporting unregulated care workers.

Bach et al.'s (2009) article focused on the role of the critical care nurse in end-of-life (EOL) decision making. The topic is meaningful to practicing nurses, and for those who are interested in understanding the role of the nurse in supporting families through difficult decisions. The researchers aimed to develop a conceptual framework to elucidate the process that occurs between nurses and clients. A qualitative approach was chosen because "little is known about the role of nurses in EOL in the critical care setting, and therefore a grounded theory study in this area is needed to further understand this important role" (p. 499). The researchers clearly identified the purpose of the study as an effort "to bring to light the role of critical care nurses in decision making at the end of life" (p. 499).

The researchers supported the need for the study through a thorough review of the extant literature. They noted that most clients spend their last days in critical care settings, and nurses play a pivotal role in supporting clients through EOL decisions. Additionally, the authors argued that critical care nurses are advocates for their patients in making their wishes known to the physician. Bach et al. (2009) stated that although some important aspects of the role of the critical nurse's role in EOL decision making have been discussed in the literature, the processes that facilitate such discussions and ultimately decision making had not been previously studied, thereby indicating the need for their research and the grounded theory approach.

Grounded theory method is specifically aimed at discovering the processes at work in the substantive area. Thus, the method is well suited for uncovering the processes used by critical care nurses when working with clients facing EOL issues. Consistent with the Straussian grounded theory approach, the researchers stated the research question as "what role do nurses have in EOL decision making in the critical care setting?" (p. 499). This question is both broad enough to allow key issues to emerge, yet narrow enough to focus the research directly on a specific issue.

Because the research question focused specifically on the role of the nurse in critical care, the sample consisted of 14 registered nurses (RNs); 10 worked in the Intensive Care Unit, and 4 worked in the Cardio-Respiratory Care Unit. The sample is appropriate for gathering data relevant to the research question. Prior to beginning data collection, the researchers obtained approval from an ethics board. The authors also noted that the nurses received a letter outlining the purpose of the study, the research method, and assurance that they could withdraw from the study at any time.

The data were gathered through individual interviews that were guided by a written interview agenda. Questions were revised as the study progressed to clarify emerging concepts or explore new theoretical leads. The interviews were transcribed verbatim. The computer program N-VIVO was used to organize and store data. The data were then analyzed using the process described by Strauss and Corbin (1998), which involved open coding, axial coding, and selective coding. Although the researchers did not specifically describe theoretical sampling, they did discuss the process of selective coding, which is related to theoretical sampling. Selective coding entails coding for the core category, and helps the researchers determine connections among the categories. Bach and colleagues explained that "through selective coding, categories were examined to discover broader relationships and identify main themes while allowing a framework to emerge and recreate data into a conceptual framework" (p. 501).

The overall theme that was discovered upon analysis of the data was "Supporting the Journey." The researchers explained that this category involved "all measures taken to support . . . life," or to "decide to support the death" (p. 503). This main category explains most of the action in the substantive area and conveys the nurses' role in EOL decision making in the critical care setting. Four major themes were also discovered, including 1. Being there, 2. A voice to speak up, 3. Enable coming to terms, and 4. Helping to let go. These four themes explained the nurses' roles in supporting both the patient and the family. In describing the development of the themes, the researchers provided data to support their inclusion. Thus, the concepts are grounded in the data.

The four main concepts appear to be important dimensions of the overarching category "Supporting the journey." The authors stated that the four main categories were developed upon "further reflection on and analysis of the data" (p. 503). Theoretical findings presented in the results of the study are significant for practicing nurses, those developing hospital policies, and those educating the public on the role of the nurse. Applicability of the findings to other areas of nursing could be explored through further research.

The researchers provided a thorough discussion of the applicability of the findings for educating members of the interdisciplinary team, and family members of critically ill clients. Further, the findings "give voice" to critical care nurses who are not typically recognized for their role in EOL care. The findings confirm the vital role of the critical care nurse in providing presence and support through EOL issues. Additionally, the participants, all critical care nurses who clearly address EOL issues regularly, had not received any EOL or palliative care education. Thus, the researchers concluded that nursing programs, and critical care orientation programs, should require education in EOL, palliative care, and bereavement.

APPLICATION TO EDUCATION

Nursing education continues to be an important area for the conduct of research and presents another context in which nurse researchers can conduct grounded theory investigations. Although relatively few grounded theory studies exist in the domain of nursing education, research studies that focus on teaching-learning offer the grounded theory researcher a rich opportunity for study. An example of the contribution grounded theory can make to nursing education is a study by Luhanga, Yonge, and Myrick (2008), "Failure to assign failing grades: Issues with grading the unsafe student."

This article serves as the reference for critique in this section and was selected because it demonstrates the use of grounded theory in studying a nursing education issue. This study illustrates a good presentation of findings from a grounded theory investigation.

Luhanga et al. (2008) "sought to determine how preceptors teach and manage unsafe students" (p. 1). The authors explained that in Canada, where the study took place, preceptors often take responsibility for a student in the clinical setting, and faculty rely on their feedback to determine the competence of the student. The topic is relevant to nursing education, and is neither too broad nor too narrow in its scope. A qualitative approach was chosen because "to date, there is little literature regarding the process of precepting students with unsafe practices" (p. 3). The researchers conducted a review of the literature which supported the need for further inquiry into the substantive area. The study was expected to provide insights into how preceptors work with students who demonstrate unsafe practice in the clinical arena.

Grounded theory method is useful for uncovering new dimensions of a research area, and is thereby appropriate for achieving the stated purpose of the research. The researchers did not state whether Straussian or Classic grounded theory method was chosen, and appear to mix the methods. For example, a research question was not explicitly stated, which is consistent with Classic grounded theory method, but an interview guide, based on the review of the literature was used, which is more consistent with Straussian grounded theory method. Data gathering commenced with a purposive sample. Permission was obtained from an Ethics Board prior to beginning data collection.

Participants were originally selected based on their experience with precepting senior-level students who exhibited unsafe practices. As data analysis began, preceptors were sought who had not had experiences with unsafe students, but had nonetheless served as preceptors. The researchers explained that these participants provided "negative cases," but did not provide the data or categories that led to the decision. Data were collected through individual interviews and review of documents such as preceptor guidelines. The researchers did not state whether field notes were gathered during the interviews or if the interviews were transcribed. The interview questions were altered based on the data collected during the interviews which is consistent with the method.

Data were analyzed through constant comparison, and entailed open coding, theoretical coding, and selective coding. Each of these processes was well described by the researchers. They specifically addressed the study's rigor in terms of credibility and fittingness. The core category was identified which "tied all other categories in the theory together" (p. 5). The core category was named "promoting student learning and preserving patient safety" and entailed five dimensions, or categories, which were empirically derived from the data. These dimensions were named: "1. hallmarks of unsafe practice, 2. factors contributing to unsafe practice, 3. preceptors' perceptions and feelings, 4. grading issues, and 5. strategies for managing unsafe practice" (p. 5). In the article, the researchers chose to focus specifically on the *grading issues*.

The category "grading issues" included three subcategories, entitled *reasons for presenting as an unsafe student, reasons for failure to fail borderline or unsafe students* and *role of the preceptor as gatekeeper to the profession.* The development of each of the subcategories was supported with data. The conceptual linkages among the core category, the category "grading issues" and its subcategories were made clear. The theoretical findings presented in the article, although mainly descriptive in nature, enhanced understanding of non-faculty involvement in evaluating nursing students' performance in the clinical setting. Variation within the data was enhanced by recruiting preceptors who had experience working with unsafe students, and those who had not.

Although the researchers recognized the importance of the role of the preceptor as "gatekeepers" in disciplines other than nursing, they were careful not to make sweeping statements about the usefulness of the findings. The conclusions they drew were confined to the results of the study, and the recommendations they made for nursing education were appropriate. Although they noted that preceptors' hesitancy to assign failing grades to unsafe students has been documented in disciplines such as social work and medicine, it is not clear whether the results of Luhanga, Yonge, and Myrick's (2008) study could be applied wholesale in other disciplines. Thus, the authors recommended the study be replicated "nationally and internationally . . . to explore the issues of professional and pedagogical accountability" (p. 12).

APPLICATION TO ADMINISTRATION

Nursing administration is an oft overlooked area of nursing practice and the extant research in this area is sparse. Few studies have explored administrative issues from a grounded theory perspective. A recent article by Sherman, Bishop, Eggenberger, and Karden (2007) provides an excellent example of the usefulness of the grounded theory approach in discovering new aspects of nursing roles. In their study, the researchers explained that the participants had "fallen into the position through assuming it as an interim assignment" (p. 86), conveying the lack of career planning for management positions. The authors further explained that the role of the nurse manager is multi-faceted and not well defined. Their grounded theory study helped to elucidate the dimensions of the role from the perspective of those who are in the position.

Sherman et al. (2007) used grounded theory method to explore the dimensions of nursing leadership. The purpose of the study was to examine the competencies needed by contemporary nurse mangers. The focus of the study is limited enough to delineate the research area, but broad enough to be meaningful. A qualitative research approach was chosen because the viewpoint of those in front line management positions was sought. The purpose of the research study was clearly stated, and the relevance of the project in relation to nursing practice was made explicit. A review of the literature was presented on the role of the nurse manager and highlighted the need for the study and a qualitative approach.

Sherman et al. (2007) stated that the study was conducted using Straussian grounded theory techniques, which is appropriate when themes and categories are sought. The themes were used by the researchers to develop a framework for a competency model. Interviews were conducted using an interview guide developed by the researchers, which is also consistent with Straussian methods of inquiry. Data collection began upon receiving approval from an ethics board, and involved recruitment of nurse managers from hospitals and public health agencies. In sum, 120 nurse managers were interviewed individually. Theoretical sampling was not explicitly described, but an effort was made to include both experienced and inexperienced nurse managers. Ninety-eight participants were experienced managers and 22 were inexperienced managers. Interviews were recorded and transcribed, and field notes were taken during interviews. Transcribed data and field notes were coded according to the procedures outlined by Strauss and Corbin (1998).

Data analysis resulted in two major themes: "The nurse manager role as a career choice," and "The stressors and challenges of the role." Six competency categories were also formed, and their development was guided by Lucia and Lepsinger's (1999, as cited by Sherman et al., 2007) framework. The competency categories developed from the data were: personal mastery, interpersonal effectiveness, financial management, human resource management, caring, and systems thinking. The investigators noted that the competencies were derived from the data, but specific examples of in vivo codes were not given. Credibility, auditability, and fittingness of the data were not explicitly addressed by the researchers. The development of the two major themes, however, was supported with data and their development was thoroughly explained.

The researchers noted that competency categories were grounded in the data, and each represents a different aspect of the role of the nurse manager. A diagram was included to visually display the connectedness of the concepts. The findings are significant in that the dimensions of the role of the nurse manager were discovered that had not been previously identified. Because only nurse managers were interviewed, there is not sufficient variation to warrant application of the findings to other disciplines without testing of the model.

Sherman et al. (2007) noted that some of their findings were consistent with depictions of the nurse manager's role in the literature. The researchers emphasized that the participants had not planned to become nurse managers, or received formal education on the role. They stressed that the results indicated that nurse executives should "assess current leadership talent, define needs for the future, and develop strategies for succession planning" (p. 93). Additionally, the investigators noted that formalized career planning was needed for those who aspire to leadership positions. Nurse educators were also charged with incorporating leadership education into academic curricula. The recommendations for nursing education and leadership were based on the findings of the study and emphasized the need for formal preparation of nurses for leadership positions.

SUMMARY

Grounded theory as a qualitative research approach provides an excellent method of investigation for phenomena important to nursing. This chapter reviewed application of the method to areas important to nursing practice, education, and administration and offered selected examples of published research that applies the methodologies described in Chapter 7. There is a substantive body of knowledge emerging from grounded theory research. Recognizing the need for middle-range theory development in nursing, investigators should continue to apply this rigorous qualitative method to the investigation of phenomena important to nursing practice, education, and administration.

References

Bach, V., Pleog, J., & Black, M. (2009). Nursing roles in end-of-life decision making in critical care settings. *Western Journal of Nursing Research, 31*, 496–512. doi: 10.1177/0193945908331178.

Bondas, T. (2009). Preparing the air for nursing care: A grounded theory study of first line nurse managers. *Journal of Research in Nursing, 14*, 351–362. doi: 10.1177/1744987108096969.

Chiovitti, R. F. (2008). Nurses' meaning of caring with patients in acute psychiatric hospital settings: A grounded theory study. *International Journal of Nursing Studies, 45*, 203–223. doi: 10.1016/j.ijnurstu.2006.08.018

Corbin, J., & Strauss, A. (2008). *Basics of qualitative research* (3rd ed.). Los Angeles, CA: Sage Publications.

Crowe, V. L. H. (2009). Unprivitizing: A bridge to learning. *The Grounded Theory Review, 8*, 31–47. Retrieved from: http://www.groundedtheory.com/booksjournals.

Glaser, B. G., & Strauss, A. (1967). *The discovery of grounded theory: Strategies for qualitative research*. New York: Aldine.

Hanson, K. J., & Stenvig, T. E. (2008). The good clinical nursing educator and the baccalaureate nursing clinical experience: Attributes and praxis. *Journal of Nursing Education, 47*, 38–42. Retrieved from: http://www.journalofnursingeducation.com/.

Luhanga, F., Yonge, O. J., & Myrick, F. (2008). Failure to assign failing grades: Issues with grading unsafe students. *International Journal of Nursing Education Scholarship, 5*, 1–14. Retrieved from: http://www.bepress.com/ijnes/.

McGilton, K. S., Bowers, B., McKenzie-Green, Boscart, V., & Brown, M. (2009). How do charge nurses view their roles in long-term care? *Journal of Applied Gerontology*, doi: 10.1177/0733464809336088.

Mills, J., Francis, K., & Bonner, A. (2008). Getting to know a stranger – rural nurses' experiences of mentoring: A grounded theory study. *International Journal of Nursing Studies, 45,* 599–607. doi: 10.1016/j.ijnurstu.2006.12.003.

Reid-Searl, K., Moxham, L., Walker, S., & Happell, B. (2008). Shifting supervision: Implications for safe administration of medication by nursing students. *Journal of Clinical Nursing, 17,* 2750–2757. doi: 10.1111/j.1365-2702.2008.02486.x.

Sherman, R.O., Bishop, M, Eggenberger, T., & Karden, R. (2007). Development of a leadership competency model. *The Journal of Nursing Administration, 37,* 85–94. Retrieved from: https://journals.lww.com/jonajournal.

Strauss, A., & Corbin, J. (1998). *Basics of qualitative research: Grounded theory procedures and techniques.* Newbury Park, CA: Sage.

Wells, J. N., Cagle, C. S., Bradley, P., & Barnes, D. M. (2008). Voices of Mexican American caregivers for family members with cancer. *Journal of Transcultural Nursing, 19,* 223–233. doi: 10.1177/1043659608317096.

Research Article

Nursing Roles in End-of-Life Decision Making in Critical Care Settings

Vicky Bach, *Fraser Health Authority*, Jenny Ploeg, Margaret Black, *McMaster University*

This study used a grounded theory approach to formulate a conceptual framework of the nursing role in end-of-life decision making in a critical care setting. Fourteen nurses from an intensive care unit and cardio-respiratory care unit were interviewed. The core concept, Supporting the Journey, became evident in four major themes: Being There, A Voice to Speak Up, Enable Coming to Terms, and Helping to Let Go. Nurses described being present with patients and families to validate feelings and give emotional support. Nursing work, while bridging the journey between life and death, imparted strength and resilience and helped overcome barriers to ensure that patients received holistic care. The conceptual framework challenges nurses to be present with patients and families at the end of life, clarify and interpret information, and help families come to terms with end-of-life decisions and release their loved ones.

Keywords: end of life; decision making; grounded theory; nursing; ICU; critical care

*T*he contemporary approach to death "diminishes our society's understanding of death as a life event" (Haisfield-Wolfe, 1996, p. 932). Today, it is rare that death or dying is encountered in the media, other than violent death, or spoken about freely during ordinary conversation. Moreover, our present technological abilities present us with many dilemmas, including the ability to postpone death, facilitating the process of "letting go" and the accompanying challenge of wondering if more could have been done (Kyba, 2002; Pattison, 2004; Prendergast & Puntillo, 2002). This article describes the nursing role in decision making at the end of life in the critical care setting.

Many patients spend their final days in critical care settings. For patients who die in institutions, such as hospitals, half spend at least the last 3 days of their lives in special care units such as the intensive care unit (ICU) and cardio-respiratory care unit (CRCU), and approximately one third spend at least 10 days in an ICU before their death (Curtis et al., 2001). A cross-sectional study of Canadian death records to determine number of deaths in special care units such as ICU and CRCU found that in teaching hospitals more than one fourth, or 27%, of deaths

Authors' Note: Please address correspondence to Vicky Bach at jvbach@shaw.ca.

From Bach V, Ploeg J, Black M. *Western Journal of Nursing Research*. vol. 31, issue 4, pp. 496–512.
Copyright © 2009 by SAGE Publications. Reprinted with permission.

occurred in critical care, whereas in nonteaching hospitals 15% died in critical care (Heyland, Lavery, Tranmer, Shortt, & Taylor, 2000).

End of life in the ICU is a challenge. Nature and spirituality have been supplanted by all that medical science has to offer by way of technology and life support, prolonging the dying process and dictating the time of death (Miller, Forbes, & Boyle, 2001). Cook, Giacomini, Johnson, and Willms's (1999) qualitative study observed ICU rounds and family meetings during which staff discussed whether to withdraw or withhold life support. Interviews were carried out with clinicians, ethicists, and those involved in pastoral services. Their study described a different rhythm to the dying process, a slowing down and controlling of the process of death to give the team, family, and clinicians time to come together and collaborate on their differing understandings and plans for the dying person. However, decision making and planning were complicated by the specifics of withdrawal sequences and which technological support would be withdrawn first. Their findings revealed that advanced planning could be overshadowed by situations that were unexpected, leaving key decisions or issues unspoken or implied, issues that could negatively affect dying.

Dawson's (2008) case study in the ICU found a focus on cure rather than improving the end-of-life experience. In her analysis, Dawson viewed critical care nurses as crucial in decision making to improve the quality of the end-of-life experience; nurses had accountabilities at the end of life including supporting family members and being aware of and acting on the goals of patients who were dying. However, as members of the ICU team, nurses could not deliver care that was responsive to patients' needs and prevent a cascade of treatment. This was in part because of a lack of education and a lack of understanding of palliative care principles as well as the team's inability to holistically identify the issues affecting patient quality of life.

Thelan (2005) examined research on end-of-life decision making in the ICU. She defined end-of-life decision making as a process into which families and patients entered, and participants included physicians and nurses. Thelan found that there was an identified decision-making role for nurses as the link between families and physicians in decisions at the end of life while interpreting and explaining information. However nurses' participation was limited as discussions and decisions were led mainly by physicians.

Baggs et al. (2007) conducted an ethnographic study in four ICUs to examine end-of-life decision making, using both observational and interview data. Their findings revealed that the nursing voice was limited in end-of-life decisions. Nurses adjusted their manner of approaching physicians when seeking decisions to obtain the care outcomes that they required for their patients. Nurses also reported waiting for particular physician rotations before making requests on behalf of their patients. These studies alone highlight the difficulties and conflicting forces that shape the dying experience.

End-of-Life Decision Making and the Nursing Role

When looking specifically at the nursing role in end-of-life decision making, there is a growing body of literature describing the methods used by registered nurses (RNs) to facilitate decision making at the end of life (Bottorff et al., 2000; Hancock et al., 2007; Norton & Talerico, 2000; Scherer, Jezewski, Graves, Wu, & Bu, 2006). However, the process of facilitation has not been described, and actually the concept is only superficially understood (Bottorff et al., 2000). Researchers' findings support the nursing role in facilitating patient and family participation in end-of-life decision making and describe this role as identifying needs and assisting patients and their families through the process of dying, supporting choices made by patients, and developing relationships of trust with patients and families while maintaining consistent communication (Bottorff et al., 2000; Norton & Talerico, 2000; Scherer et al., 2006). However, the specific ways in which RN roles are played out in end-of-life care remain poorly defined and described.

A number of qualitative studies have looked at end-of-life decision making in the ICU, specifically the nursing role (Jezewski & Finnell, 1998; Norton & Talerico, 2000). These studies help to shed light on the impact of the nursing role in the ICU and also nursing interaction with other members of the ICU team. Jezewski and Finnell (1998) used a grounded theory approach and interviewed 21 oncology nurses working in an acute care setting in an attempt to clarify the nursing role in the decision-making process, in this case specifically related to advanced directives. The authors found that communication was a key role for nurses, with the nurse acting as mediator to reduce conflict and support cohesion and understanding.

Norton and Talerico (2000) described specific strategies that nurses and physicians used to facilitate end-of-life decision making in a variety of settings including the ICU. This grounded theory study found that certain issues such as a willingness to initiate and enter into the discussion were central to the process of decision making for nurses.

Little is known about the role of nurses in end of life in the critical care setting, and therefore a grounded theory study in this area is needed to further understand this important role. Previous studies have focused more narrowly on advanced directives (Jezewski & Finnell, 1998) and on communication in a variety of practice settings (Norton & Talerico, 2000). Some of the strengths of a grounded theory approach to this topic include (a) a focus on the complexity of phenomena and human actions, (b) the recognition that people take active roles in responding to problematic situations, (c) the acknowledgement that people act on the basis of meaning that is defined through interaction, and (d) the development of a relevant framework or theory, grounded in the data, that serves as a basis for action (Strauss & Corbin, 1998).

Purpose

The purpose of this study is to bring to light the role of critical care nurses in decision making at the end of life. A grounded theory approach as described by Strauss and Corbin (1998) was used. The research question was, what role do nurses have in end-of-life decision making in the critical care setting?

Method

Sample and Setting

Participants were recruited from an ICU and a CRCU in a large teaching hospital in southwestern Ontario, Canada. These settings were chosen because, as previously indicated, approximately 42% of patients spend their last days in complex care settings (Heyland et al., 2000), and yet the role of nurses in end-of-life decision making in such settings has not been extensively studied. Together, these two units have 17 beds and admit patients with a mean age of 60 years. Patients admitted to this particular ICU and CRCU experience complex medical, surgical, and cardiac issues and often require mechanical ventilation, dialysis, and fluid resuscitation related to drug overdose; the mortality rate is approximately 22% per year.

Participant recruitment involved the use of a variety of methods, including posters, informal meetings, and direct requests for participation. All clinical managers were given a poster, which briefly outlined the purpose of the research study and gave the researcher's name and contact information, to place in their units. A more personal approach was also used, where the researcher was present in the unit on several occasions to identify and gather groups of three to four nurses to speak with informally. It was hoped that this more personal approach, rather than a poster, would encourage some of the nurses to participate, would express the value of hearing their voices, and would emphasize the importance of understanding their nursing role at the end of life. Over the next several weeks, with little response to the above methods, nurses were effectively recruited through the researcher spending time on the units and identifying nurses who would be available for a spontaneous interview. The charge nurses also supported recruitment by posting a schedule and asking nurses to choose their interview times.

Potential participants were identified by purposive sample techniques. Participants had to be working in their unit for at least 2 years and therefore had to have reached a level of competence and had to have an awareness of the overall goals of their working environment (Benner, 1984). Consistent with Strauss and Corbin (1998), theoretical sampling was used to deliberately choose individuals who could contribute to the evolving conceptual framework. The participants would be able to provide rich descriptions of the phenomenon being explored and through their experience could further our understanding of the emergent themes. Sampling continued until saturation of categories and their properties was reached.

Data Collection

Data were collected and analyzed concurrently throughout the research process (Strauss & Corbin, 1998). Data collection occurred through a process of guided, semistructured interviews lasting from 18 to 40 minutes. Interviews were conducted at the work setting in a quiet meeting room, which ensured privacy, and were digitally recorded and transcribed verbatim.

An interview guide was used to provide a starting point for data collection. Interview questions were derived from the first author's (V.B.) own work experiences and a review of the literature. Interview questions addressed demographic data and the nurses' views of their own experiences with end-of-life care. Questions explored their involvement in end-of-life decisions and their thoughts on this role. Examples of questions asked include the following: "Describe some of the situations that you have been involved in with patients who are dying" and "Describe any decisions or situations that you would like to have been involved in but were unable to." Participants were encouraged to share their stories and experiences and given the opportunity at the end of the interview to add further information that was not specifically asked through the interview process. As new concepts and gaps in understanding were identified, the interview guide was revised (see Table 1 for the final version of the interview guide). The computer program N-VIVO was used to help organize the data.

Table 1 • Interview Guide—Final

Phase 1—Establishment

Intent: Open communication and dialogue; make the participant at ease. Establish context through brief description of nursing role, continuing education.

1. How long have you been a nurse? How long in this unit?

2. Have you attended workshops or participated in further education having to do with palliative care?

Phase 2—Decision exploration

3. Describe a situation that you have been involved in with an older patient who was dying.

4. Can you tell me what end-of-life decisions are?

5. Who has been involved in these decisions?

6. Describe your actions or involvement related to these decisions.

Phase 3—Registered nursing role

Intent: Explore the registered nursing role in health-related decisions as well as the types of decisions registered nurses are being asked to facilitate.

7. Do you think there is a specific role for registered nurses related to decision making at end of life?

8. If no, why not? If yes, what is that role?

9. Was there a decision or situation that you would like to have been involved in but were unable to?

10. Is there anything that you would do differently?

Phase 4—Conclusion

11. Is there anything else you would like to add?

If you have nothing else to add, I will now turn the tape recorder off. Thank you again for agreeing to participate in this research.

Data Analysis

A three-phase process of open, axial, and selective coding was used to examine and interpret the data by isolating words and phrases to discover meaning and create connections (Strauss & Corbin, 1998). Open coding identified main concepts or phenomena in the data through a line-by-line review to examine parts of the data for variation and associations (Priest, Roberts, & Woods, 2002) and disclose concepts and categories. The most useful method of coding was one that used the actual words and phrases of the participants.

Analysis continued through axial coding, which began the "process of reassembling data that were fractured during open coding" (Strauss & Corbin, 1998, p. 124). At this point in the analysis, categories were grouped together and relationships related to the nurses' role in end-of-life decision making were constructed as a new and deeper understanding of the data emerged (Priest et al., 2002).

Through selective coding, categories were examined to discover broader relationships and identify main themes while allowing a framework to emerge and recreate data into a conceptual framework. Four main themes were identified, and an ongoing data analysis identified the central theme (Supporting the Journey) that was referred to by all but one of the participants and was integral to each of the main themes. From the data analysis, the substantive grounded conceptual framework of the nursing role in end-of-life decision making in critical care settings was generated. Data analysis was conducted by the first author (V.B.), with ongoing review by the other authors. Although V.B. determined the themes and defined and expanded meanings, all of the authors reviewed the coding, read transcripts to understand the reality of the interpretation, and give appropriate feedback, and all authors reached consensus on the final themes.

A number of strategies were used to address the criteria for evaluation of grounded theory studies described by Strauss and Corbin (1998). First, to promote credibility of study findings, negative case analysis was used to test for rival hypotheses. Selected interview transcripts were reviewed by two investigators during the development of categories. The main themes were reviewed by all research team members, and consensus was reached on the final themes. The research process was also clearly described, including sample selection, theoretical sampling, analysis procedures, and identification of the overall theme and major categories.

The first author's (V.B.) own experiences also informed the study. V.B. worked with a palliative care team in a large teaching hospital at the same time that V.B.'s 89-year-old father was admitted to a hospital and died 3 weeks later. The conjunction of these two experiences led to the development of this research topic, specifically the role of nurses in decision making at the end of life.

Ethics

Prior to the interview, all nurses received a detailed information letter outlining the purpose and methods of the study as well as a consent form informing them that they could withdraw from the study at any time. The study was approved by the Hamilton Health Sciences/Faculty of Health Sciences Research Ethics Board.

Results

Participants

The sample consisted of 14 RNs, including 12 women and 2 men. In all, 10 worked in the ICU and 4 in the CRCU. Their nursing experience ranged from 5 to 32 years, with an average of 13 years. Their experience in their respective units ranged from 2 to 20 years, with an average of 9 years spent in critical care. Ten participants had not received any palliative care education.

Supporting the Journey

The overall theme or basic social process related to the nursing role in end-of-life decision making, as identified from the perceptions of the nurses, was Supporting the Journey. In examining the collected data, 13 out of the 14 nurses interviewed talked about support. Support was described as an ongoing process that accommodated itself to the needs of each situation. Support was a bridge between life and death, which the nurses talked about as "all measures taken to support . . . life" or acknowledging that the time had come to "decide to support the death." Through giving of themselves in a range of capacities, the nurses endeavored to journey with patients and families where it was difficult for others to go and to support the patients to reach end of life peacefully and in comfort.

Helping to Let Go

The final theme identified by participants was Helping to Let Go. This theme involved nurses helping the patient and family to acknowledge and accept the conclusion of the patient's journey toward death. Nurses helped families emotionally release their loved ones and helped them to understand what the future might look like. Nurses then advocated for patients and families, although this was a complex and delicate task. The nurses advocated for the patient with the family and the medical team and also advocated for the family with the medical team. Laura discussed physicians who had difficulty "letting go" when she said, "Often doctors have a hard time, the nurses seem to be more accepting of these things 'cause they see the suffering that goes on."

Nurses also described the challenges they faced in helping families let go of their loved ones, in particular those challenges created by machines: the IVs, monitors, and life support. As Rose said, "A lot of families . . . don't want to stop treatment, even though . . . there's probably not much that can be done and they just want to hang on. . . . They want everything done." Laura spoke about families not understanding life support or the implications of having a family member on life support. She thought that families often felt guilty that there was "so much [technology] available and they can be saved so we should do it, at all cost."

Discussion

This research makes a number of important contributions to the literature of end-of-life decision making in critical care settings and the role of nursing. First, study findings revealed the critically important role of nurses in supporting the journey to end of life in critical care settings. Nurses played a number of key roles in being present to help patients to die in comfort and in helping patients and families come to terms with the expected death and to let go. Maxwell (2006) discussed comfort as an ICU nursing focus to ensure that comfort and dignity are maintained. Previous studies have acknowledged that there is limited evidence of how nurses are actually performing end-of-life roles (Scherer et al., 2006) or of their actual participation in end-of-life decision making (Thelan, 2005).

Second, this study revealed that one of the most fundamental roles nurses play is being present at the bedside, providing comfort, a caring touch, and a listening ear. Other literature has also talked about the importance of a nursing presence. Ciccarello (2003) described the use of presence by nursing as "one of the most powerful albeit simple interventions at end-of-life" (p. 219). The main elements of presence are being attentive, being open and sensitive to experience, being accountable, and consistently remaining in the moment. Shaw (2008) described the need for recognition of the nursing practice of being with patients that is separate from tasks and technology. Rather, it is a human interaction that supports being intimate and connected. In this study, nurses were present with their patients and families, not only actively attending family meetings but also simply being with and letting patients and families express their emotions while actively listening and supporting. The results of this study are supported by the theoretical framework of Rushton (2005), which blends the concepts of being and doing. Although it is from a pediatric perspective, Rushton's framework can be applied to adults and families in palliative care as she stated that nursing presence requires action, which includes helping patients to cope and endure and supporting families in their need to understand the dying experience.

Third, this study confirmed the vital end-of-life role nurses have in explaining and interpreting. In a study of communication at the end of life, Hancock et al. (2007) stated that patients did not recall up to half of the information they received because of stress, misunderstanding related to terminology, or blocking of information as a method of coping. The nursing role of giving or clarifying information is well supported in the literature. Wilkin and Slevin's (2004) study supported this role as part of caring actions, which included information giving as well as explaining. Scherer et al. (2006) expanded this role to giving information to patients to help them define their illness experience so that when they were no longer able to speak for themselves the nurses could communicate with families to assist in decision making.

Also seen in this study is the issue of truth telling, which involved differences in ⟩ nursing approach. In being truthful, the nurses endeavored to balance honesty with hope. Telling the truth can be interpreted as giving information to help patients and/or families make informed care decisions. Therefore, language must be understandable. From an ethical perspective, not telling the truth denies trust and denies the patient or family an ethical and legal right (Hebert, Hoffmaster, Glass, & Singer, 1997). In their article on hope and truth telling, Begley and Blackwood (2000) identified hope as having a positive effect on health and stated that promoting hope in patients is significant for nursing. However, the two concepts, hope and truth telling, need a careful and deliberate balance, with full collaboration and agreement within the care team to ensure that patients and families receive the care they need and deserve (Vivian, 2006).

Fourth, study findings affirm tensions experienced by nurses between caring for the patient and family and taking care of technology in a critical care setting. Baggs et al. (2007) described an "overuse of technology" as problematic and not compatible with patient preferences. Pattison (2004) described delaying death through sustaining life with technology, however at a cost to the patient, through care that is highly medicalized and not holistic.

Finally, this study emphasizes the lack of preparation critical care nurses receive to provide skilled, sensitive end-of-life care in a critical care setting. Only 4 of the 14 nurses interviewed had received any palliative care education. In their qualitative studies, both Ciccarello (2003) and Dawson (2008) stated nurses in critical care settings are poorly prepared to deliver holistic, supportive care.

There are several important implications for nursing practice based on the findings of this research. This model of Supporting the Journey fosters and creates value for nursing care at the end of life in critical care settings. Nurses are involved in decision making at the end of life, but it is time to stop "leading quietly" and become part of an active, knowledgeable, and caring force. Nurses can accomplish this through (a) being fully present with the patient and family during end of life; (b) advocating for the patient's end-of-life wishes; (c) advancing their practice with patients, families, and other members of the health care team by actively participating in family meetings and strengthening working relationships with health care staff; (d) mentoring novice nurses and encouraging them to value their own "voice" and develop their holistic practice; and (e) participating in ongoing learning related to leading practices in end-of-life care.

Nursing education can evolve to support the development of nursing practice in end-of-life decision making. Education in both palliative care and end-of-life care, including grief and bereavement, should be included in the nursing curriculum. In addition, education on the role of the critical care nurse in the ICU and CRCU is needed to understand the implications of combining humanistic care with technology.

Miller, P. A., Forbes, S., & Boyle, D. K. (2001). End-of-life care in the intensive care unit: A challenge for nurses. *American Journal of Critical Care, 10*(4), 230–237.

Norton, S. A., & Talerico, K. A. (2000). Facilitating end-of-life decision-making: Strategies for communicating and assessing. *Journal of Gerontological Nursing, 26*(9), 6–13.

Pattison, N. (2004). Integration of critical and palliative care at end of life. *British Journal of Nursing, 13*(3), 132–139.

Prendergast, T. J., & Puntillo, K. A. (2002). Withdrawal of life support: Intensive caring at end of life. *Journal of the American Medical Association, 288*, 2732–2740.

Priest, H., Roberts, P., & Woods, L. (2002). An overview of three different approaches to the interpretation of qualitative data. Part 1: Theoretical issues. *Nurse Researcher, 10*(1), 30–42.

Rushton, C. H. (2005). A framework for integrated pediatric palliative care: Being with dying. *Journal of Pediatric Nursing, 20*(5), 311–325.

Scherer, Y., Jezewski, M. A., Graves, B., Wu, Y.-W. B., & Bu, X. (2006). Advance directives and end-of-life decision making: Survey of critical care nurses' knowledge, attitude, and experience. *Critical Care Nurse, 26*(4), 30–40.

Shaw, S. (2008). Exploring the concepts behind truth-telling in palliative care. *International Journal of Palliative Nursing, 14*(7), 356–359.

Strauss, A. L., & Corbin, J. (1998). *Basics of qualitative research: Techniques and procedures for developing grounded theory* (2nd ed.). Thousand Oaks, CA: Sage.

Thelan, M. (2005). End-of-life decision making in intensive care. *Critical Care Nurse, 25*(6), 28–37.

Vivian, R. (2006). Truth telling in palliative care nursing: The dilemmas of collusion. *International Journal of Palliative Nursing, 12*(7), 341–348.

Wilkin, K., & Slevin, E. (2004). The meaning of caring to nurses: An investigation into the nature of caring work in an intensive care unit. *Journal of Clinical Nursing, 13*, 50–59.

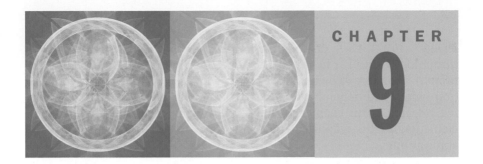

Ethnography as Method

*E*thnography is considered to be the oldest of the qualitative research methodologies" (Roberts, 2009, p. 291). As nursing practice has broadened so too have the research methods used to study practice, particularly the meanings of health and illness as lived by individuals, families, and groups. Nurses have used ethnography to study a variety of topics important to nursing, including children's quality of life after heart transplant (Green et al., 2007); the culture of a Taiwanese nursing home (Chuang & Abbey, 2009); and decision-making by hospice professionals (Waldrop & Rinfrette, 2009). These are just a few examples of how nurses are using ethnography to better serve those individuals who are entrusted to their care. To fully understand why there is a demonstrated commitment to ethnographic research, it is important to look at the foundations of ethnography as a research method.

Social scientists share an interest in and a commitment to discovery. Anthropologists, as a particular group of social scientists, are committed to the discovery of cultural knowledge. Early in the history of the social sciences, individuals interested in culture found that the ways of traditional science were inadequate to discover the nuances of people who live together and share similar experiences. This inadequacy led to the beginnings of *ethnography*, a means of studying groups of individuals' lifeways or patterns. Sanday (1983) reports that ethnographic methods are not new. The ancient Greek Herodotus was an ethnographer who recorded variations in the cultures to which he was exposed. According to Sanday, Franz Boas's (1948) ethnographic examination of the Eskimo culture signaled the contemporary beginning of ethnographic study.

Anthropology is synonymous with the term *ethnography*. The product of anthropologists' work is ethnography (Muecke, 1994). As early as the 1960s, references can be found regarding the value of an ethnographic approach as a means to study nursing culture (Boyle, 1994; Leininger, 1970;

Ragucci, 1972). Early nurse ethnographers embraced the methods of anthropology to study phenomena they perceived were irreducible, unquantifiable, or unable to be made objective. Leininger (1985) went beyond the borrowing of ethnographic methods to develop what she called "ethnonursing research." This chapter explores ethnography and discusses common elements of ethnographic methodology and its uses, interpretations, and applications.

ETHNOGRAPHY DEFINED

A ccording to Spradley (1980), "Ethnography is the work of describing culture" (p. 3). The description of culture or the cultural scene must be guided by an intense desire to understand other individuals' lives so much that the researcher becomes part of a specific cultural scene. To do this, Malinowski (1961) believed that researchers must learn the "native's point of view" (p. 25). Spradley, however, warned that ethnography is more than the study of the people; rather, "ethnography means learning from people" (p. 3). Spradley also pointed out that "the essential core of ethnography is this concern with the meanings of actions and events to the people [ethnographers] seek to understand" (p. 5).

Beyond Spradley's (1980) discussion of ethnography, there is a long-standing debate about what constitutes ethnography. Muecke (1994) suggested, "there is not a single standard form of ethnography" (p. 188). Boyle (1994) proposed that "the style and method of ethnography are a function of the ethnographer, who brings her or his own scientific traditions, training, and socialization to the research project" (p. 182). This debate has led to a certain amount of confusion about ethnography as a method and has further fueled arguments about the relative value of ethnography as rigorous science (Savage, 2000). More recently, Brink and Edgecombe (2003) suggested that there has been a "bastardization of [qualitative] research designs" (p. 1028), in particular, ethnography. Despite the disagreements and controversies surrounding the method, ethnography has and will continue to provide important information about the meanings, organization, and interpretations of culture.

According to Muecke (1994), the four major ethnographic schools of thought are (1) classical; (2) systematic; (3) interpretive or hermeneutic; and (4) critical. classical ethnography requires that the study "include both a description of behavior and demonstrate why and under what circumstances the behavior took place" (Morse & Field, 1995, p. 154). Regardless of the school of thought or type of ethnography, use of the method requires considerable time in the field, constantly observing and making sense of behaviors.

The objective of *systematic ethnography* is "to define the structure of culture, rather than to describe a people and their social interaction, emotions, and materials" (Muecke, 1994, p. 192). The difference between classical and systematic ethnography lies in scope. Classical ethnography aims to describe everything about the culture. Systematic ethnography takes a focused look at the structure of the culture—what organizes the study groups' lifeways. Systematic ethnography is the framework used by Spradley, whose method of ethnographic inquiry is explored fully in this chapter.

The aim of *interpretive* or *hermeneutic ethnography* is to "discover the meanings of observed social interactions" (Muecke, 1994, p. 193). According to Wolcott (cited in Muecke, 1994), "Ethnography is quintessentially analytic and interpretive, rather than methodological" (p. 193). Interpretive ethnographers are interested in studying the culture through analysis of inferences and implications found in behavior (Muecke, 1994).

Critical ethnography is another type of ethnography Muecke (1994) described. It "draws on cultural studies, neo-Marxist and feminist theories and research on critical pedagogy" (Gordon, Holland, & Lahelma, 2001, p. 193). Critical ethnographers do not believe there is a culture out there to be known but, rather, that researchers and members of a culture together create a cultural schema. Ethnographers subscribing to this tradition account for "historical, social and economic situations" (Fontana & Frey, 1994, p. 369) when reporting. Germain (2001) adds that "critical ethnography . . . is distinguished from conventional approaches by its focus on issues of injustice and social oppression" (p. 279). "Inherent in a critical approach is the understanding that through communicative practices and reflection, researchers and participants discern an absolute truth of the culture" (Manias & Street, 2001, p. 235).

Carspecken (1996) has become a popular model for the conduct of critical ethnography. His five-stage method has been utilized by nurses. The steps which he suggests are not necessarily sequential include: compiling the primary record via observations and recordings; undertaking the primary "reconstructive analysis"; using dialogical data generation—describing the insiders view through the use of interviews and focus groups; subjecting the data to systems analysis; and, seeking explanation through social–theoretical models. Researchers interested in learning more about Carspecken's work should read the primary source.

These four types of ethnographies represent four philosophic positions. "All research proceeds from philosophy, articulated or not" (Germain, 2001, p. 279). Therefore, it is essential that researchers define their position before embarking on an ethnographic study. A researcher's philosophic stance determines what he or she will study as well as the framework for data collection and analysis.

In addition to the four types of ethnographies described, it is important to add the work of Leininger. Leininger (1985) identifies a specific approach to ethnography she calls ethnonursing that allows nurses to "study explicit nursing phenomena from a cross-cultural perspective" (p. 38). The goal is "to discover nursing knowledge as known, perceived and experienced by nurses and consumers of nursing and health services" (p. 38). The most

to a greater understanding of the dynamics of particular phenomena and relationships found within cultures.

When choosing ethnography as the approach to study a particular culture or subculture, the nurse should ask several important questions. Do I have the knowledge and skill necessary or the research support available to conduct a credible study? Do I have the time to conduct this study? Do I have the resources to carry it out? Will the data collected bring new insights to the profession? If the nurse researcher answers *yes* to these questions, then his or her study has the potential to contribute significantly to the nursing profession.

In addition to answering the preceding questions, nurses interested in ethnography should know why the approach may be useful. Spradley (1980) identified four primary reasons for using ethnography to study a particular culture. The first is to document "the existence of alternative realities and to describe these realities in [the terms of the people studied]" (p. 14). Much of what individuals know about other cultures they interpret based on their own culture. This way of thinking is limiting in that it promotes the idea that one truth—and thus, one reality—exists. For ethnographers, a description of alternative realities provides a rich and varied landscape of human interaction. Coming "to understand personality, society, individuals, and environments from the perspective of other than professional scientific cultures . . . will lead to a sense of epistemological humility" (Spradley, 1980, p. 15).

A second reason, according to Spradley (1980), for using the ethnographic approach is to discover grounded theories. Through description of culture, researchers are able to discover theories that are indigenous to the culture (Grant & Fine, 1992). Foundational to grounded theorists' research is a belief that the only useful theory is one that is grounded in the beliefs and practices of individuals studied. The principle that research should be based on the beliefs and practices of individuals (cultural groups) studied is also foundational to the work of ethnographers. The major difference between the conduct of ethnographic and grounded theory research is that ethnographers wishing to develop grounded theory will advance the description and interpretation of cultural observations to a level that yields a description of basic social-psychological process. For a full discussion of grounded theory, see Chapter 7.

Germain (2001) supports the development of theory as a natural outcome of ethnographic study. She offers that "ethnography contributes descriptive and explanatory theories of culture and cultural behaviors and meaning. Within the ethnography may be identified other middle-range theories such as typologies and hypotheses for further study" (p. 281).

A third reason for choosing ethnography is to better understand complex societies. Early anthropologists believed that the ethnographic method was ideally suited to the study of non-Western cultures. Today, anthropologists see the value of using ethnography to study subgroups of larger cultures—both

Western and non-Western. Examples can be found in nursing in the works of Green et al. (2007) and Chuang and Abbey (2009).

The fourth reason Spradley (1980) offers for using the ethnographic approach is to understand human behavior. Human behavior has meaning, and ethnography is one way to discover that meaning. Such discovery becomes particularly important when nurses look at the clients' health and illness behaviors. Understanding how and why cultural groups such as Hispanic immigrants, elderly citizens, abused women, or the Amish behave in health and illness situations can assist nurses who care for these groups to better provide interventions to enhance the health-related strategies already in use by the groups.

When nurses decide they will use ethnography to study a culture of interest, a parallel consideration will be whether they will conduct a micro- or macro-ethnographic study. Leininger (1985) called these study types "mini" or "maxi," respectively. Regardless of the terminology, the intent has to do with the scale of the study. A *micro-* or *mini-ethnography* is generally of a smaller scale and is narrow or specific in its focus. Schulte's (2000) ethnographic study of the culture of public health nurses in a large, Midwestern, urban health department is an example of a micro-ethnography. The study focused on one organization, a particular group of employees, and occurred during a 6-month period. Therefore, the study was considered a micro-ethnography because of its description of only one group, public health nurses, within one health department, and with a limited time in the setting.

Increasingly, nurse researchers are using the term *focused ethnography* to identify their small-scale ethnographies. Focused ethnographies have as their focal point a distinct problem that is studied within a single context with a limited number of individuals.

> Focused ethnographies share with classical ethnographies a commitment to conducting intensive participant observation activities within a naturalistic setting, asking questions to learn what is happening, and using other available sources of information to gain as complete an understanding as possible of people, places and events of interest. (Roper & Shapira, 2000, p. 7)

Green and coresearchers' (2007) study of quality of life for school-aged children following a heart transplant is an example of a focused ethnography. In this study, the researchers focused on a small group of 11 children who had received heart transplants in a large children's hospital in Arkansas. The researchers reported that pediatric heart transplant patients and their families make up a subculture of transplant patients. The individuals interviewed and the subject matter were very focused.

A *macro-* or *maxi-ethnography* is a study that examines the culture in a broader context, extends over a longer period, and is most often reported in book form. Magilvy and Congdon's (2000) and Lipson's (2001) ethnographies are examples of this type of study. These researchers observed a significant number of individuals over a period of several years with a larger scope.

Spradley (1980) further delineated the scope of ethnographic studies by placing them on a continuum. On one end are micro-ethnographic studies that examine a single social situation (nurses receiving report on one unit); multiple social situations (critical care nurses participating in a report on three intensive care units); or a single social institution (the American Cancer Society of Philadelphia). Moving on the continuum closer to macro-ethnographic studies, Spradley included multiple social institutions (American Cancer Societies of Florida); a single community study (Chinatown in San Francisco); multiple communities (Hispanic communities in East Los Angeles); and a complex society (tribal life in Africa).

ELEMENTS AND INTERPRETATIONS OF THE METHOD

A number of individuals have described ethnographic research methods. Early ethnographic reports were written by individuals who documented their observations of the cultures they encountered. Although many of these individuals were not trained anthropologists, they gave rich and vivid accounts of the lives of the people they met. Sanday (1983) pointed out that these recorders were not participants in paradigmatic ethnography. *Paradigmatic ethnography* consists of the range of activities completed by a trained ethnographer, including observing, recording, participating, analyzing, reporting, and publishing experiences with a particular cultural group. Sanday offered three traditions within paradigmatic ethnography: (1) holistic; (2) semiotic; and (3) behavioristic.

The *holistic ethnographic interpretation* is the oldest tradition. The commitment of researchers in this tradition is to "the study of culture as an integrated whole" (Sanday, 1983, p. 23). According to Sanday, the ethnographers who ascribed to this approach included Benedict (1934), Mead (1949), Malinowski (1922), and Radcliffe-Brown (1952). Although all four ethnographers varied in their focus, their underlying commitment was to describe as fully as possible the particular culture of interest within the context of the whole. For instance, "Mead and Benedict were interested in describing and interpreting the whole, not in explaining its origin beyond the effect of the individual on it" (Sanday, 1983, p. 25). Radcliffe-Brown and Malinowski were not committed to the "characterization of the cultural whole but to how each trait functions in the total cultural complex of which it is part" (Sanday, 1983, p. 25). Although the focus of both sets of ethnographers was different, the underlying commitment to viewing the culture as a whole was preserved.

The *semiotic interpretation* focuses on gaining access to the native's viewpoint. Like the researchers committed to holistic interpretation, the major anthropologists in this tradition did not share epistemologies. The two major followers of this tradition are Geertz (1973) and Goodenough

(1970, 1971). According to Sanday (1983), Geertz views the study of culture not as a means to defining laws but as an interpretative enterprise focused on searching for meaning. Furthermore, Geertz believes that the only way to achieve cultural understanding is through *thick descriptions*, large amounts of data (descriptions of the culture) collected over extended periods. According to Geertz, the analysis and conclusions offered by ethnographers represent fictions developed to explain rather than to understand a culture.

Goodenough (1970, 1971) is an ethnographer who embraces the semiotic tradition. He does so through what has been described as *ethnoscience*, "a rigorous and systematic way of studying and classifying emic (local or inside) data of a cultural group's own perceptions, knowledge, and language in terms of how people perceive and interpret their universe" (Leininger, 1970, pp. 168–169). "Ethnoscience [is] viewed as a method of developing precise and operationalized descriptions of cultural concept" (Morse & Field, 1995, p. 29). Ethnoscience is also called ethnosemantics or ethnolinguistics to emphasize the focus on language.

According to Sanday (1983), Geertz's commitment is to the "notion that culture is located in the minds and hearts of men" (p. 30). Culture is described by writing out systematic rules and formulating ethnographic algorithms, which make it possible to produce acceptable actions such as the "writing out of linguistic rules that makes it possible to produce acceptable utterances" (Sanday, 1983, p. 30).

"The differences between Geertz and Goodenough are not in aim but in the method, focus, and mode of reporting" (Sanday, 1983, p. 30). Both ethnographers are committed to the careful description of culture. Geertz's method and reporting are viewed as more of an art form compared with Goodenough's method, in which the focus is on rigorous, systematic methods of collecting data and reporting findings.

The third interpretation is the *behaviorist approach*. Ethnographers using this approach are most interested in the behavior of members of a culture. The main goal "is to uncover covarying patterns in observed behavior" (Sanday, 1983, pp. 33–34). This approach is deductive. Ethnographers subscribing to this interpretation look specifically for cultural situations that substantiate preselected categories of data. Use of this interpretation deviates radically from the intent of the other two interpretations, which rely solely on induction.

Leininger (1978, 1985), a nurse anthropologist, developed her own interpretation of ethnography: ethnonursing. *Ethnonursing*, according to Leininger, is "the study and analysis of the local or indigenous people's viewpoints, beliefs, and practices about nursing care behavior and processes of designated cultures" (Leininger, 1978, p. 15). The goal of ethnonursing is to "discover nursing knowledge as known, perceived and experienced by nurses and consumers of nursing and health services" (Leininger, 1985, p. 38). The primary function of Leininger's approach to ethnography is to focus on nursing and related health phenomena. This approach has been an important contribution to the nursing field. Many nurse ethnographers subscribe to Leininger's philosophy and apply her method of inquiry. A recent article by Prince (2008) on resilience in African American women formerly involved in street prostitution is a good example of the use of Leininger's method to analyze data.

SELECTING ETHNOGRAPHY

When nurses choose to conduct ethnographic research studies, usually they have decided there is some shared cultural knowledge to which they would like access. The way individuals' access cultural knowledge is by making *cultural inferences*, which are the observer's (researcher's) conclusions based on what the researcher has seen or heard while studying another culture. Making inferences is the way individuals learn many of their own group's cultural norms or values. For instance, if a child observes another child being scolded for talking in class, the observer—without being told—concludes that talking in class can lead to an unpleasant outcome. Therefore, the child learns through cultural inference that talking in class is unacceptable. Ethnographers follow this same process in their observations of cultural groups. According to Spradley (1980), ethnographers generally use three types of information to generate cultural inferences: cultural behavior (what people do); cultural artifacts (the things people make and use); and speech messages (what people say).

A significant part of culture is not readily available. This information, called *tacit knowledge*, consists of the information members of a culture know but do not talk about or express directly (Hammersley & Atkinson, 1983; Spradley, 1980). In addition to accessing explicit or easily observed cultural knowledge, ethnographers have the responsibility of describing tacit knowledge.

Understanding the Researcher's Role

To access explicit and tacit knowledge, researchers must understand the role they will play in the discovery of cultural knowledge. Because the researcher becomes the instrument, he or she must be cognizant of what the role of instrument entails. The role requires ethnographers to participate in the culture, observe the participants, document observations, collect artifacts, interview members of the cultural group, analyze, and report the findings. This role requires a significant commitment to the research that should not be taken lightly. In addition, it requires that researchers regularly reflect on the impact their participation in the culture has on the data and analysis.

The step-by-step method of collecting, analyzing, and presenting ethnographic research, according to Spradley (1980), is presented to educate readers. Although Spradley's is not the only ethnographic approach available, it is presented because of its explicitness, clarity, and utility for novice ethnographic researchers.

Box 9-1

Steps for Conducting Ethnographic Research

1. Do participant observation.
2. Make an ethnographic record.
3. Make descriptive observations.
4. Make a domain analysis.
5. Make a focused observation.
6. Make a taxonomic analysis.
7. Make selected observations.
8. Make a componential analysis.
9. Discover cultural themes.
10. Take a cultural inventory.
11. Write an ethnography.

Spradley (1980) identifies 11 steps in the conduct of ethnographic research. Box 9-1 summarizes these steps. The processes for data generation, treatment, analysis, and interpretation are discussed within the context of the steps identified.

Gaining Access

One of the first considerations when initiating an ethnographic study is to decide on the *aim*. Based on the *aim* of the inquiry, researchers can decide the scope of the project. Will the aim be to focus on a particular group or a particular problem of a group? Will you use a focused, micro- or mini-ethnography approach? Will you examine a single social situation? Multiple social situations? A single social institution? Multiple social institutions? A single community study? Multiple communities? Complex societies?

Once researchers have decided on the scope of the project, their next step is to gain access to the culture. Because ethnography requires the study of people, the activities in which they are involved, and the places in which they live, to conduct the study, researchers will need to gain access to the culture. This may be the most difficult part of the study. Because researchers are not usually members of the group studied, individuals in the culture of interest may be unwilling or unable to provide the access required. In other instances, researchers may be studying social situations that do not require a group's permission. For instance, if researchers are interested in the culture of individuals who come to the local pharmacy to obtain their medications, permission may not be required. However, if they are interested in studying the culture of health professionals in an outpatient clinic, permission is necessary.

Access is easiest when researchers have clearly stated the study purpose and have shared how they will protect the participants' confidentiality.

In addition, offering to participate in the setting may enhance researchers' abilities to gain entry to social situations. If, for example, a researcher wishes to study the culture of health professionals working in an outpatient clinic, his or her willingness to participate by offering "volunteer" services while in the setting may improve the chances of obtaining admission. As a "volunteer," the researcher not only has the opportunity to make observations but will also become part of the culture after remaining on the scene for an extended period. Each organization or institution will have its policies and procedures, some more clearly delineated than others. It is strategically important that you ascertain early what those involved require both formally and informally to gain access. Gaining access using the appropriate procedures will begin to build the trust needed to be successful in the field.

Making Participant Observations

The role of rapport has not been talked about a great deal in the literature. However, the rapport the researcher establishes with those being studied is critical. "Rapport is often cited as a central tenet of research relationships, it has but, in a similar vein to that of insider status, it is perhaps something taken for granted in the literature" (McGarry, 2007, p. 11). The relationships that are developed during the early fieldwork period will provide the doorway to that which comes later.

Actual fieldwork begins when researchers start asking questions about the culture chosen. Initially, the ethnographer will ask broad questions of the setting. Using the outpatient clinic as an example, the researcher might ask: Who works in the clinic? Who comes to the clinic for care? What is the physical set-up of the clinic? Who provides the care to clients who come to the clinic?

In addition to asking questions, the researcher will begin to make observations. There are three types of observations: descriptive, focused, and selective (Spradley, 1980). *Descriptive observations* start when the researcher enters the social situation. The ethnographer will begin by describing the social situation, getting an overview of the situation, and determining what is going on. After completing this type of observation, the researcher will conduct more focused descriptive observations. These observations are generated from questions the researcher asked during the initial descriptive phase. For example, while in the clinic the researcher discovers that nurses are responsible for health teaching. A *focused observation* is required to look specifically at the types of health teaching done by the nurses in the setting. Based on this focused observation, the researcher conducts a more *selective observation*. For example, the researcher observes that only two out of the seven nurses in the clinic conduct any health teaching with clients with acquired immunodeficiency syndrome (AIDS). A selective interview or observation involving the two nurses will address additional questions about why clinic staff members behave as they do.

Neophyte ethnographers should not be led to believe that they conduct observations and interviews in the linear manner just described. Rather, broad, focused, or selective questions may arise out of any observation. Furthermore, the intent of an observation is not to merely "look at" something. More accurately, through observation while in the setting, researchers look, listen, ask questions, collect artifacts, and analyze data collected in a cyclic manner.

At any given time, ethnographers may be more or less involved in the social situation. For example, when the outpatient clinic is busy, the researcher as volunteer may be quite involved as a participant in the culture. At times of lesser traffic, the researcher may spend more time observing or interviewing. Explicit rules for when to participate and when to observe are not available. Researchers, the *actors* (members of the culture studied), and the activity determine the degree of participation in the social situation.

Roper and Shapira (2000) offer that "relying on personal observations alone can be misleading" (p. 70). It will be essential that all interpretations of observations be validated through other collected information. The researcher must be always aware of the fact that all individuals view social situations through their own cultural lenses. Therefore, cross-comparison of data is fundamental. Brink and Edgecombe (2003) observed the number of published ethnographic studies that use only one data collection strategy. It is critical for the neophyte ethnographer to understand the necessity of using varying data collection strategies to provide a rich cross-comparison of information collected.

More recently, there is a growing body of literature describing the *practitioner ethnographer*. Barton (2008) describes the practitioner ethnographer as "a member of the investigated phenomena, a practitioner in the field, a reactive part of the event with insider knowledge and an historical perspective" (p. 12). "They are more than just participants; they live and have lived the experience that they want to investigate" (p. 11). Practitioner ethnographers are focused on the dynamics between the data, the self, and the practice environment (Barton). There are particular principles which should be considered if one wishes to conduct a study as a practitioner ethnographer. The researcher interested in this role should carefully consider the pros and cons of engaging in an ethnography using this approach.

Making the Ethnographic Record

On completion of each observation, ethnographers are responsible for documenting the experience. Documents generated from the observations are called *field notes*. Field notes are generally made during or immediately after an observation or interview. These are generally written "more or less *contemporaneously* with the events, experiences and interactions they describe or recount" (Emerson, Fretz, & Shaw, 2001, p. 353). Field notes may be managed by handwriting and storing them manually or by using computer programs to store and categorize data. A number of data storage, retrieval, and analysis software programs are available (see Chapter 3). Researchers who do not have a computer or are more comfortable documenting their observations in writing may use handwritten notes they organize in file boxes. These notes will chronicle what the researchers have seen and heard, answers to questions they asked, and created or collected artifacts. In addition, the field notes can be used to describe the researchers' reflections on what is seen and heard and how their presence may be affecting the data collection.

In the clinic, for example, the researcher may observe the physical layout. Based on the observation, the researcher may ask questions related to what happens in each room. A floor plan (artifact) may become part of the record. The researcher may also take photographs to document the colors of the clinic or the decorations used. These artifacts may offer important insights as the study continues.

It is important throughout the study—but especially in the beginning—not to focus too soon and also not to assume that any comment, artifact, or interaction is incidental. Researchers should document experiences to create a thick or rich description of the culture. In the outpatient example, the researcher should document the colors of the clinic. This observation may seem incidental; however, if a staff member later reports that it is important to maintain a calm atmosphere in the clinic because of the types of clients seen, then the choice of the color may be an artifact that supports this belief system.

In addition to recording explicit details of a situation, ethnographers will also record personal insights. A wide-angle view of the situation will provide the opportunity to detail what participants have said and to share what may be implicit in the situation. Using a wide-angle lens to view a situation provides ethnographers with a larger view of what is actually occurring in a social situation. For example, if an ethnographer is interested in observing a change-of-shift report and attends the report with the purpose of investigating the nurses' interactions, the researcher may miss valuable information regarding the report. With a wide-angle approach, the ethnographer would observe all individuals, activities, and artifacts that are part of the social situation, rather than merely focus on the interactions between the nurses in the report. Attention to all parts of the social situation will contribute to a richer description of the cultural scene. Once the researcher has a good grasp of the *wide-angle view*, then more focused and selective observations can take place.

Spradley (1980) offers three principles researchers should consider as they document their observations: "the language identification principle, the verbatim principle, and the concrete principle" (p. 65). The *language identification principle* requires that ethnographers identify in whose language the text is written. Spradley has pointed out that the most frequently recorded language is the *amalgamated language* (see Example 9-2), that is, the use of the ethnographer's language as well as the informants' language. For example, a nurse ethnographer recording his or her observations of aclinic day might choose to mix the answers to questions with personal observations. Such mixing may create problems when data analysis begins because the researcher can lose sight of the cultural meaning of the observation. To minimize the potential of this happening, entries should identify the person making the remarks. Example 9-1 illustrates the correct way to record field notes. In Example 9-2, the record does not describe how the researcher obtained specific information. It is difficult to decipher whether the notes are the researcher's interpretations or whether the researcher obtained the information directly from the informants.

Example 9-1

Field Note Entry No. 1	July 2, 2005

Ethnographer   Today when I visited the clinic, I noticed that the walls were painted blue. I asked the receptionist who had done the decorating.

Receptionist   "We had several meetings with the decorator."

Example 9-2

Field Note Entry No. 1	July 2, 2005

Today I observed the clinic waiting area. The area is painted in a pale blue. The chairs are wood and fabric. The fabric is a white-and-blue print, which contrasts with the wallpaper. The waiting area is very busy. The colors have an effect on the clients. They come in looking very harassed, then they fall asleep. A decorator helped with the colors.

Although Example 9-1 is a limited notation, readers can get a sense of how researchers should report field notes to facilitate analysis. In this example, the receptionist's response gives the ethnographer clear information about the decorating. The use of the word *we* in Example 9-1 gives the researcher insight into the interactions occurring among staff members. Although Example 9-2 offers significant information, the researcher will find it difficult, after long months of data collection, to return to this note and distinguish his or her insights from factual information obtained from the informants.

The reporting of the receptionist's comments in Example 9-1 reflects the *verbatim principle*, which requires ethnographers to use the speaker's exact words. To adhere to this principle, researchers may use audiotaping, which not only offers ethnographers verbatim accounts of conversation but also affords them an extensive accounting of an interaction that will provide the material for intensive analysis. Documenting verbatim statements also provides researchers with a view of native expressions. In Example 9-1, the use of verbatim documentation allows the researcher to gain insight into the language. The receptionist's use of the word *we* to describe the activities with the decorator may provide valuable insights into the culture of the clinic. The *concrete principle* requires that ethnographers document without interpretation what they have seen and heard. Generalizations and interpretations may limit access to valuable cultural insights. To reduce interpretation, researchers should document observations with as much detail as possible.

Example 9-3 offers an example of concrete documentation without interpretation or generalization. In this example, documentation is clear. The researcher has recorded facts and conversation verbatim.

Example 9-3

Field Note Entry No. 1	July 2, 2005

The clinic waiting area is painted ocean blue. The ladder-back chairs are light brown wood with upholstered seats. The fabric on the seats is an ocean blue-and-white checkered pattern. There are two small 2-ft by 3-ft by 2½-ft brown wooden tables between the six chairs in the waiting room. There are two chairs along one wall with a table in the corner. Then, two chairs along the second wall with another table in the corner. The third wall has the two remaining chairs. The room is an 8-ft by 9-ft rectangle. Each table has a ginger jar lamp. The lamp base and shade are white. The fourth wall has a door and window in it. The draperies on the window are floor length and match the pattern on the chairs.

Individuals enter the clinic, approach the receptionist, state their names, sit in the chairs, and close their eyes. Some patients snore.

Ethnographer	"The colors in this room are great. Everything seems to go together so well. Who did the decorating?"
Receptionist	"We had several meetings with the decorator."

Making Descriptive Observations

Every time ethnographers are in a social situation, they generally will make descriptive observations without having specific questions in mind. General questions, which guide this type of observation, are *grand tour questions*. For example, a grand tour question that might initiate a study of a particular clinic is the following: How do people who live in this neighborhood receive health care? Remembering that the primary foci of all observations include the actors, activities, and artifacts will assist in the development of grand tour questions.

Spradley (1980) has identified nine major dimensions to any social situation:

1. *Space* refers to the physical place or places where the culture of interest carries out social interactions. In the outpatient clinic example, space would include the physical layout of the care delivery site.
2. *Actors* are people who are part of the culture under investigation. In the clinic example, the nurses, physicians, clients, maintenance workers, secretarial and receptionist staff, and family members of clients in the clinic would be the actors.
3. The *activities* are the actions by members of the culture. In the clinic example, activities would include the treatments provided to clients and conversations between cultural group members.
4. *Objects* in the clinic example would include artifacts such as implements used for care, pamphlets read by clients, staff records, and

meeting minutes. Any inanimate object included in the space under study may give insight into the culture.

5. Any single action carried out by group members is an *act*. An example of an act observed in the clinic would be the locking of the medicine cabinet.

6. An *event* is a set of related activities carried out by members of the culture. In the clinic example, the ethnographer one day may observe the staff giving a birthday party for a long-time client.

7. It is important that the researcher document the *time* he or she made observations and when activities occurred during those times. In addition to recording time, the researcher must relate the effect time has on all nine dimensions of social situations.

8. *Goal* relates specifically to what group members hope to achieve. The clinic example illustrates how painting the clinic blue may be a way for the staff to relate their intention to create a calming effect on clients, who often must wait long periods.

9. The researcher should also record *feelings* for each social situation, including the emotions expressed or observed. For example, during the staff-given birthday party for a long-time client, the ethnographer might observe tears from the client, cheers by the staff, and anger by a family member. Recording feelings provides a rich framework from which to make cultural inferences.

The nine dimensions can be useful in guiding observations and questions related to social situations. It is beneficial to plot the nine dimensions in a matrix (Spradley, 1980) to contrast each dimension. For example, in addition to describing the space where the culture carries out its interactions, researchers should relate space to object, act, activity, event, time, actor, goal, and feelings. What does the space look like?

> What are all the ways space is organized by objects? What are all the ways space is organized by acts? What are all the ways space is organized by activities? What are all the ways space is organized by events? What spatial changes occur over time? What are all the ways space is used by actors? What are all the ways space is related to goals? What places are associated with feelings? (Spradley, 1980, pp. 82–83)

Critical ethnographers would add the dimensions of social and political climate to Spradley's (1980) list. It is extremely important that researchers consider issues of power, social class, and politics to get a full view of the culture. In the clinic example, the researcher might ask the following questions: Why are women the providers of intimate care? Does the male doctor ultimately make all the decisions? If so, why? Once researchers have collected data on all dimensions and have related each piece of data to other information, they can begin to focus on further observations.

On completion of this analysis, ethnographers will look for relationships among the parts or relationships to the whole. Based on these new categories, researchers will make additional observations and ask more questions. In the clinic example, the researcher might ask, Why do the RNs have the primary responsibility for care of the clients with AIDS and sexually transmitted diseases (STDs)? Are there different types of AIDS clients, and are they cared for by specific RNs? Are AIDS clients treated differently from the clients with STDs? Are other nurses consulted regarding the care of these two groups of clients? Are the nurses able to select the types of clients for whom they care?

Clearly, the researcher will generate a number of questions from this taxonomic analysis of the concept *nurse*. In addition to using a reductive exercise, ethnographers should try to discover whether there are larger categories for which they have not accounted. In the clinic example, are the people in the clinic part of a larger system? If the clinic is affiliated with a hospital or a community-based organization, then the answer is *yes*. The nurse ethnographer will then need to ask further questions based on this association and conduct focused interviews to validate whether the previously derived larger or smaller categorizations are accurate.

Making Selective Observations

Through selective observations, researchers will further refine the data they have collected. Selective observations will help to identify the "dimensions of contrast" (Spradley, 1980, p. 128). Spradley offers several types of questions that will help researchers discern the differences in the dimensions of contrast. The *dyadic question* seeks to identify the differences between two domains. The question is, In what way are these two things different? In the clinic example, one of the questions the researcher should ask is, In what ways are NPs and CNSs different? *Triadic contrast questions* seek to identify how three categories are related. The researcher in the clinic example might ask, Of the three—NPs, CNSs, and RNs—which two are more alike than the third? *Card-sorting contrast questions* allow ethnographers to place the domains on cards and sort them into piles based on their similarities. This also can be managed by specific computer software applications (see Chapter 3). By identifying the similarities, the contrasts become easily recognizable. Asking these questions of the available data will lead ethnographers to the setting to ask still other questions.

Making a Componential Analysis

"Componential analysis is the systematic search for attributes associated with cultural categories" (Spradley, 1980, p. 131). Boyle (1994) indicates that componential analysis has two objectives: to specify the conditions under which participants name something and to understand under what

Table 9-1 • Dimensions of Contrast			
	Dimensions of Contrast		
Domain	*Licensed*	*Supervised Personnel*	*Health Care Provider*
Doctors	Yes	No	Yes
Nurses	Yes	Yes	Yes
Receptionist	No	Yes	No
Maintenance staff	No	Yes	No
Secretaries	No	Yes	No

conditions the participants give something a specific name. Componential analysis is language driven.

During this stage of analysis, researchers are looking for units of meaning. Each unit of meaning is considered an attribute of the culture. Again, researchers are searching for missing data. During componential analysis, they examine each domain for its component parts and ask questions to identify the dimensions of contrast. Based on the identification of missing data, the researchers will make selected observations. Table 9-1 is an example of simple componential analysis that illustrates dimensions of contrast based on the sorting of people who work in the outpatient clinic. In the clinic example, the ethnographer is able to determine that unlicensed personnel do not provide health care. This analysis helps the researcher to begin to identify a hierarchical structure. He or she must validate conclusions through selective interviews and observations. The purpose of using this process is to search for contrasts, sort them out, and then group them based on similarities and differences. This activity provides ethnographers with important information regarding the culture under study.

To fully carry out a componential analysis, ethnographers should move through the process in a sequential manner. The eight steps of the procedure are as follows: (1) select a domain for analysis (people who work in the clinic); (2) inventory previously discovered contrasts (some members are licensed, have supervisors to whom they report, and provide health care); (3) prepare the worksheet (this is called a *paradigm*); (4) classify dimensions of contrast that have binary values (licensed, yes or no); (5) combine related dimensions of contrast into ones that have multiple values (doctors and nurses are licensed personnel who provide health care); (6) prepare contrast questions for missing attributes (Are doctors the owners of the clinic because they appear not to have a reporting relationship?); (7) conduct selective observations and interviews to discover missing data and confirm or discard hypotheses; (8) prepare a complete paradigm (Spradley, 1980). "The final paradigm can be used as a chart in [the] ethnography" (p. 139). Although every attribute will not be discussed on the chart, important ones

ETHICAL CONSIDERATIONS

*T*he protection of study participants is important regardless of the research paradigm, whether it is a qualitative or quantitative approach, phenomenology, grounded theory, ethnography, action, or historic. Because ethics is covered broadly in Chapter 4, this section shares unique ethical issues specific to ethnography.

When conducting ethnographic research, researchers by virtue of their roles as participant-observers are in a unique position to fit in. Researchers live among the people and therefore have the ability to be invisible at times in the researcher capacity. The invisible nature of researchers has significant value in data collection but can present potential dilemmas from an ethical standpoint. The important elements in conducting any type of research study are to inform participants fully about the matter to which they are consenting, inform participants that they can withdraw from the study at any time for any reason, reduce all unnecessary risks, ensure that the benefits of the study outweigh the risks, and ensure that the researchers who will be conducting the study have appropriate qualifications (Lipson, 1994).

Informed consent is an ethical principle that requires researchers to obtain voluntary consent, including description of the potential risks and benefits of participation. Munhall (1988) recommends using "process consent" (p. 156) rather than the traditional consent signed in the beginning of most studies and not revisited unless participants question their obligations related to the study. *Process consent* or "consensual decision-making" (Ramos, 1989, p. 61) means that researchers renegotiate the consent as unforeseen events or consequences arise (Munhall, 1988; Ramos, 1989). By providing the opportunity to renegotiate the consent and be part of the decision making as the study develops, ethnographers afford participants the chance to withdraw or modify that to which they initially agreed.

Lipson (1994) suggests that consent in the field becomes somewhat more difficult. For instance, the researcher secures consent before formal fieldwork begins. Some time passes, and the researcher is in the field at the time an unexpected event occurs, such as the birth of a child. Although it is important that the researcher inform the group that he or she is chronicling this event for research purposes, it would be intrusive to address consent at that point. One way to handle this situation would be for the researcher to inform participants at a later time that the birth experience gave him or her insight into cultural values. If objections are raised, the researcher would be unable to erase the memory of the event; however, to protect the informants, he or she would not include those data in the study. Covert participation in all research is regarded as a violation of individuals' rights. Therefore, ethnographers should always be forthright with their intentions.

Risk is another major concern. Researchers should never put a participant group in danger for data collection purposes. For example, the researcher in the field may discover that some young men are staging a gang fight in which they plan to use weapons. Believing that it would be important to learn more about conflict and how the group handles it, the researcher plans to go as an observer. In this situation, the risk to the people involved far outweighs the goal to observe how the group handles conflict. Intervention is necessary. How the researcher intervenes should be determined by a number of factors. A research mentor is invaluable in helping the novice researcher sort out when and how to intervene. Too many variables are involved to offer a simple answer. The important principle is that the researcher should not engage in data collection to achieve his or her own goals when significant risk to research participants is involved.

Another principle described by Lipson (1994) is the researcher's qualifications. Usually, institutional review boards will assess the researcher's qualifications based on review of the submitted research proposal. An unqualified researcher can do substantial damage to a culture. It is essential that, even as a neophyte ethnographer, one clearly understands what it is he or she is doing and the potential risks in conducting a study without adequate sensitivity and knowledge.

Roper and Shapira (2000) also suggest that researchers adopt specific strategies to address ethical dilemmas. The ones recommended are to

deliberately evaluate their own effects on the research process by consciously identifying biases brought to the field and also emotional responses resulting from their experiences.

Next, . . . come up with an explicit description of their role during data collection. Finally, . . . establish mechanisms that guarantee honest and trustworthy research relationships. (p. 114)

Goodwin et al. (2003) also address the inherent problems for researchers who conduct research in a setting in which they have worked or have familiarity. In this case, the authors suggest that the role of researcher is frequently overlooked. When this occurs, sensitive information may be shared in the presence of the researcher when viewed as a practitioner rather than in the role of researcher. As a practitioner, other professionals may consider sensitive information confidential. As a researcher, however, the level of confidentiality may be compromised. There is no "right" way to handle this situation. However, Goodwin and colleagues suggest that the researcher has the responsibility to be as overt as possible in the research role.

It is important that all qualitative researchers—but, in particular, ethnographers—be aware of and knowledgeable about their responsibilities to research participants. Specifically, because of the intimate nature of the relationships that develop when ethnographers live among study participants, these researchers have a duty to inform and protect informants.

Lee, B. K., & Gregory, D. (2008). Not alone in the field: Distance collaboration via the Internet in a focused ethnography. *International Journal of Qualitative Methods, 7*(3), 30–46.

Leininger, M. (1970). *Nursing and anthropology: Two worlds to blend.* New York, NY: Wiley.

Leininger, M. (1978). *Transcultural nursing: Concepts, theories and practices.* New York, NY: Wiley.

Leininger, M. (1985). Ethnography and ethnonursing: Models and modes of qualitative data analysis. In M. Leininger (Ed.), *Qualitative research methods in nursing* (pp. 33–71). Orlando, FL: Grune & Stratton.

Lipson, J. G. (1994). Ethical issues in ethnography. In J. M. Morse (Ed.), *Critical issues in qualitative research methods* (pp. 333–355). Thousand Oaks, CA: Sage.

Lipson, J. G. (2001). We are the canaries: Self-care in multiple chemical sensitivity sufferers. *Qualitative Health Research, 11*(1), 103–116.

Magilvy, J. K., & Congdon, J. G. (2000). The crisis nature of health care transitions of rural older adults. *Public Health Nursing, 17*(5), 336–345.

Malinowski, B. (1922). *Argonauts of the Western Pacific.* London: Routledge & Kegan Paul.

Malinowski, B. (1961). *Argonauts of the Western Pacific.* New York, NY: Dutton.

Manias, E., & Street, A. (2001). Rethinking ethnography: Reconstructing nursing relationships. *Journal of Advanced Nursing, 33*(2), 234–242.

McGarry, J. (2007). Nursing relationships in ethnographic research: What of rapport? *Nurse Researcher, 14*(3), 7–14.

Mead, M. (1949). *Coming of age in Samoa.* New York, NY: New American Library, Mentor Books.

Morse, J. M., & Field, P. A. (1995). *Qualitative research methods for health professionals.* Thousand Oaks, CA: Sage.

Muecke, M. A. (1994). On the evaluation of ethnographies. In J. M. Morse (Ed.), *Critical issues in qualitative research methods* (pp. 187–209). Thousand Oaks, CA: Sage.

Munhall, P. L. (1988). Ethical considerations in qualitative research. *Western Journal of Nursing Research, 10*(2), 150–162.

Omery, A. (1988). Ethnography. In B. Sarter (Ed.), *Paths to knowledge: Innovative research methods for nursing* (pp. 17–31). New York: National League for Nursing.

Pellat, G. (2003). Ethnography and reflexivity: Emotions and feelings in fieldwork. *Nurse Researcher, 10*(3), 28–37.

Prince, L. M. (2008). Resilience in African American women formerly involved in street prostitution. *The ABNF Journal, 19*(1), 31–36.

Radcliffe-Brown, A. R. (1952). *Structure and function in primitive society.* London: Oxford University Press.

Ragucci, A. T. (1972). The ethnographic approach and nursing research. *Nursing Research, 21*(6), 485–490.

Ramos, M. C. (1989). Some ethical implications in qualitative research. *Research in Nursing and Health, 12,* 57–63.

Roberts, T. (2009). Understanding ethnography. *British Journal of Midwifery, 17*(5), 291–294.

Roper, J. M., & Shapira, J. (2000). *Ethnography in nursing research.* Thousand Oaks, CA: Sage.

Rowe, J. H. (1965). The Renaissance foundation in anthropology. *American Anthropologist, 67,* 1–20.

Sanday, P. R. (1983). The ethnographic paradigm(s). In J. Van Maanen (Ed.), *Qualitative methodology* (pp. 19–36). Beverly Hills, CA: Sage.

Savage, H. (2000). Ethnography and health care. *British Medical Journal, 321*(7273), 1400–1403.

Schulte, J. (2000). Finding ways to create connections among communities: Partial results of an ethnography of urban public health nurses. *Public Health Nursing, 17*(1), 3–10.

Spradley, J. P. (1980). *Participant observation.* New York, NY: Holt, Rinehart & Winston.

Spradley, J. P., & McCurdy, D. W. (1972). *The cultural experience: Ethnography in complex society.* Prospect Heights, IL: Waveland Press.

van Maanen, J. (1983). The fact of fiction in organizational ethnography. In J. van Maanen (Ed.), *Qualitative methodology* (pp. 36–55). Beverly Hills, CA: Sage.

Waldrop, D. P., & Rinfrette, E. S. (2009). Making the transition to hospice: Exploring hospice professionals' perspectives. *Death Studies, 33*, 557–580.

Waters, A. L. (2008). An ethnography of a children's renal unit: Experiences of children and young people with long-term renal illness. *Journal of Clinical Nursing, 17*, 3103–3114.

Wolf, Z. R. (1988). *Nurses' work, the sacred and the profane.* Philadelphia, PA: University of Pennsylvania Press.

Woods, P. (1992). Symbolic interactionism: Theory and method. In M. D. LeCompte, W. L. Millroy, & J. Presale (Eds.), *The handbook of qualitative research in education.* San Diego, CA: Academic Press.

Wolcott, W. F. (2003). Ethnographic research in education. In C. F. Conrad, J. G. Haworth, & L. R. Lattuca (Eds.), *Qualitative research in higher education: Expanding perspectives* (2nd ed.). Saddle River, NJ: Pearson Education.

Wright, D. J. (2002). Researching the qualities of hospice nurses. *Journal of Hospice and Palliative Nursing, 4*(4), 210–216.

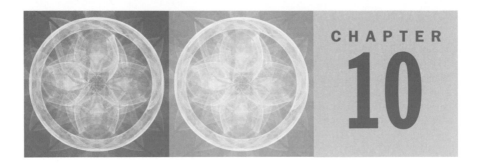

Ethnography in Practice, Education, and Administration

As I reviewed the literature for this chapter, I was struck by the limited number of studies that are classified as ethnography. Pondering the scarcity of studies, I found myself asking—have we become so results oriented that the study of culture has been limited to mini studies of some aspect of nursing because of the time it takes to conduct a good ethnography? I hope not because ethnography is an important way of studying nursing and the cultural practices imbedded within it. The study of patterns within a culture provides an excellent opportunity to describe the practices of the people for whom nurses care, to understand the health-related phenomena of people within various cultures, and to examine nursing's own unique culture. Ethnography provides a chance to explore both the clinical aspects of nursing and its administrative and educative patterns and lifeways.

This chapter provides an overview of ethnographic studies that have explored cultures of interest to nursing. In addition, it critiques ethnographic studies that reflect clinical nursing practice, nursing education, and nursing administration to provide readers with examples of published works and the contributions these works have made to the field. The ethnographic studies examined in this chapter have been critiqued using the guidelines in Box 10-1. The critiquing guidelines offer specific directives for determining the quality of the ethnographic works presented in this chapter and in the literature. The questions in Box 10-1 are specific to ethnographic research

Box 10-1

Criteria for Critiquing Ethnographic Research

Focus

1. What is the culture being studied?
2. What is the focus or scope of the study?
3. What is the purpose of the study?

Method

1. How does ethnography fulfill the purpose of the study?
2. Is the study conducted in the field?
3. What guidelines have been established for participant consent?
4. How has the researcher protected study participants' rights?

Sampling

1. Why is the group selected to inform the study appropriate?
2. Does the researcher discuss how key informants are selected and why?

Data Collection

1. What strategies were used to collect data?
2. How do the strategies selected fully inform the study?
3. What was the researcher's role in the study?
4. How has triangulation of data sources (observation, interview, collection of artifacts) enhanced credibility of findings?
5. Is time in the field adequate to meet the purpose of the study?

Data Analyses

1. What strategies were used to analyze data? Were they consistent with the method?
2. How is the cyclic nature of data collection or data analyses reported?
3. Based on the report, can another researcher follow the logic of the researcher's conclusions?

Rigor

1. How has the researcher maintained his or her "objectivity"?
2. How has the researcher documented the authenticity of the data?
3. What role do the informants play in validating the researcher's findings?

Findings

1. Do the findings make clear a description of the culture studied?
2. In what context are the findings presented?
3. Are findings presented in a rich narrative format providing readers with a "feel" for the culture?
4. Do the findings go beyond the description to explain why particular aspects of the culture are as they are?
5. Are the findings reported in a systematic way, such as by themes?

Conclusions

1. How do the conclusions relate to the findings of the study?
2. What is the relevance of the findings to nursing, and how can they be used in practice?
3. What future directions for research are offered?

and reflect the most important aspects researchers must evaluate in an ethnographic report. A reprint of Chuang and Abbey's (2009) article found at the end of this chapter assists readers in understanding the critiquing process. Table 10-1 summarizes a recent series of ethnographic studies representing the areas of nursing education, administration, and practice.

APPLICATION TO PRACTICE

"The purpose of classical ethnography is to describe a whole culture" (Grbich, 2007, p. 40). Although often not addressed as such, the clinical setting by its very existence is a culture of its own. Clinical practice takes place within a cultural context. Therefore, using ethnographic methods to study the culture found in professional caring environments is appropriate. Whether the interest is in studying humor in critical care (Dean & Major, 2008), postoperative pain assessment decisions (Harper, Ersser, & Gobbi, 2007) or the culture of a Taiwanese nursing home (Chuang & Abbey, 2009), ethnographic research provides the framework for exploring the richness of nursing and nursing-related phenomena. Chuang and Abbey is the reference for critique in this section.

You can tell from the title of this study that Chuang and Abbey (2009) focused their research on Taiwanese nursing homes. The authors state that this is an important study because admission to a nursing home is very recent in Taiwan. Institutionalizing the elderly runs counter to cultural norms in this country. The scope of the study is one nursing home located in southern Taiwan which is managed by a government hospital. As stated by the authors, the purpose is to describe the culture of nursing home life for older residents in Taiwan. The purpose, focus, and reason for the study are appropriate. The authors have included enough detail so that the reader knows that there may be differences between different types of nursing home management.

Although the researchers do not explicitly answer the question, why ethnography, it is clear from the introduction to the method that they plan to study the culture of the nursing home and so by inference the reader can be satisfied that the method is appropriate. The report indicates that the research will be conducted onsite and the informants will be nursing personnel, orderlies, a clerk, and residents of the facility.

Chuang and Abbey (2009) report that they obtained approval through a human subjects review board. The authors do not state the method used to obtain informed consent from the residents. However, in addition to obtaining approval from the university human subjects review board, the researchers also gained permission from the governing body of the facility and the director of the department of nursing. Gaining formal consent is important because in addition to fulfilling the expectations of strong research, it also begins to build rapport with the organizational staff.

Initially, the informants for this study included 1 head nurse; 8 nurses; 18 nursing assistants, including 2 orderlies and a clerk. Chuang and Abbey

Table 10-1 • Selective Sampling of Ethnographic Studies

Author(s)	Domain	Culture	Focus	Data Collection Strategies	Data Analyses
Bland (2007)	Practice/ Administration	Three nursing homes in New Zealand	The concept of comfort in residential aged care	Interviews Participant observation Documents	A range of analytical approaches
Chuang and Abbey (2009)	Practice	Taiwanese nursing home	Culture of the nursing home for older residents	Participant observation Interview Related documents	NVivo 7
Clabo (2008)	Practice/ Administration	Two post-op units	Pain assessment	Participant observation Interviews Focus groups	Bourdieu's approach to ethnography
Dean and Major (2008)	Practice/ Administration	Healthcare setting: palliative care and ICU	Sustaining humor in critical and palliative care	Semi-structured interviews Participant observation	Line by line analysis Identification of codes—themes
Green et al. (2007)	Practice	Eleven children who had received a transplant	Quality of life after a transplant	Critical self reflection Semi-structured interviews	Content analysis, constant comparative method
Harper et al. (2007)	Practice/ Administration	Military nurses working in surgical and orthopedic units	Post op pain decision-making	Artifacts Semi-structured interviews	Ethnomethodology, NUDIST6
Prince (2008)	Practice	African American women who were formerly involved in prostitution	Resilience	Observations Interviews Reflection	Leininger's Ethnonursing

(Continued)

Table 10-1 • (Continued)

Author(s)	Domain	Culture	Focus	Data Collection Strategies	Data Analyses
Hunter et al. (2008)	Education	Neonatal intensive care unit (NICU)	Nurses learning from each other in the NICU	Participant observation In-depth interviews	Inductive ETHNOGRAPH5
Scott and Pollack (2008)	Administration	Pediatric intensive care unit	The role of nursing unit culture related to research utilization	Observation Interview Personal reflection	Pattern identification
Sorensen et al. (2008)	Administration	ICU	Nursing leadership in contemporary healthcare	Interview Focus group	Content analysis
Waldrop and Rinfrette (2009)	Practice/ Administration	Hospice unit	Professional decisions about moving patients to hospice	Observation Focus groups Survey data	Constant comparative
Waters (2008)	Practice	Children experiencing long-term renal illness	Quality of life	Participant observation Interviews Drawings Document analysis	Spradley (1979)

(2009) do not fully explain why these individuals were included. As the study progressed, a purposive sample was employed. This sample included 16 residents, 8 nurses, 6 nursing assistants (one private), 1 physician's assistant, 1 orderly, and 4 family members (p. 1642). It is unclear why these individuals were selected for the first or second group.

Chuang and Abbey (2009) used interview, participant observation, and examination of important documents to inform the study. The use of multiple methods of data collection is important. It adds to the credibility of the findings.

During the eight months of the study, the researchers offer that they conducted observations on different days of the week, including weekends and during all three shifts. Both participant-as-observer and observer-as-participant strategies were used. In addition, interviews and analyses of documents were used to gain a richer understanding of the setting. The researchers also reported using reflexive practices to maintain self awareness and to gain a better understanding of their actions throughout the data collection phase. The use of multiple methods to collect data, time in the field, and variability of time of observations are all important components of reaching a rich understanding of the culture.

Transcripts and field notes were analyzed using NVivo7. NVivo7 is a data analysis program which organizes data into manageable units of analysis to facilitate understanding of the raw data. The authors do not offer documentation of the cyclic nature of data collection and data analyses which is so very important in the implantation of ethnography. The statements referring to two different interview groups provides some insight into the possibility that, in fact, the cycle of data collection and analyses did exist since the researchers report that after the initial interviews, a *purposive* sample was used to continue the interview.

The report of the findings includes a table which defines the process used to analyze the data. It also includes a table illustrating the themes and the categories of data that support the themes. These give the reader an eye into the analysis process. Further, the results section provides informant statements which helps to support that the findings do emanate from the stories of the informants.

As stated earlier, time in the field and use of multiple methods of data collection support the rigor of the research. In addition, Chuang and Abbey (2009) report that the process used for data analyses—a compare and contrast method, further verified their findings as did the use of a decision trail and the thick descriptions by informants. Informants' verification of the findings is not included in this report.

Chuang and Abbey (2009) report three major themes: collective life, care rituals, and embedded beliefs. The subcategories under each of these themes tell the story for the informants. Clearly, statements reflecting living in a public space, mealtime as highlight, everyday is the same, and the ceiling is my best mate (p. 1643), captures the culture of life in this nursing facility. The researchers offer examples of similar data reported by other researchers.

The researchers' conclusions are not overstated. They state clearly that this is the situation in this Taiwanese nursing home. The contribution that the study makes is that it illustrates from the informants' perspectives what it is like to live in this space. The findings have the potential to inform nursing practice. Chuang and Abbey (2009) conclude their report by stating, "a change in nursing home culture would be appropriate to promote a more resident-centered form of care and to enhance the provision of individualized care" (p. 1647). It is clear that these authors have added to the body of nursing knowledge focused on care of the elderly, particularly those living in a nursing home. It also provides valuable insights into changes Taiwanese health care providers are making as the number of elderly in institutionalized settings grows. The authors' work provides the groundwork for future studies in this and related areas.

APPLICATION TO EDUCATION

Nursing education presents another context in which nurse researchers can conduct ethnographic studies. The teaching and learning environment, including the way students, faculty, health care providers, and clients relate to one another in clinical settings, creates its own culture. Few published studies have specifically illustrated the lifeways of students and faculty. Since the last publication of this text, the trend continues. Few ethnographic studies of nursing education were found despite an extensive electronic literature search. Clearly, ethnographic research has a role in the teaching and learning process and offers the qualitative education researcher rich opportunities.

The article "Learning How We Learn: An Ethnographic Study in a Neonatal Intensive Care Unit" (Hunter et al., 2008) serves as the reference for critique in this section. The study does not represent a traditional academic research focus but does reflect how the concept of education can be studied using and ethnographic approach.

In the article, Hunter et al. (2008) clearly identifies that the aim of the study is to "identify how nurse clinicians learn with and from each other in the workplace" (p. 657). The culture being studied is that of an Australian neonatal intensive care unit (NICU). Why this particular NICU is selected is unclear. The researchers do make an excellent case for studying NICUs based on the complex subculture which they believe exists. The focus of this particular study is a 20 bed NICU in Australia.

The researchers do not explain why they selected ethnography to achieve their aim. However, they do report spending 12 months onsite conducting interviews and observations on all three shifts. Participation by informants was voluntary. Ethics committees at both the university and hospital reviewed and approved of the study. In addition, Hunter et al. (2008) used two different consent forms, one for participation and the other for recording. In situations when engagement in the site is for a long period of time, researchers would be best served to use process consent.

Process consent allows individuals to reassess their willingness to continue in the study at some point after their initial agreement.

The participants in this study were 32 nurse clinicians, 14 medical registrars, 5 allied health workers, a nurse educator, a clinical nurse consultant, a nurse manager, 5 senior medical specialist, and one administrative worker (Hunter et al., 2008, p. 659). Hunter et al. report that 57% of those working on the unit participated. One could assume from this that appropriate individuals participated. The report would be stronger if the researchers discussed who the key informants were and how they were selected.

In-depth interviews and observations were the strategies used to conduct the study. The researchers do not make reference to how the two methods supported the credibility of the findings.

Data analyses were conducted using ETHNOGRAPH 5. Qualitative data analysis packages such as this one help to organize, retrieve, and identify key themes. There is no description in this report of how rigor was assured. Generally, ethnographers use time spent within the culture and cross checking of data to assure that the findings are credible.

The researchers offer four major "dimensions." These include: Orientation of nurses or "learning to do things the way we do things here," orientation of medical registrars (The term medical registrar in Australia refers to medical practice), through nurses' eyes, preceptoring—moving up the ladder, and decision-making. These four dimensions speak to what is required to be learned in order to be an effective nursing clinician. The descriptions offered by Hunter et al. (2008) provide informant's words to illustrate the dimensions identified. The reader can easily see the relationship between the subjective comments included and the dimensions identified.

"This study offers insight into bedside clinical teaching, which is advantageous because it is reality-based" (Hunter et al., 2008, p. 663). According to the authors, using ethnography gives researchers and clinicians the opportunity to look closely at the interactive context in which learning occurs in the NICU. Looking carefully at learning within the context of the NICU provides a framework for future planning of unit level education. The researchers do not overstate their findings. Significant page space is taken up in this article to *tell the story*. This should not be viewed as a limitation of the report, but rather as the focus of an ethnographic study. Researchers engaged in this approach focus heavily on the story telling when the number of pages is controlled by the publication guidelines. Hunter et al. (2008) provide the reader with the opportunity to view how ethnography can be used to guide the learning process.

APPLICATION TO ADMINISTRATION

*I*n previous editions of this text, it was challenging to find research articles which focused exclusively on nursing administration. It is indeed true again. However, what has become apparent is many of the articles you will find in Table 10-1 focus on practice issues but are not exclusively practice.

For a example, a report by Clabo (2008) focuses on pain assessment in two postoperative units. Although the focus is on a particular practice issue, clearly the implications of the research are in the area of nursing administration. For this reason, you will find that several of the articles in the table are identified as both practice and administration.

It is important to point out that it is not unusual for researchers who publish ethnography in a research journal to focus on only one facet of a larger study. Because of the significant amount of information generated in a long-term cultural study, many ethnographies are published as books. When researchers choose to publish their ethnographic work in a journal, the scope of the report must meet the page guidelines of the selected journal. Sorensen, Iedema, and Severinsson (2008) research on nursing leadership in contemporary health care is a report of one part of a larger 3-year study of an intensive care unit. This study entitled "Beyond Profession: Nursing Leadership in Contemporary Healthcare is critiqued to demonstrate the application of ethnography in nursing administration. Table 10-1 offers additional examples of ethnographic research studies.

Sorensen et al. (2008) share that the current report is part of a larger 3-year study which has been conducted in an intensive care unit in Australia. This publication is one part of the study which focuses on nursing leadership within the unit. It is reported that the 3-year study focused on this topic as well as end of life care. There is no explanation as to why ethnography is the method of choice. The researchers share that nursing leadership became symbolic of many of the concepts that emerged during the study.

The research does take place in the field which is characteristic of ethnography. There is no report on how human subjects were protected or how informed consent was obtained. Given that this study is part of a larger study, the reader might find documentation of informed consent in the report of the larger study. This is not meant to suggest that the reader is required to determine whether this is the case. Each sub-account of a larger investigation should be treated as though it is an independent research report.

Focus groups and interviews were conducted over a period of three years with nurses in the study. Based on the report, these were successful strategies for data collection. Also important is the amount of time, the researchers spent in the field. Using more than one data collections strategy and time in the field are two important ways to assure the credibility of the findings. The data generated from the focus groups and interviews were analyzed using the constant comparative method. This is an appropriate method of analysis for ethnographic studies.

There is no explicit description of rigor, however, as noted above, time in the field and triangulation of data collection strategies are two ways to exploit the findings. Similar to the study reported in the *Education Section* of this chapter, the authors utilize the pages of the report to tell the story of nursing leadership in this ICU. The three major units of analysis emerged. These included: nursing care at the end of life, barriers to enacting nursing's professional role, and opportunities for nursing leadership in the organization. These subunits were illustrated by informants' descriptions of what it is like to lead and manage in an intensive care unit, specifically as it relates to end of life care. The final themes which emerged included: (1) nursing care at the end of life; (2) barriers to enacting nursing's professional role and (3) opportunities for nursing leadership in the organization.

Sorensen et al. (2008) place their findings in the context of what is already known about end-of-life care—specifically nursing leadership. The conclusions offered in the research article are relevant and do not overstate the findings. The implications are clear. Nurses have an important role to play in organizational strategy and patient advocacy. Ultimately, Sorensen and colleagues believe that nurses need to be equal partners in healthcare.

SUMMARY

*T*his chapter reviewed samples of published ethnographic research in the areas of nursing practice, education, and administration. Each critique presents the strengths and limitations of the ethnographic research included. The reviewed authors have contributed to the literature and provided readers with an opportunity to become part of the culture or subculture they studied.

Ethnographic research and the studies that use ethnography as a method add to the richness and diversity of the human experience by allowing readers to share in the lives of the people studied. As nurse researchers become more comfortable with multiple ways of knowing and multiple realities, they will benefit by participating in the creation and dissemination of the knowledge imbedded in the cultural realities that are a person's life.

References

Bland, M. (2007). Betwixt and between: A critical ethnography of comfort in New Zealand residential aged care. *Journal of Clinical Nursing, 16*, 937–944.

Chuang, Y., & Abbey, J. (2009). The culture of a Taiwanese nursing home. *Journal of Clinical Nursing, 18*, 1640–1648.

Clabo, L.M.L. (2008). An ethnography of pain assessment and the role of social context on two postoperative units. *Journal of Advanced Nursing, 61*(5), 531–539.

Dean, R.A.K., & Major, J.E. (2008). From critical care to comfort care: The sustaining value of humour. *Journal of Clinical Nursing, 17*, 1088–1095.

Grbich, C. (2007). *Qualitative data analysis: An introduction.* London: Sage.

Green, A., McSweeney, J., Ainley, K., & Bryant, J. (2007). In my shoes: Children's quality of life after heart transplantation. *Progress in Transplantation, 17*(3), 199–208.

Harper, P., Ersser, S., & Gobbi, M. (2007). How military nurses rationalize their postoperative pain assessment decisions. *Journal of Advanced Nursing, 59*(6), 601–611.

Hunter, C.L., Spence, K., McKenna, K., & Iedema, R. (2008). Learning how we learn: An ethnographic study in a neonatal intensive care unit. *Journal of Advanced Nursing, 62*(2), 657–664.

Prince, L.M. (2008). Resilience in African American women formerly involved in street prostitution. *The ABNF Journal, 19*(1), 31–36.

Scott, S.D., & Pollock, C. (2008). The role of nursing unit culture in shaping research utilization behaviors. *Research in Nursing and Health, 31*, 298–309.

Sorensen, R., Iedema, R., & Severinsson, E. (2008). Beyond profession: Nursing leadership in contemporary healthcare. *Journal of Nursing Management, 16*, 535–544.

Spradley, J.P. (1979). *The Ethnographic Interview.* New York: Holt, Rinehart and Winston.

Waldrop, D.P., & Rinfrette, E.S. (2009). Making the transition to hospice: Exploring hospice professionals' perspectives. *Death Studies, 33*, 557–580.

Waters, A.L. (2008). An ethnography of a children's renal unit: Experiences of children and young people with long-term renal illness. *Journal of Clinical Nursing, 17*, 3103–3114.

Research Article

The Culture of a Taiwanese Nursing Home

Yeu-Hui Chuang and Jennifer Abbey

Aim. *To explore and understand the culture of nursing home life for older residents in Taiwan.*

Background. *The environment, the care providers and the residents all influence how the nursing home operates and performs. The literature has shown that there has been a move from understanding nursing home culture to changing it. However, there is no literature illustrating nursing home culture in Taiwan. It is appropriate to understand the phenomenon before making any changes.*

Design. *Ethnographic methodology was used to understand this phenomenon.*

Methods. *Three methods, participant observation, in-depth interviews and examination of related documents, were used to collect information from July 2005–February 2006. All the data were recorded in either field notes or verbatim transcripts and were analysed concurrently.*

Results. *Three themes have been generated including collective life, care rituals and embedded beliefs. 'Living in a public area', 'mealtime is the highlight', 'every day is the same', and 'the ceiling is my best mate' are used to explain the collective life. Under care rituals, there are 'the perception of inadequate staffing in spite of legal requirements being met' and 'task-oriented care'. The embedded beliefs can be described by the notions of 'patients and hospitalisation' and 'compromise'.*

Conclusions. *A tedious, monotonous, idle and lonely life is experienced by the residents, and insufficient staffing is obvious, despite the legal staffing requirements being met. This is exacerbated by the provision of care that is task-oriented rather than individual driven. The residents, whether consciously or not, consider themselves to be the patients of a hospital. They easily compromise to maintain harmony and balance in the nursing home life.*

Relevance to clinical practice. *The findings contribute to the understanding of Taiwanese nursing home culture and filling the gaps in nursing knowledge for the purpose of improving care of residents.*

Keywords: cultural issues, elderly, ethnography, nurses, nursing, Taiwan

Accepted for publication: 1 October 2008

Authors: *Yeu-Hui Chuang,* PhD, MSN, MS, RN, Assistant Professor, Department of Nursing, Chung Hwa University of Medical Technology, Tainan, Taiwan; *Jennifer Abbey,* PhD, FRCNA, RN, Professor of Nursing (Aged Care) at Queensland University of Technology (QUT) and Director of the QUT Dementia Collaborative Research Centre for Consumers, Carers and Social Research, Brisbane, Australia

Correspondence: Yeu-Hui Chuang, 89, Wen-Hwa 1st Street, Jen-Te Hsiang, Tainan 717, Taiwan. Telephone: +886 6 2674567. E-mail: yeuhui@mail.hwai.edu.tw

From Chuang Y-H, Abbey J. *Journal of Clinical Nursing.* vol. 18, pp. 1640–1648. Copyright © 2009 by Blackwell Publishing Ltd. Reprinted with permission.

Introduction

Any nursing home, over time, develop its own culture (Price 2004). Those inside the nursing home will interact with each other, combining their values, beliefs and assumptions in everyday practice. Each of these individuals will not only bring an influence on the culture, the culture will but also influence them. Nursing home culture was frequently discussed during the 1980s and early 1990s, particularly in the US (Vladeck 1980, Tisdale 1987, Shield 1988, Savishinsky 1991, Diamond 1992, Farmer 1996). However, the major focus of research has shifted from exploring culture itself to focusing on cultural change to improve the performance of nursing homes (Gibson & Barsade 2003, Deutschman 2005). It is reasonable to make any appropriate changes in order to improve the care of residents after understanding the culture.

Institutionalisation of the older people has usualy been viewed in Taiwan as conflicting with the traditions of filial piety and generational responsibility (Wu et al. 1997). However, as Taiwanese society shifts from an agricultural to an industrialised and urbanised society, the dependent and frail elders are becoming more likely to be placed in an institution. The first nursing home in Taiwan was established on a pilot basis in 1991 by the Department of Health. Since then, the number of licensed nursing homes has increased to 311 (17,392 beds) in 2006 (Taiwan Long-Term Care Professional Association 2005).

Although the number of the nursing homes is increasing, nursing home cultures have never been adequately explored and understood in Taiwan. The majority of the Taiwanese literature on the issues related to residential care used quantitative analysis to describe the prevalence of cognitive impairment, residents' morale, quality of life or care, continuing education needs and restraint reduction program (Lin et al. 1998, Wu et al. 1998, Chen 2001a, Yeh et al. 2001, 2003, Lo et al. 2002, Tseng & Wang 2002), the decision process of nursing home admission (Liu & Tinker 2003, Huang & Chang 2006), and cost and care quality amongst different types of ownership (Lee et al. 2002a, Chen et al. 2003). The qualitative studies focused on examining the relocation and adaptation process underscoring the transition to institutionalise (Chen 2002), on exploring the indicators or dimensions of the care quality (Yang 2000, 2001, 2002, Chao & Roth 2005), and comparing the residents' daily lives in America and Taiwan (Chang & Fang 2004). Due to the lack of literature related to nursing home culture, the aim of this study is to describe the culture of nursing home life for older people residents in Taiwan.

The Study

Methodology

Ethnography is a qualitative methodology, with origins in anthropology, which generally seeks to understand and interpret the behaviours of groups of people (Atkinson et al. 2001). In an ethnographic approach, understanding culture is gained in the setting in which it occurs. For a better understanding of the phenomenon under consideration, the researcher was 'immersed' in the research setting to gain holistic information about the nursing home culture.

Methods

Research setting

The selected nursing home, Gingin Nursing Home (a pseudonym), is located in southern Taiwan. It is managed by a government hospital, and offers nursing care to all chronically ill, dependent and frail persons. The physical layout is hospital oriented and each room houses three to five residents with 90 beds in all. During the observation period, the occupancy rate was around 70–91%. The major diagnosis of the residents was Cerebrovascular Accident, and half of the residents were moderately or severely dependent on care defining by the scores of the Barthel index. The nursing personnel include one head nurse, eight nurses, eighteen nursing assistants (NAs), including two orderlies, and a clerk. This nursing home was selected for four reasons:

1. Its residents include both native-born Taiwanese and mainlanders, the two major groups within the older population of Taiwan;
2. It is an accredited nursing home with standard staffing levels and is equipped according to government regulations;
3. The setting was unfamiliar to the researcher prior to data collection;
4. The setting's governing body granted permission to undertake this study.

Ethical considerations

Ethical approval was obtained from the Queensland University of Technology Ethics Committee before commencing the study. An approval letter from the Director of the department of nursing was also received due to their being no ethical committee in the nursing home. The participants' rights of self-determination, autonomy, privacy and anonymity were ensured throughout the study.

Data collection

Three methods, participant observation, in-depth interviews and examination of related documents, were used to collect data. All the data were recorded in either field notes or verbatim transcripts.

In this study, participant, observations were undertaken on different days of the week, including weekends, and on different shifts, including the day (8 a.m. to 4 p.m.), evening (4 p.m. to 12 a.m.) and night shifts (12 a.m. to 8 a.m.) for better understanding the real situations. Both the participant-as-observer and observer-as-participant roles were used. Seventy-seven observations were made from a total of 350 hours of observation in eight-month period.

Field notes were used to record the behaviours, conversations and activities seen and heard in the field and also included experiences, feelings, confusions and thoughts that arose during the fieldwork, which assisted an understanding of the personal thoughts and feelings brought to the study.

Beyond this, purposive sampling was employed to select sixteen older residents, eight nurses, six NAs, one private NA, one physician's assistant, one orderly and four family members who were interviewed. Sixty formal interviews were conducted.

Residents' charts were reviewed and their medical histories were obtained. This information was collected to enable descriptions of the sample to be made and to enrich, and to support or validate the data from interviews or observations.

The nursing protocols and nursing care guidelines which provided a clear description of the insights and philosophy of the nursing home culture were also reviewed.

In ethnographic studies, as with most qualitative research, the researcher is the primary instrument for data collection (Streubert Speziale & Carpenter 2003). Additionally, it is impossible for the researchers to escape the study field to investigate it (Hammersley & Atkinson 1995). As an instrument of data collection and an inevitable participant in the study context, I conducted reflexive practices to remain self-aware and monitor interactions between myself and the participants in the nursing home through use of field notes.

Data Analysis

The verbatim interview transcripts and the field notes were converted to a format accessible by the NVivo7 qualitative software to facilitate data management. We used the analysis method summarised from Graneheim and Lundman (2004), LeCompte and Schensul (1999), and Miles and Huberman (1994) as the major guideline for systematic analysis of the data (Table 1). Furthermore, 'thick descriptions' (Geertz 1973, p. 27) were given to provide meaning and explanation of the phenomenon under investigation. Excerpts from interviews and field notes were used to illustrate and validate the categories and themes that emerged.

Rigour

The rigour was ensured though the following strategies. First, the time frame of eight months of interviews and observations enabled us to develop trusting relationships with the participants and allowed in-depth data to be gathered. Second, the accuracy of the information was ensured by undertaking multiple formal or informal interviews with the participants on the same topic, and making repeated observations of the same activities in their natural context. These strategies enabled clarification of

Table 1 • The Process of Data Analysis	
Steps	*Description*
1 Order and organise the collected data	Transcribe digitally recorded interviews and type up the field notes
2 Read the data repeatedly	Read through all the data several times in order to obtain a general sense of the information
3 Search for meaning units and label the meaning units into codes	A meaning unit is words, sentences or paragraphs
4 Group codes together to create subcategories and then group subcategories to create categories	Examine each code and then combine them to generate broader and more abstract subcategories and then categories. Each of these categories includes several discrete codes
5 Generate themes	A theme is a thread of a core meaning among meaning units, codes and categories on an interpretative level. Group the categories together to generate the theme

incomplete or unclear issues. Third, the use of thick descriptions of the information gathered from three methods provided rich and deep insights into nursing home culture. Fourth, when I coded or sorted data into categories or themes during the data analysis phase, comparing and contrasting existing data verified the coherence of the data. Finally, a decision trail which included verbatim transcripts and a description of how the data were analysed was maintained and documented for future audits.

Results and Discussions

Three major themes regarding the nursing home culture have emerged from the interview transcripts, field notes and documents. These are 'collective life', 'care rituals' and 'embedded beliefs'. A variety of categories have also emerged, which expand on each theme (Table 2).

Collective life

Life in the nursing home is overwhelmingly collectivist. The residents have no choice but to live with a group of people, and everyday life is marked by a number of regularly repeated patterns. These are that the residents felt they were living in a public area, that the mealtime is the highlight, that every day is the same, and that the 'ceiling is my best mate'.

Living in a Public Area. In their daily lives, the residents live with not only a number of other residents, but also with staff and a variety of other people. Additionally, no security guard or locks bar the entrance and a high percentage of occupancy is characteristic of this nursing home. All of these facts make the environment crowded, and expose the residents to a variety of different people. The residents are forced to live in a public place. In the field notes:

> While I was talking to Mr. Ging, the NA came in without any greeting. She just passed by and went to check Mr. Chen who was sleeping in the next bed . . . Mr. Ging said that he was used to this. 'If they want to come in then they come. If they want to leave then they leave'.

Additionally, several foreign NAs lived in the nursing home to take care of the residents. The foreign NAs were hired by the residents or their families. They provided

Table 2 • Themes Regarding the Nursing Home Culture	
Themes	*Categories*
Collective life	Living in a public area
	Mealtime is the highlight
	Every day is the same
	The ceiling is my best mate
Care rituals	Perception of inadequate staffing in spite of legal requirements being met
	To do rather than to be: task-oriented care
Embedded beliefs	Patients and hospitalisation
	Compromise

total personal care for the residents who employed them. The residents or their families felt that the employment of a personal assistant would ensure that the residents would have full attention and care while living in the nursing home. Meanwhile, the family would feel less guilty due to the lack of time they were able to give to the residents. The foreign NAs usually slept beside the residents using a foldable bed. This, of course, made the room more crowded than it otherwise would have been.

This finding matches with Fiveash's (1998) finding that residents consider nursing home life like living in a public domain. There is no doubt that whilst they live in such a 'public' area, residents have only limited forms of privacy. Meanwhile, the underlying emphasis on the collective can be considered as directly at odds with the concept of privacy, which emphasises the individuality of human beings and one's right to a private life (Schopp et al. 2003). The staff in the nursing home deal with the private issues of the residents every day. They enter the residents' rooms and bedsides, deal with their personal items and touch their bodies. Body care and bathing, the most private of activities, are treated as public acts (Twigg 2002). There are no private rooms in this nursing home, so each resident has very limited personal space, shared to some extent with other residents in the same room. On this point, Bauer (1994) has emphasised that knocking on patients' doors can contribute a symbol supportive of privacy. This issue became only more important when considered in the light of fact that the nursing home is a communal environment.

Mealtime is the Highlight. Eating is an activity essential to the nursing home residents and, in particular, there is nothing more important than having a meal in Chinese culture. One common sayings describe this importance: 'While you are eating, you are the same as an emperor'. The residents, staff and the family members all, consciously or unconsciously, paid a significant attention to food and meals. This emphasis was apparent in both their conversations and their behaviours, as the following transcripts show: 'I think I only do two things here. The most important one is eating and the other is sleeping' (Mr. Tai). 'Life? Here? It is something regarding meals' (Mr. Bao).

Three mealtimes were the most important regular activities conducted in the nursing home. Even though they might avoid other social activities, most residents would never skip a meal. The quote, 'You can forget to take medicines, but you cannot forget to eat food' (Ms. Lu), evokes the importance with which mealtimes were held. The residents sought to gain both physical energy and psychological satisfaction from their meals. 'It is blessed and it means a very good fortune, if you still can eat', said one resident, Mr. Yu.

Without any official announcement at mealtimes, the residents routinely transferred themselves to their eating locations in the corridor outside the nursing station, at the desks of the nursing station or at their bedsides in their rooms. The residents came from different directions, walking, pushing themselves in wheelchairs or with assistance from the NAs.

Although little literature has directly discussed the notion of mealtimes being the highlight of nursing home life, several studies have shown the importance of mealtimes in nursing homes (Kayser-Jones 2000, Nijs et al. 2005). Additionally, the Chinese cultural emphasis on meals contributes further to the importance of mealtimes. As Li and Hsieh (2004) and Wu (1995) have suggested, mealtimes are one of the most important daily activities of Chinese people. The older residents would inevitably act according to this belief and pay significant attention to food.

Every Day is the Same. A fixed schedule and environment, relatively fixed housemates, and a regular routine of care tasks made life in the nursing home seem immutable and frozen. 'Nursing home life is nothing but routine' said Mr. Han. From the moment the residents opened their eyes in the morning, the same routine tasks were performed every day. Everyone seemed to follow an unseen timetable marking the patterns of their days. Sadly, the timetable was not set by the residents, but was the timetable of the staff. The residents passively obeyed the care provider's order and schedule. Based on the field notes, an A0 sized poster placed on the bulletin board in the corridor indicated the daily routine. Interestingly, what was indicated was only the timetable for an ordinary day, not a weekly or monthly schedule. This implied that each day's activities would be almost the same as that of every other day.

> I am doing the same things every day . . . They told me when to eat then I eat. They told me when to sleep then I sleep. (Mr. Chi)

A fixed schedule, set in advance for each task, dominates life in the nursing home: the residents and staff live almost entirely according to the routine of the nursing home. This in turn lends an overwhelming sameness to the pattern of life experienced in the nursing home. However, this way of providing care is heavily focused towards the group, and the needs of individuals are easily neglected.

Without any choice or control over everyday matters, the residents seldom felt valued, and tended to have low levels of self-esteem (Kane 2001). One study has responded to this problem, suggesting that providing residents with more opportunities to make their own decisions concerning their care is necessary (Mullins & Hartley 2002). The fact that the timetable for each day is driven by the schedule of the staff matches with Lo *et al.*'s (2002) fiindings, where it was indicated that nursing homes tend to have schedules fixed for the convenience of the staff. This behaviour has been shown to have a negative impact on residents' feelings of autonomy (Mattiasson *et al.* 1997). Two other studies have also described the relatively fixed everyday events and activities of residents in nursing homes (Liukkonen 1995), Chang & Fang 2004). This suggests that the phenomenon of 'everyday is the same' appears to be present in a variety of nursing homes internationally.

The Ceiling is My Best Mate. Feelings of loneliness and isolation often marked the faces of the residents, and regularly filled their conversations and behaviours. Although the residents lived in a nursing 'home' with a large number of people, they still felt 'home alone' in their minds.

During a typical day, few people voluntarily came to the residents' sides to provide them company or talk to them, except when a necessary task was performed by the staff. It was difficult for the staff to stay with each resident after completing the tasks, because they had to hurriedly move to the next resident to continue their routine care. Most of the time, the residents were all alone. In the field notes I recorded that:

> Mr. Chen sits in the wheelchair in front of a desk in the nursing station . . .
> His face keeps toward the ground and seldom looks up. Sometimes, he
> grabs the water in the baby's bottle with a straw inside the hole of the nipple
> to sip the water. Then, he puts the bottle back to the desk and looks down
> again. He has been sitting there for 1½ hours, and no one had talked with
> him until one NA brought his food tray and said two words 'It's mealtime'.

Two female residents described their feelings of loneliness. 'I just lie here all day. No one. No one will come to talk to me. I am all alone' (Ms. Mu). 'The ceiling is my best mate. I stare at the ceiling when I am lying in the bed. The ceiling is the only one who will not leave me alone' (Ms. Lu).

Making friends was also not easy in the nursing home. Internal factors, such as hearing difficulties, marked accents, conservative personalities and declining physical functions, as well as external factors, such as fewer arranged social activities and no dining room, tended to affect the residents' social relationships with the other residents. One resident described the difficulty of making friends in the nursing home:

> He does not understand what I am talking about because of the marked accent and I do not understand what he is talking about due to my difficulties hearing. (Mr. Ken)

Feelings of loneliness are experienced by the older nursing home residents. This matches with the findings of several earlier studies (Bondevik & Skogstad 1996, Chan & Kayser-Jones 2005). Bergman-Evans (2004) argued that feelings of loneliness may be twofold amongst the cognitively intact residents. Despite the fact that the nursing home is collective and that there may be many opportunities to interact with others, the residents still felt alone. The inadequate numbers of staff, difficulty of making friends and the infrequency of visits from friends and families also contribute to the feelings of loneliness experienced by the residents. As Thomas (1996) has pointed out, the feeling of loneliness is exacerbated by a lack of companionship. As well, several studies have indicated that companionship and emotional support provided by families, friends and staff can dilute the feelings of loneliness experienced by nursing home residents (Bondevik & Skogstad 1998, Chan & Kayser-Jones 2005).

Care Rituals

Care rituals describe and interpret both the care provided for the residents of the nursing home, and the actions that the nurses perform whilst providing care. It suggests that nursing staff deliver care in a rationalised, ritualistic and unthinking way, and that they do this because this is the way it has always been done. The staff tend to follow a fixed tempo of routines and practices without thinking too much. Two categories of 'perception of inadequate staffing in spite of the legal requirements being met', and the 'to do rather than to be' attitude are used to expand on the theme of care rituals.

Perception of Inadequate Staffing in Spite of the Legal Requirements Being Met. According to the Nurses' Act 2000, the nurse-to-resident ratio is 1:15, and nursing assistant-to-resident ratio is 1:5 in Taiwanese nursing homes. These ratios, however, are based on the numbers of nursing staff to beds in a 24-hour period, meaning that the numbers do not reveal how many residents a nurse must provide care for during each shift. As the total number of beds in this nursing home is 90, according to the regulations there should be at least six nurses and 18 NAs. On the surface, the total number of staff clearly matched the requirements, but the number of staff on-duty was insufficient based on my observations and the interviews with the staff, residents and family members. Ms. Lee, one NA, remarked, 'We are busy, just like a rotating top. Just keep moving and no time to stop. One thing after another after another'.

It was obvious that the theoretically adequate numbers of staff did not tally with the practical realities. The nursing station would usually be empty in a regular morning and all the nursing staff would be engaged with their daily tasks. The problem appears to rest in the fact that the legal requirements lack a holistic and realistic approach to nursing home needs. A variety of practical problems, illnesses, dependency levels and conditions of the residents have not been appropriately taken into account in the current requirements for 'adequate' staffing.

Other studies have shown that the time devoted to each resident by NAs is between 92-02 and 137-4 minutes direct resident care per day in long-term care facilities (Chen *et al.* 2003, Li & Yin 2005). However, no Taiwanese studies have reported nursing time. In this study, the range of the nurse time per resident per day was 29–38 minutes and NA time was 87–115 minutes. These figures are based on the calculation of the number of on-duty nurses and NAs in relation to the number of elderly residents cared for in the nursing home during the observation period. However, the exact time of direct care for each resident might be less than these figures, given the time nursing staff need to spend handing over, doing paperwork, and arranging medicines. Even without taking this into account, these figures are lower than the 168 minutes of care provided by NAs (Centers for Medicare and Medicaid Services 2001) and 75 minutes of care provided by registered nurses (Health Care Financing Administration 2000) reported in the USA; the NA time is, however, similar to that found in the Taiwanese studies stated above.

'To Do Rather than to be': Task-Oriented Care. Due to the heavy work load, both nurses and NAs were inclined to interact with the residents in a formal manner, allowing them to deliver the mandatory and instrumental tasks efficiently. Spending time to do the assigned job rather than to be with the residents was the obvious fact in the nursing home. As one NA, Ms. Wu, said, 'Right after you begin to work, you just want to finish the assigned tasks as soon as possible. That's your job'.

The nursing home is hospital based, and has a medical-oriented care model toward the provision of physical rather than emotional care, might also contribute to the task-oriented approach to care evidenced in the nursing staff. The staff paid significant attention to 'completing their tasks'. Finishing all the assigned tasks indicated to the staff that the duty of the work shift was complete. Furthermore, physical tasks were easy to identify and monitor, so were given careful attention. In the field notes:

> One NA, Ms. Sun, was nasogastric feeding Mr. Goom. She earnestly focused on the diet, the feeding syringe . . . She followed the right procedures and carefully injected the food into the tube. Mr. Goom watched her. However, she didn't talk with Mr. Goom or regularly make eye contact with him. It was very quiet. She just concentrated on finishing the feeding.

As well, the nurses completed the documentation of the Activities of Daily Living (ADL) scale and fall assessment tool once a week, because these were required by the nursing home. However, no cognitive or psychological assessments, such as the Mini-Mental State Examination (MMSE) or geriatric depression scales, were ever used to screen the residents' problems. It appeared as though the nurses worked solely to finish their assigned tasks, while ignoring any care requirements that were not assigned.

A task-oriented approach to care has been observed in a variety of long-term care settings (McCormack 2003, Swagetty *et al.* 2005). Kane (2001) has suggested that those providing care need to prioritise persons before tasks. Such a change in emphasis would move a task-oriented form of care towards a more resident-centred approach to care (Chu 2004, Robinson & Rosher 2006), in turn providing a more flexible and individualised form of care (Gnaedinger 2003).

Embedded Beliefs

The values and beliefs of the residents and staff of the nursing home can be described by the notions of 'patients and hospitalisation' and 'compromise'. The residents and staff rarely expressed these concepts in their conversations, but they were clearly evident in their behaviours and practices.

Patients and Hospitalisation. The concepts of being a patient and hospitalisation were embedded in the minds of several residents and staff. This nursing home has a hospital-like appearance. All staff wear uniforms and provide major physical and medical-oriented care. These factors combine to make it difficult for the nursing home to have truly homelike atmosphere. The residents usually claimed that they were hospitalised rather than living in a 'home'. They frequently called themselves or the other residents 'patients' rather than 'residents'. However, living in a hospital-like environment also allowed them to feel they have safe access to medical care. Moreover, the residents tended to accept the role of being a patient to excuse their admission to the nursing home.

The hospital-based layout of the nursing home could easily contribute to feelings amongst the residents of institutionalisation and a non-home-like atmosphere. Similarly, one study has found that Taiwanese nursing homes are designed to be more like hospitals than American nursing homes (Chang & Fang 2004). However, various studies have suggested that modern long-term care facilities need to remove their traditional hospital-like image and work towards more home-like settings (Wang & Kuo 2006, Woodhouse 2006).

Furthermore, the traditional Confucian value of filial piety also contributes to this notion. Families felt that they had the moral responsibility to take care of their dependent elders (Liu *et al.* 2003), and that admission to the nursing home somehow violated that duty (Lee *et al.* 2002a,b). Consequently, it appears that families used the idea of hospitalisation to protect themselves from feeling 'guilty' about the violation of this duty. The residents also embraced such an understanding, persuading themselves that their admission was to improve their conditions, and not because of their family's failure to practice filial piety. They tended to internalise the role of being a patient in order to maintain their self-esteem and a good relationship with their families. Accordingly, this traditional Chinese concept helps to account for why the residents thought they were hospitalised.

Compromise. Compromise for the sake of harmony is considered, in Chinese culture, a kind of virtue. It emphasises traditions of balance, harmony and collectivism. For satisfying their social identities, Chinese people are often told to be cooperative, well-mannered, compromising, self-suppressive and non-confrontational. Beyond this cultural impetus, some residents were retired from the military and were used to obeying orders. All of this combined to create an environment of obedience in the nursing home. Newly admitted residents would be told the house rules. They would view these rules as the 'law of the land', which they would try to obey in order to cause less trouble for the staff. They also observed other residents' behaviours and activities, adapting their own to the norm to achieve balance and harmony in the nursing home. They tried to hide their feelings, not saying or doing what they thought was the wrong thing so as not to harm the balance of the nursing home. They also tried to tolerate any difficulties or discomforts that were forced upon them, and shied away from asking or bothering the staff.

Mr. Chang . . . had difficulty eating his meal . . . After 30 minutes, there was still a lot remaining . . . Later, his wife told me that, 'He is shy to ask for help and feels embarrassment for doing it'.

As the residents said, 'I don't want to say anything to make trouble and make the relationships worse. If it is not gone too far and I still can tolerate it, I will make no complaint' (Mr. Gu).

If something or someone might damage the harmony of the institution or the relationship between the residents and the staff, the residents would try to avoid them. They silently accepted all things that happened to them. They then rationalised this behaviour, providing reasons such as the business of the nursing staff, karma, or a group life. They tried to compromise and practice their benevolence to achieve their own goal: maintaining harmony while living in the nursing home.

This finding matches with the findings of Kuo and Kavanagh (1994), who suggested that social conflicts in nursing homes would often be avoided to prevent 'losing face'. Similarly, Chao and Roth (2005) found that nursing home residents often attempted to suppress their voices, and worry about making trouble for their care providers. Passive acceptance was another strategy the residents used to cope with life in the nursing home. For many residents, the way to fit into a new nursing home environment was to accept the established routines and norms (Lee *et al.* 2002a,b).

Additionally, in Chinese culture, it is considered inappropriate to challenge experts (Chen 2001a). The staff are often regarded as professional experts by the residents, which means the residents would avoid challenging their views.

Conclusions

This study gives unique insight into health care culture by describing the nursing home members' thoughts, behaviours and practice. A tedious, monotonous, idle and lonely life is experienced by the residents in the nursing home, and insufficient staffing is obvious, despite the legal staffing requirements being met. This is exacerbated by the provision of care that is task-oriented rather than individually driven. The residents, whether consciously or not, consider themselves to be the patients of a hospital, and will compromise to maintain harmony and balance in the nursing home life.

This study makes a strong contribution to the existing literature on the nursing home culture. It provides practical information for nursing staff, managers, educators and policy-makers, such as improving the existed care protocols. In the future, a change in nursing home culture would be appropriate to promote a more resident-centred form of care and to enhance the provision of individualised care.

Contributions

Study design, data analysis and manuscript preparation: Y-HC, JA; data collection: Y-HC.

References

Atkinson P, Coffey A, Delamont S, Lofland J & Lofland I. (2001) *Handbook of Ethnography.* Sage, Thousand Oaks.

Bauer I (1994) *Patients' Privacy; An Exploratory Study of Patients' Perception of Their Privacy in a German Acute Care Hospital.* Avebury, Aldershot, UK.

Bergman-Evans B (2004) Beyond the basics: effects of the Eden alternative model on quality of life issues. *Journal of Gerontological Nursing* 30, 27–34.

Bondevik M & Skogstad A (1996) Loneliness among the oldest old, a comparison between residents living in nursing homes and residents living in the community. *International Journal of Aging & Human Development* 43, 181–197.

Bondevik M & Skogstad A (1998) The oldest old, ADL., social network, and loneliness. *Western Journal of Nursing Research* 20, 325.

Centers for Medicare and Medicaid Services (2001) *Report to Congress: Appropriateness of Minimum Nurse Staffing Ratios in Nursing Home Phase II Final Report*. Department of Health and Human Services. Washington: US.

Chan J & Kayser-Jones J (2005) The experience of dying for Chinese nursing home residents: cultural considerations. *Journal of Gerontological Nursing* 31, 26–32.

Chang SH & Fang MC (2004) The elderly living in nursing homes: cross-culture comparison. *Tzu Chi Nursing Journal (Chinese)* 3, 41–49.

Chao SY & Roth P (2005) Dimensions of quality in long-term care facilities in Taiwan. *Journal of Advanced Nursing* 52, 609–619.

Chen S (2001a) A model to assess perceptions of need for nursing homes in community settings. *Journal of Theory Construction and Testing* 5, 15–18.

Chen YC (2001b) Chinese values, health and nursing. *Journal of Advanced Nursing* 36, 270–273.

Chen M (2002) *The Adaptation Process of the Elderly in Long-term Care Facilities*. National Chi-Nan University, Puli.

Chen CJ, Su HF, Hsieh PC & Wang M (2003) The relationship between facility characteristics and the quality of care in nursing homes. *The Journal of Nursing (Chinese)* 50, 62–67.

Chu E (2004) A pluralistic approach to resident centred care. *Perspectives (Gerontological Nursing Association (Canada))* 27, 14–16.

Deutschman MT (2005) An ethnographic study of nursing home culture to define organizational realities of culture change. *Journal of Health and Human Services Administration* 28, 246–281.

Diamond T (1992) *Making Gray Old: Narratives of Nursing Home Care*. University of Chicago Press, Chicago, IL.

Farmer BC (1996) *A Nursing Home and Its Organizational Climate*. Auburn House, London.

Fiveash B (1998) The experience of nursing home life. *International Journal of Nursing Practice* 4, 166–174.

Geertz C (1973) *The Interpretation of Cultures*. Basic Books, New York.

Gibson DE & Barsade SG (2003) Managing organization culture change: the case of long-term care. In *Culture Change in Long-Term Care* (Weiner AS & Ronch JL. eds). The Haworth Press, New York, pp. 11–34.

Gnaedinger N (2003) Changes in long-term care for elderly people with dementia: a report from the front lines in British Columbia, Canada. *Journal of Social Work in Long-Term Care* 2, 355–371.

Graneheim UH & Lundman B (2004) Qualitative content analysis in nursing research: concepts, procedures and measures to achieve trustworthiness. *Nurse Education Today* 24, 105–112.

Hammersley M & Atkinson P (1995) *Ethnography: Principles in Practice*, 2nd edn. Routledge, London.

Health Care Financing Administration (2000) *Report to congress: Appropriateness of minimum nurse staffing rations in nursing homes*. US Government Printing Office, Washington, DC.

Huang HL & Chang M (2006) Analysis and Implementation of research findings on the decision making in institutionalization of the elderly: a family-centered perspective. *The Journal of Nursing (Chinese)* 53, 58–64.

Kane RA (2001) Long-term care and a good quality of life: bringing them closer together. *The Gerontologist* 41, 293–304.

Kayser-Jones J (2000) Improving the nutritional care of nursing home residents. *Nursing Homes: Long Term Care Management* 49, 56.

Kuo CL & Kavanagh KH (1994) Chinese perspectives on culture and mental health. *Issues in Mental Health Nursing* 15, 551–567.

LeCompte MD & Schensul JJ (1999) *Designing and Conducting Ethnographic Research.* Altamira, New York.

Lee C., Liu T, Wu L, Chung U and Lee L (2002a) Cost and care quality between licensed nursing homes under different types of ownership. *Journal of Nursing Research* 10, 151–160.

Lee DTF, Woo J & Mackenzie AE (2002b) The cultural context of adjusting to nursing home life: Chinese elders perspectives. *The Gerontologist* 42, 667–675.

Li JR & Hsich YHP (2004) Traditional Chinese food technology and cuisine. *Asia Pacific Journal of Clinical Nutrition* 13, 147–155.

Li JC & Yin TJ (2005) Care needs of residents in community-based long-term care facilities in Taiwan. *Journal of Clinical Nursing* 14, 711–718.

Lin L, Ou M & Wu S (1998) Factors influencing morale among the elderly in long-term care. *Kaohstung Journal of Medical Sciences* 14, 357–366.

Liu LF & Tinker A (2003) Admission to nursing homes in Taiwan. *Social Policy and Administration* 37, 376–394.

Liu J. Ng SH, Loong C, Gee S & Weatherall A (2003) Cultural stereotypes and social representations of elders from Chinese and European perspectives. *Journal of Cross-Cultural Gerontology* 18, 149–168.

Liukkonen A (1995) Life in a nursing home for the trail elderly. *Clinical Nursing Research* 4, 358–372.

Lo J, Huang S, Mao H, Tsai Y, Lin H, Lee S & Chang J (2002) The current status and needs of residents in nursing home facilities. *Journal of Occupational Therapy Association, R O C* 20, 95–106.

Mattiasson A, Andersson L, Mullins LC & Moody L (1997) A comparative empirical study of autonomy in nursing home in Sweden and Florida, USA. *Journal of Cross-Cultural Gerontology* 14, 299–316.

McCormack B (2003) A conceptual framework for person-centred practice with older people. *International Journal of Nursing Practice* 9, 202–209.

Miles MB & Huberman AM (1994) *Qualitative Data Analysis: An Expanded Sourcebook,* 2nd edn, Sage, Thousand Oaks.

Mullins LC & Harley TM (2002) Residents' autonomy: nursing home personnel's perceptions *Journal of Gerontological Nursing* 28, 35–44.

Nijs KAND, de Graaf C, Kok FJ & van Staveren WA (2005) Effect of family style mealtimes on quality of life, physical performance and body weight of nursing home residents: cluster randomized controlled trial. *BMJ* 332, 1180–1184.

Price B (2004) Ethnographic research and older people. *Nursing Older People* 15, 22–27.

Robinson SB & Rosher RB (2006) Tangling with the barriers to culture change: creating a resident-centered nursing home environment. *Journal of Gerontological Nursing* 32, 19–25.

Savishinsky J (1991) *The Ends of Time. Life and Work in a Nursing Home.* Bergin and Garvey, New York.

Schopp A, Leino-Kilpi H, Vaimaki M, Dassen T, Gasull M, Lemonidou C, Scott PA, Arndt M & Kaljonen A (2003) Perceptions of privacy in the care of elderly people in five European countries. *Nursing Ethics* 10, 39–47.

Shield RR (1988) *Uneasy Endings.* Cornell University Press, Ithaca NY.

Streubert Speziale HJ & Carpenter DR (2003) *Qualitative Research in Nursing: Advancing the Humanistic Imperative,* 3rd edn. Lippincott Williams & Wilkins, Philadelphia, PA.

Swagerty DL, Lee RH, Smith B & Taunton RL (2005) The context for nursing home resident care. *Journal of Gerontological Nursing* 31, 40–48.

Taiwan Long-Term Care Professional Association (2005) *The Book of the Resources of Long-Term Care in Taiwan.* Taiwan Long-Term Care Professional Association, Taipei.

Thomas WH (1996) *Life Worth Living* Vander Wky and Burnham Acton, MA.

Tisdale S (1987) *Harvest Moon: Portrait of a Nursing Home*, Holt New York.

Tseng SZ & Wang RH (2002) Quality of life and related factors among elderly nursing home residents in southern Taiwan. *Public Health Nursing* 18, 304–311.

Twigg J (2002) The body in social policy: mapping a territory. *Journal of Social Policy* 31, 421–439.

Vladeck BC (1980) *Unloving Care.* Basic Books, New York.

Wang CH & Kuo NW (2006) Zeitgeists and development trends in long-term care facility design. *The Journal of Nursing Research (Chinese)* 14, 123–132.

Woodhouse M (2006) Making a new home: the importance of a home-like setting in nursing homes. *Sociological Viewpoints* 22, 103–110.

Wu YM (1995) Food and health: the impact of the Chinese traditional philosophy of food on the young generation in the modern world. *Nutrition and Food Science* 95, 23–27.

Wu SC., Lai HL & Chiang TL (1997) The influence of intergenerational exchange on nursing home admission in Taiwan. *Journal of Cross-Cultural Gerontology* 12, 163–174.

Wu SC, Ke D & Su TL (1998) The prevalence of cognitive impairment among nursing home residents in Taipei, Taiwan. *Neuroepidemiology* 17, 147–153.

Yang C (2000) Indicators of quality of care in nursing homes from the perspective of elderly residents' families. *The Journal of Long-Term Care (Chinese)* 4, 33–41.

Yang C (2001) Indicators of quality of care for nursing homes: from the perspectives of residents, family and nurses. *Taiwan Journal of Public Health (Chinese)* 20, 238–247.

Yang C. (2002) Indicators of quality of care for nursing homes: nurses' perspectives. *The Journal of Nursing (Chinese)* 49, 39–54.

Yeh S, Lin L, Wang W, Wu S, Lin J & Tsai F (2001) The outcomes of restraint reduction program in nursing homes. *The Journal of Nursing Research (Chinese)* 9, 183–193.

Yeh S, Lin L & Lo SK (2003) A longitudinal evaluation of nursing home care quality in Taiwan. *Journal of Nursing Care Quality* 18, 209–216.

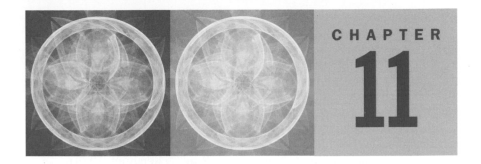

Historical Research Method

Nursing care for patients always includes acquiring a nursing history. If nurses did not collect background data, they would—through ignorance—greatly jeopardize decisions regarding a client's current health care needs and future chance of achieving a higher level of wellness. A historical understanding is also crucial to providing nursing care because of nursing's essential holistic nature. Looking at the whole person requires recognition of multiple factors that influence the individual. Similarly, decisions related to the nursing profession, such as the current shortage, risk failure, and inadequacy of response if the profession ignores its history.

In an editorial in *Nursing History Review* (*NHR*), D'Antonio (2004) questions whether nurse historians are "in the process of proclaiming history as an overarching intellectual paradigm for a practice discipline that draws its strengths from its contextual specificity and ideological flexibility" (p. 1). History may serve as a "new paradigm for nursing knowledge" (p. 1). D'Antonio's editorial sets the stage for this chapter on historical research method. Nurses need knowledge to practice. Their social contract with society and commitment to provide culturally competent care requires in-depth knowing and understanding. History allows us to look at events in the past from a variety of lenses, thus allowing us to interpret data in a number of different ways. The ability to examine past events gives meaning and texture to the care nurses provide, influences the way we educate new nurses, and provides the background to influence public and political support. Moreover, history can provide important evidence for the health care decisions being made today (Lewenson, 2008).

All knowledge has a historical dimension; conversely, history provides individuals with a way of knowing. Tholfsen (1977) explained that "the past is present in every person and in the cultural and institutional world that surrounds [them]" (p. 248). This means, Tholfsen continued, that historians must know the historical conditions of the period they are studying. Knowledge of the past helps to inform research designs that include explanatory background necessary to establish an understanding of the phenomenon under study. Selecting historical research design as the research method of choice requires that researchers understand what history is; possess an understanding of various social, political, and economic factors that affect events, ideas, and people; have interest in the subject; and be creative in their approaches (Christy, 1978; Rines & Kershner, 1979).

Historical research provides a critical way of knowing. There are, however, many ways to study the past, and, depending on the framework used, the understanding will differ. For example, the way we have studied nursing over time has changed, alternating from the presentation of nursing heroines to the more recent use of a social feminist framework. Buck (2008) describes how the "practice of history has gone through changes over time, and the influence of the methods and theories of social, political, and cultural inquiry to its evolution during the 20th century has been significant" (p. 45). Connolly (2004) asks us to broaden the study of history and writes that political history along with social history can provide important data needed for arguing the case from a political perspective for more nurses and other important related health care issues. "Nurse historians have expertise linking the stories of individual patients and nurses to their larger institutional framework, a natural link to the broader political context" (Connolly, 2004, p. 18).

Yet, historians can more easily explain why they do historical research than the steps involved in doing it. Even with the various tools and approaches available, there remains a certain "inexactness with which historians define, delineate and defend their particular research methodology" (D'Antonio, 2005, p. 1). The inability to clearly explain the process leads to a "methodological vulnerability" (p. 1) that in turn makes it more difficult to explain and understand what a historian does, ultimately jeopardizing the ability to pass this knowledge on to future historians (D'Antonio, 2005).

Throughout this chapter and Chapter 12, the reader will learn about the steps involved in historical research methodology including a brief discussion about the use of oral history and biography. Learning to do historical research requires an understanding and acceptance of the often circuitous nature of the process. In an attempt to demonstrate the number of ways historical research has been defined, refined, and applied over time, the sections "Historical Research Defined" and "Historical Research Traditions" will help to illustrate the iterative and nonlinear aspects of the process.

HISTORICAL RESEARCH DEFINED

*M*any definitions and explanations exist related to the meaning and nature of history. Austin (1958) defined *history* as "an integrated, written record of past events, based on the results of a search for the truth" (p. 4).

Kruman (1985) explained history as "facts (ideas, events, social, and cultural processes) filtered through human intelligence" (p. 111). Kruman referred to an *objective relativism* that permits the objective reality of one historian to coexist with different historical interpretations of others, thus promoting change in ideas and advances in historical inquiry. Matejski (1986) conceived of history "as a past event, a record, or account of something that has happened" (p. 175). Furthermore, Matejski described history as a field of study with its own set of criteria and methods that enable researchers to collect data and interpret findings. Having its own method that has often borrowed from other disciplines, historical inquiry examines the interactions of people, activities, and "multiple variables" (Matejski, 1986, p. 177) that affect human thought and activity. The narrative that results from a historian's findings must creatively weave many factors into a readable and interesting story.

Historical research opens windows into the past, creating new ideas and reshaping human thinking and understanding. Ashley (1978) explained the crucial role historical research plays in the foundation of nursing scholarship by defining history as "the study of creative activity in human behavior [that] gives one the courage to create and respond to what is new without fear of losing one's identity with the whole of humanity" (p. 28). As Lynaugh (1996) suggested, history becomes "our source of identity . . . it helps us gain identity and personal meaning in our work, improves our comprehension and our planning, and validates social criticism" (p. 1).

Like nursing, history is an art and science. Olson (2000) stresses the link between the art and science of history and calls for a dialogue among historians to include quantifiable data along with qualitative data. Olson further notes that "quantifiable information from public and private records is often crucial to uncovering the seemingly hidden history of women" (p. 138). Demonstrating the use of numbers to explain past phenomena, Olson examined the school records of the St. Luke's Hospital Training School for Nurses between the years 1892 and 1937. These records provided the quantifiable data that told a "story" about those who attended this Midwest school. The discipline of history requires the use of scientific principles to study the interrelationship of social, economic, political, and psychological factors that influence ideas, events, institutions, and people. Yet, to explain the findings of historical inquiry while balancing the rigors of scientific inquiry and the understanding of human behavior, historical researchers must revert to the "art of contemplation, speculation, and of interpretation" (Newton, 1965, p. 24).

Researchers who choose historical methods must exhibit more than just a curiosity about the past. Researchers formulate a thesis about the relationship among ideas, events, institutions, or people in the past. Chronologically ordering events over time does not explain the established links and ties. Probing for explanations between historical antecedents requires questioning, reasoning, and interpreting. Christy (1978) explained that "healthy skepticism becomes a way of life for the serious historiographer" (p. 6). Historians seeking to discover meanings in the past must sift through data and examine each piece closely for clues.

D'Antonio (1999) speaks of the use of cross-disciplinary interpretation in the writing and rewriting of nursing history. This "'two-way street' between the historical traditions of nursing and those of the liberal arts" (p. 268) has led to significant change in the understanding of nurses' work. For it is the historians' "active engagement in the process of theorizing—of generating and testing broader ideas about meaning and significance that might ultimately change our perception of the work and worth of nursing" (D'Antonio, 2008, p. 20). Most historical nursing research in the late 20th century will include some kind of reference to issues related to gender, class, race, and politics of professionalism (D'Antonio, 1999). Yuginovich (2000) states, "history is probably a stronger force than language in molding our social consciousness" (p. 70). Examining nurses' roles as women, caregivers, leaders, administrators, educators, and practitioners in light of a multidisciplinary framework provides the historian with a variety of useful sources, broad interpretations, and necessary tools in which to examine data.

When studying the past, historical researchers use a variety of sources, such as private letters, personal and professional journals, books, magazines, and newspapers. Researchers travel in time and explore these materials, seeking a relationship among ideas, events, institutions, or people. The purpose of a historical study is not to predict but, rather, to understand the past in order to explain present or future relationships. From historical documents, historical researchers derive insight from past lived experiences that they can adapt to generate new ideas (Barzun & Graff, 1985).

Researchers use a historical design if they believe something from the past will explain something in the present or the future. Conflict between what the researcher thinks and what he or she may have read about a particular topic also influences the decision to do historical research. For example, a misconception regarding nurses' participation in the late 19th century women's movement led Lewenson (1990, 1996) to study the relationship between the women's suffrage movement and the four nursing organizations that formed in America between 1893 and 1920. Lewenson conducted a historical inquiry to dispel the tension resulting from a contemporary understanding of the past, also called a present-mindedness, which omitted nursing's political response to the events of the late 19th and early 20th centuries.

Present-mindedness refers to using a contemporary perspective when analyzing data collected from an earlier period. Such data analysis is stigmatized as unhistorical and leads to inaccurate conclusions when ideas and lived experiences of people in the past are compared with later events (Tholfsen, 1977, p. 247). Although Tholfsen warned historians to be careful of absolutes and the dangers of present-mindedness, he has argued that "the best history is rooted in a lively interest in the present" (p. 247).

Nevertheless, history refers to constant change, and it is this change that "produces the endless diversity characteristic of the historical world" (p. 248). Researchers must study each period within the context of its age to avoid judging or interpreting the past without respect to changes made over time. Hence, difference found in every age must "be understood in its own terms" (p. 248).

Nursing is a field ripe for historical research. Nurses come from rich, diverse backgrounds that are useful in helping to better understand and explain human behavior. Nurses, who are adept at studying human behavior, are well suited to conduct historical inquiry in which they study human behavior in the context of an event, a place, a person, an institution, or an idea in the past. Like historians, nurses identify and interpret patterns of behavior that occur over time.

HISTORICAL RESEARCH TRADITIONS

*M*orse and Field (1995) identified two traditions or schools of thought in historical research: the positivistic or neopositivistic and the idealist schools. In the *neopositivistic school*, historians take a more quantitative posture. The focus is on "reducing history to universal laws" (p. 33). Historians use data analysis to verify or categorize information. "There is a strong effort to show cause–effect relationships" (p. 33).

In the *idealist school*, historians are most concerned with getting inside an event and trying to understand the thoughts of individuals involved in the event while considering the time, place, and situations (Fitzpatrick, 2001; Morse & Field, 1995). The idealist school is more closely aligned with the values of qualitative research represented in the present text.

Regardless of the tradition observed by historical researchers, the intent is always the "interpretation and narration of past events" (Morse & Field, 1995, p. 33). Historical researchers must clearly identify the focus of the study and then make a commitment to a philosophic position.

Historical research design is being distinguished from other qualitative designs that build on positivistic traditions (D'Antonio, 2005). D'Antonio briefly describes Gaddis's (2002) four methodological practices that structure historical research and separate this design from that of others. Historians look for interactions between and among variables and how these interactions might effect change. The historian plays with the idea of what might have happened if the variables changed. For example, what would have happened if Nightingale did not go to the Crimean War or if Lavinia Dock did not advocate women's suffrage? This helps historians sharpen their focus on "other events, actors, social themes, or political processes that might otherwise remain hidden" (D'Antonio, 2005, p. 2). Historians look for "contextual specificity" and do so by placing an event within a specific time frame and then examining the time leading up to the event, as well as following the course of the event. Judgments are made about the various factors or variables that contribute to the story. D'Antonio believes that this is where the distinction between historical research and other methods exists. Historians must "consider and assess the significance of the work completed by other historical methods and make judgments" (p. 2).

FUNDAMENTAL CHARACTERISTICS OF HISTORICAL RESEARCH

Although no single historical method exists, Lynaugh and Reverby (1987) have offered essential guideposts and rules of evidence to ensure the credibility and usefulness of the historian's findings. Lusk (1997) has identified several methodological stages, including selecting "a topic and an appropriate theoretical framework, finding and accessing the resources, and analyzing, synthesizing, interpreting, and reporting the data" (p. 355). In search of an approach, Barzun and Graff (1985) wrote that, "without form in every sense, the facts of the past, like the jumbled visions of a sleeper in a dream, elude us" (p. 271).

The next section offers beginning historical researchers a guide to developing a historical study. As in any process, researchers must allow fluidity between the steps of the guide, that is, they must easily move from one step to another, in both directions. For example, the data collected may direct the literature review, and the literature review, in turn, may determine the thesis.

SELECTION OF HISTORICAL RESEARCH AS METHOD

To understand the wholeness of the past, nurse historians select a framework to guide the study. However, as Lynaugh and Reverby (1987) have warned, no one formula or specific method exists for doing historical research. Tholfsen (1977) contends that "history lacks a coherent theoretical and conceptual structure" (p. 246). No one theoretical framework exists for the study of history. Although there is no "set methodology . . . some methodological consensus exists" (Lusk, 1997, p. 355). History is a discipline with many structures that Cramer (1992) describes as "permanent or semipermanent relations of elements that determine the character of the whole" (p. 6). Superimposed structure enables researchers to organize data. For example, when using geography to frame a study, the researcher may write a regional history, or when using a particular topic to organize a study, the researcher may focus on women's work (Cramer, 1992).

Society asks historians to analyze experiences and use the information gained to explain and prepare society for similar events in the future. For example, historians study the records of war so that society will learn what may help in future wars (Hofstadter, 1959). Writing for a specific purpose creates further tension between the dual natures that exist within the historian's role: the writing of a historical narrative and the writing of a historical monograph. According to Hofstadter, the historical narrative tells a story but often is disappointing in the analysis, and the historical monograph approximates a scientific inquiry but lacks literary style and frequently offers insufficient analytic data. However, both functions are enriched by interrelating social sciences and historical inquiry. Hofstadter believes that a combination of social sciences and historical research produces fresh ideas and new insights into human behavior.

Historians look at other disciplines to help inform and structure their work. To understand the development of nursing education in North America and to provide a theoretical framework, historians might use research from women's and educational history in the United States. Knowledge of U.S. labor history, which is important to nursing history because of nurses' apprenticeship role in hospitals, would also be a useful framework for historiographers to conceptually organize data. To study history using a variety of approaches, such as philosophic, national, psychohistorical, or economic, allows researchers to explore a point in time with a conceptual guide from a particular discipline (Ashley, 1978; Matejski, 1986).

Nurse historians consider different theoretical frameworks to structure their historical studies. They may select from theoretical approaches such as biographical, social, and intellectual histories. A *biographical history*, the study of an individual, opens a wide vista to an entire period (Brown, D'Antonio, & Davis, 1991). Biography uses the story of a person's life to understand "the values, expectations, tensions and the conflicts of the time and culture within which he or she lived" (Brown et al., 1991). Interpretation requires historians to familiarize themselves with a period so that they may derive meanings from within the particular time frame rather than superimpose them from a later, contemporary distance. For example, to understand the life of the early 20th-century nurse and birth control activist Margaret Sanger, it is essential to understand society's attitudes about women's roles and beliefs about procreation. Biographical research lends itself to uncovering stories about nurses who participated in the profession. These studies do not need to be limited to the study of more famous nursing leaders (Grypma, 2005, 2008). By studying the lives those who may not have been considered "worthy" of attention in previous periods, historical researchers can enrich and inform the history of nursing.

Social history explores a particular period and attempts to understand the prevailing values and beliefs by examining the everyday events of that period. Connolly (2004) uses a definition of social history that examines the "experience, behavior, and agency of those at society's margins, rather than its elite" (p. 5). Buck (2008) further explains that social history provides "an inclusive framework for reinterpreting the past and experiences of ordinary people, movements, and events through the thematic prisms of class, gender, and race" (p. 46). Exploration into the lives of women, for example, provides a richer understanding of events than were previously available from a "consensus" framework. Individual stories about those outside of the mainstream of American ideas have not been routinely included in historical accounting of events. Historian Vern Bullough recommended a strategy for doing social history. She suggested including the use of specific quantitative data to understand the life experiences of "'ordinary' men and women" (Brown et al., 1991, p. 3). An analysis of census data, court records, and municipal surveys, for example, assists historians to go beyond the boundaries of class, ethnicity, economics, and race—hence enabling them to gain a broader understanding of the study subject. In an example of a social history, Melchior (2004) studied the evolution of nursing history in Canada, utilizing nursing and feminist historical research methods. Melchior argued for "new directions" (p. 340) in nursing history that focus attention on the everyday experience of nurses and nursing students.

Intellectual history, in which *"thinking* is the event under analysis," lends itself to several approaches (Brown et al., 1991, p. 2). Historians may explore the ideas of an individual considered to be an intellectual thinker of a period; for example, they might study the ideas of public health nurses such as Lillian Wald. Or, they may explore the history of ideas over time, such as nursing leaders' ideas that influenced the development of nursing education in the United States. Another approach may be to explore the attitudes and ideas of people who are not considered major intellectual thinkers of the period, such as the ideas of practicing nurses (Hamilton, 1991). While conducting their research, historians must be aware that conflict may arise between the ideas and the contextual backgrounds that gave rise to them (Hamilton, 1993).

Historical researchers must be ready to "live in permanent struggle with conceptual ambiguities, missing evidence and conflicting viewpoints" (Lynaugh & Reverby, 1987, p. 4). Historians continually face a methodological polarity whereby tension exists between the "general and the unique, [and] between the particular and the universal" (Tholfsen, 1977, p. 249). However, these tensions and uncertainties are essential to history because they mirror human experience with all of life's contradictions and ambiguities (Tholfsen, 1977). When approaching historical research, researchers must expect ambiguity of design as well as data. Researchers must decide on a particular theoretical framework and understand the conflicting views and ideas regarding the approach. Keeping this information in mind helps historians construct creative designs that address their particular research interest.

DATA GENERATION

Developing a Focus

To apply a historical design, researchers must first define the study topic and prepare a statement of the subject (Kruman, 1985). A clear, concise statement tells readers what researchers have studied and their reasons for selecting particular subjects. Researchers must explain their interest in the topic and justify its relationship to other topics. In addition, researchers establish the purpose and significance of the study to nursing and nursing research in the statement (Rines & Kershner, 1979). According to Lusk (1997), topics "should be significant, with the potential to illuminate or place a new perspective on current questions" (p. 355).

When selecting a topic, Austin (1958) suggests that the subject be "part of a larger whole, and one which can be isolated" (p. 5). Isolating a part of the topic makes the study more manageable. For example, it may be easier to study the curriculum of three nurse training schools in 1897 than to tackle nursing education in the late 19th century.

Because historical study does not predict outcomes, there is no hypothesis. A researcher's interest and hunches about the topic guide the study and move the research toward a particular field or discipline. Researchers base their ideas on background information they have obtained. Patterns that emerge in the initial fact-finding and knowledge-building steps aid in the creative formation of a thesis. For example, instead of predicting the effect of apprenticeship training on the development of nursing education, historians might identify themes or ideas about nursing education and use those themes to relate their findings. An example is Hanson's (1989) study of the emergence of liberal education in nursing education.

To successfully focus the study, researchers must gather information regarding the period to be studied. They must have a working knowledge of the social, cultural, economic, and political climate that prevailed and how these factors influenced the subject. This knowledge helps researchers establish patterns and identify relevant points regarding the subject and justifies the selection of the historical method. Moreover, when selecting a topic, researchers need to be aware of the accessibility of the sources, the relevance of the topic to the audience, and its potential to enhance understanding (Lusk, 1997).

Selecting a Title

Once historians have identified the focus of the study, it is helpful to delimit the project by titling it. The title tells readers what to expect from the study and narrows the topic for the historian. Typically, the title includes the time frame and purpose, for example, "A Review of Critical Thinking in Nursing: 1990–2000." The title also should entice the reader to read the study and can be creative in using direct quotes from the study to attract readers. One word of caution when using creative titles, such as Flynn's (2009) "Beyond the Glass Wall: Black Canadian Nurses, 1940–1970" or Sampson's (2009) "Alliance of Cooperation: Negotiating New Hampshire Nurse Practitioners' Prescribing Practice" is to be sure that any electronic search on the Internet or databases will locate the work. If the title is too creative, the search engines cannot find the research and, thus, "may lose its potential impact on a large number of readers (Lewenson, 2008, p. 31).

Although the title appears first in a completed study and concisely describes the research topic, it may be the researcher's final step. The advantage of titling a study early in the project is to assist in focusing the work. Historians can always modify the title as the project develops and should be open to change based on newly uncovered data. A well-focused and delimited study will focus the literature search, making it effective and meaningful. It is essential, however, that historians do not prematurely close the literature search because the materials discovered fall outside of the predetermined time frame. Historians should continue their review of materials until they are comfortable that they have fully examined the thesis. It is easier to adjust the title than to risk conducting a poorly developed study.

Conducting a Literature Review

A good starting point for a literature review is to identify major works published on the selected topic. If historians want to study the history of critical thinking, then they must assess what has been written on the subject and identify the themes and inconsistencies related to critical thinking that exist in the literature. Part of the review includes identifying the problems connected with the topic. For example, the ambiguities that have arisen over defining and evaluating critical thinking would be important to the inquiry. A conclusive search of the literature for references from contiguous periods allows for a greater understanding of the subject. Computer databases provide a means by which researchers can obtain data needed in the literature review. Lorentzon (2004) found that the "newly digitalized journal" dating from 1888 until 1956 of the *Nursing Record/British Journal of Nursing* provides an important new avenue for searching topics published in this journal. The *American Journal of Nursing*, first published in 1900, is also digitalized and offers nurse researchers incredible insight into nursing practice since the journal's inception.

A literature review helps researchers formulate questions that need to be addressed, delineate a time frame for the study, and decide on a theoretical framework. In addition, the review affords researchers opportunities to learn what types of materials are available. For example, through the literature review, a researcher will learn whether he or she can obtain primary sources or firsthand accounts of an event, such as the letters written by an individual living during the period of study. The researcher also learns of secondary sources or secondhand accounts of events, such as histories or newspaper articles that have already been written on the particular study subject.

Based on the literature review, historians formulate questions regarding events that influenced the chosen subject. To elucidate the subject, researchers ask questions beginning with "How," "Why," "Who," and "What" in light of the ideas, events, and institutions that existed and individuals who lived during a particular period. If, for example, a researcher narrows a topic such as U.S. public health nursing to the study of public health nurses living at the Henry Street Settlement, then questions such as the following may guide the direction of the literature search: How did the Henry Street Settlement begin? Who began the Henry Street Settlement? What is a settlement house? Why was the settlement located on Henry Street? These questions may prompt the researcher to examine biographies of people who participated in the settlement house movement during the late 19th and early 20th centuries. Or, to better understand life at that time, the historian might read city records regarding population statistics or examine published materials to comprehend another historian's perception of women's roles, education, work, and life during the study period. Newspaper accounts, written histories, proceedings of minutes, photographs, biographies, letters, diaries, and films may help historians seeking a greater understanding of a particular subject.

During the literature review, historians must develop an organizing strategy that will help them analyze the data. Some facts obtained may seem trivial in the beginning of the project but may become crucial to explaining or connecting events learned later in the study. Thus, careful documentation using an index card filing system or a directory in a word processing program will help researchers retrieve the information at a later time (Austin, 1958; Barzun & Graff, 1985). Bibliographic data should be recorded precisely. The bibliographic entry should include the author, title, and abstract, place of publication, date, and particular archive or library where the researcher found the information. Researchers must include all pertinent information in the notes so that, during data analysis, they will be able to easily retrieve important information or go back to the original source, if necessary.

The literature review will serve as the bibliography for the research. Using historical source materials from libraries, archives, bibliographies, newspapers, reviews, journals, associations, and the Internet, researchers begin to comprehend the extent of the subject under investigation (Matejski, 1986). To accomplish this important step, historians use collections in libraries and archives. Libraries and archives contain different types of reference materials that require different methods of storage and classification. To enable researchers to use each method appropriately, it is necessary to become familiar with both.

Libraries contain published materials that researchers often use as secondary materials. To locate these materials, researchers use a card catalog, computerized catalog system, or computerized database that allows them to locate particular works. A call number, usually given in the catalog, designates the unique location of each volume in the library. Volumes are usually arranged by subject. Libraries purchase books and thus permit the use for them to circulate (Termine, 1992), whereas archival materials remain on-site.

Archives differ from libraries in their holdings, cataloging, and circulation policies. Archives contain unpublished materials that are considered primary source materials, such as the "official records of an organization or persons . . . [that] are preserved because of the value of the information they contain" (Termine, 1992). Instead of using a card catalog to find a book, researchers use a *finding aid*, a published book or catalog that lists what is in the archive or repository. The finding aid identifies a collection using a record group, a series, and a subseries. However, instead of material being stored according to these designations, collections are often stored haphazardly within aisles, shelves, and box numbers. Libraries contain a discrete number of volumes, whereas archives contain linear (cubic) feet of records. Archives acquire their material by collections. Many organizations cannot store or maintain their records and transfer this task to archives. For example, a college of nursing may acquire the historical records, including boxes of meeting minutes, curricula, and pictures, of a diploma program that existed in the city before the opening of the collegiate program.

Unlike libraries, where books are circulated, archives require that researchers use the materials on-site. In most archives, researchers may only use pencil and paper to collect data; other archives permit the use of laptop computers. Newer technologic advances have enabled researchers to use handheld scanners in conjunction with their laptop computers. Scanners provide a safe method for copying materials (Lusk, 1997). To gain access to archives, researchers are usually required to make appointments with an archivist to discuss their project. Besides offering researchers primary source references needed in historical research, archives provide materials and memorabilia that researchers may use in exhibitions to illustrate the history of an organization or the life of a person. Because primary source materials may be fragile, archivists will only permit scholars engaged in historical research to use the collections (Termine, 1992). A frequently updated listing of archives containing rich resources for nurse historians can be found on the American Association for the History of Nursing Web site (http://www.aahn.org).

Archivists and librarians assist researchers to access materials, thus rendering an important data gathering service. However, because of the differences between libraries and archives, the work of professional archivists and librarians varies. Whereas archivists work with the records, papers, manuscripts, and nonprinted materials found in the collections, librarians manage books and publications (Termine, 1992). Table 11-1 summarizes the differences between libraries and archives.

The powerful connection between historians and archival materials was part of a discussion during the preconference for the 2004 annual meeting of the American Association for the History of Nursing. Archives provide a setting for nurse historians to relate closely to the subject under study. For historians, the ability to hold the original letters of nursing leaders like Lavinia Dock or Florence Nightingale inspires an almost reverent feeling toward the material and the archives (Rafferty, 2004). Other historians, like Lorentzon (2004), explain that the "musty smell" of paper archives provides

Table 11-1 • Differences between Libraries and Archives		
	Libraries	*Archives*
Holdings	Published materials	Unpublished materials: records, manuscripts, papers
Locators	Card catalog	Finding aid
	Call number	Record group, series, subseries
	Unique location by subject	Haphazard location of "boxes" by aisle, shelf, box number
Stored	Volumes (titles)	Linear (cubic) feet
Acquired	Purchased by volume or issue	Donated or purchased collections
Use of materials	Circulation	Noncirculation; use of paper and pencil only or laptop computer to collect data

Adapted from Termine, J. (1992, March). Paper presented at the State University of New York, Health Science Center at Brooklyn, College of Nursing, Brooklyn, NY, with permission.

the historian with a reassuring sense of ambiance that cannot be replaced by "cold" microfilm readers and computer screens (p. 280). The archives connect historians to vital pieces of data that researchers must read, assess, interpret, and place within the context of the study.

DATA TREATMENT

Identifying Sources

Historians must find some way to understand what actually occurred during a particular period. To research historical antecedents, researchers must identify sources from the period. Primary sources give firsthand accounts of a person's experience, an institution, or an event and may lack critical analysis. However, primary sources, such as personal letters or diaries, may contain the author's interpretation of an event. Thus, researchers must analyze and interpret the meaning of the primary sources. Cordeau (2009) selected a multitude of primary source material dating from the U.S. Civil War period in order to historicize the lived experiences of nurses during this period of time. Examples of primary sources included "letters, diaries, reports, journals, government records, art as well as nursing, medical, and allopathic textbooks" (p. 77).

Ulrich (1990) wrote about Martha Ballard, an 18th-century midwife from Hallowell, Maine. Using Ballard's diary as a primary source, Ulrich wrote a rich biographical account of Ballard, as well as a historical rendering of everyday life during this period. Ballard's diary, which she kept daily for more than 27 years, connected "several prominent themes in the social history of the early Republic" (p. 27). More important, Ulrich explained, "It [the diary] transforms the nature of the evidence upon [which] much of the history of the period has been written" (p. 27). Earlier historians did not consider the potential the diary had for uncovering historical data about this period in the United States. Rather, they perceived Ballard's daily record as trivial and too filled with daily life to be of any importance—because she documented the births at which she assisted, the travel she endured to reach laboring women, the stories she wrote about other people, and the accounts of her own family. However, on viewing the same diary, Ulrich believed that it reached directly to the "marrow of eighteenth century life" (p. 33). The "trivia that so annoyed earlier readers provides a consistent, daily record of the operation of a female-managed economy" (p. 33).

Oral histories also serve as primary source material. Boschma, Scaia, Bonifacio, and Roberts (2008) explain that oral history is both a "framework or analytic model and a methodology" (p. 81). Collection of this kind of data can provide "objective information" closing the gaps where other primary source documentation leaves incomplete, and oral history can also be viewed as part of a "social history" (p. 81). As a social history, collecting interviews of ordinary lives "creates history," from the "bottom up" by capturing a different perspective than of those in power (Boschma et al., 2008, p. 81). Unlike primary sources that are written by people directly involved in an event, secondary sources are materials that cite opinions and present interpretations. Secondary sources use primary sources to tell a story (Mages & Fairman, 2008). Newspaper accounts, journal articles, and textbooks from the period being studied are secondary sources that place researchers within the context of a period. For example, newspaper accounts of the 1893 Columbian World Exposition held in Chicago added authenticity to the story about the founding of the American Society of Superintendents of Training Schools for Nurses (known today as the National League for Nursing). However, researchers may use secondary sources as primary sources, depending on the researchers' questions or the purpose of the study (Austin, 1958). Mages and Fairman (2008) note that "the lines between primary and secondary sources can become blurred" (p. 131). For example, although newspaper articles from the late 19th century offered secondary accounts of what happened, they also provided insight into what was considered important during that period. Thus, if researchers are studying the insights of individuals present at a particular point in history, then they may use newspaper accounts as primary as well as secondary sources. Chaney and Folk (1993), for example, used cartoons found in the American Medical Association journal *American Medical News* as a primary source in the study "A Profession in Caricature: The Changing Attitudes Towards Nursing in the *American Medical News*, 1960–1989."

Mages and Fairman (2008) organize primary sources into categories that range from "personal documents, government documents, organizational documents, media communications, artifacts and realia, audio/visual materials, and dissertations" (p. 131). While these categories help the researcher to understand the range of possible primary sources, there are "no rigid groupings. Some items uncovered may fit into more than one, and alternatively a few primary sources may not seem to fit into any" (p. 130). Primary sources can be found anywhere starting from someone's collection of their grandmother's letters found in an attic or garage, or materials located in archives, special collections, museums, and historical societies (Mages & Fairman, 2008).

Herrmann (2008) considers the use of artifacts as an additional source historians can use that is rarely included in the literature. The author defines an artifact as an "inanimate physical object from an earlier time, produced by human workmanship, and carried out with a view to subsequent use, but without the conscious intent of imparting connected information" (p. 159). The artifact tells a story. Herrmann gives the example of the evolution of the manikin "Mrs. Chase," which served as a teaching tool for nursing students since the early 1900s. From the early manikins that supported student learning allowing them to practice such nursing interventions as the basic bed bath and bandaging to the SimMan manikin of today, the legacy of Mrs. Chase and the changing technology over the years provide rich data for historians to examine.

Confirming Source Genuineness and Authenticity

When selecting primary sources, the genuineness and authenticity of those sources become an important issues. Barzun and Graff (1985) explained that historians are responsible for verifying documents to ensure they are genuine and authentic. *Genuine* means that a document is not forged; *authentic* means that the document provides the truthful reporting of a subject (Barzun & Graff, 1985). Authenticating sources requires several operations, none of which is fixed in a specific technique. Researchers rely on "attention to detail, on common-sense reasoning, on a 'developed' field for history and chronology, on familiarity with human behavior, and on ever-enlarging stores of information" (p. 112). Authenticity of letters or journals becomes even more important when researchers find them in a nursing school attic or closet. More than likely, primary sources within archival collections have already been found to be genuine and have been authenticated by the institution in which they are housed. Nevertheless, researchers are responsible for the final authenticity of a document. A careful reading of the document, an examination of the type of paper and the condition of the material, and an extensive knowledge of the period can help researchers verify the document as authentic.

The validity of historical research relies on measures that address matters concerning external and internal criticism. *External criticism* questions the genuineness of primary sources and ensures that the document is what it claims. *Internal criticism* of data is concerned with content authenticity or truthfulness. Kerlinger (1986) suggests that internal criticism "seeks the 'true' meaning and value of the content of sources of data" (p. 621). Researchers must ask, Does the content accurately reflect the period in which it is written? Do the facts conflict with historical dates, meanings of words, and social mores from the time?

Spieseke (1953) emphasizes that when determining the reliability of the contents, researchers must evaluate when authors of primary sources wrote their account—whether it was close to the event or 20 years later. Other questions researchers must ask are, Did a trained historian or an observer write the story? Were facts suppressed? If so, why? To ensure the accuracy of the writer, Spieseke suggests that researchers check for corroborating evidence, look for another independent primary source that supports the data, and identify any disagreements between sources. Ulrich (1990), for example, authenticated Ballard's diary by corroborating some of Ballard's entries regarding feed bills with other sources from the town in which she lived.

The data that researchers can validate externally as genuine, however, may be inconsistent when researchers examine the data contents. For example, an individual may have written letters in the 19th century, but the content may conflict with known facts of that period and pose serious questions regarding the truth of the content (Kerlinger, 1986). Nevertheless, external criticism "ultimately . . . leads to content analysis or internal criticism and is indispensable when assessing evidence" (Matejski, 1986, p. 189). Austin (1958) illustrated this point by explaining that learning the date of a source (external criticism) helps researchers determine whether the content reflects the period in which it was written (internal criticism), and vice versa.

In historical studies for which the story can be enhanced or explained by someone who is still alive and who has lived through a period of time, an oral history provides a useful data source. Collecting oral histories provides an important primary source for many historical studies in nursing and adds to the understanding of nursing's history. Kirby (1997/1998) speaks about the use of oral history to illuminate the "hidden worlds" of areas such as nursing, childhood, and family that are often not represented in archival collections. Kirby notes that "oral history offers an alternative form of evidence through which historians can discover the form and structure of these hidden worlds" (p. 15). For example, a collection of stories told by nurses who have experienced changes in the hospital or the way we care for the terminally ill provides depth and richness to nursing's historical tapestry. "Over the past 20 years, research using oral history method has played a significant role in retrieving and recording historical experiences of 'non-elite' nurses and their patients who have no record of their lives or historical documents" (Biedermann, 2001, p. 61).

To do an oral history, the historian uses many of the same steps used in doing a history. One of the key differences in collecting oral histories is that living subjects are used and thus require consideration afforded to all research using human subjects. The Oral History Association (2000) Web page (http://omega.dickinson.edu/organizations/oha/pub_eg.html)

provides detailed explanations of the responsibilities of the interviewer, the interviewee, and the organization sponsoring the oral histories, the archive that stores oral histories, and transcribers. Readers interested in using an oral history method in their study are referred to other sources such as the Oral History Association for a more comprehensive understanding of this method. In addition, Boschma et al. (2008) explore the use of oral history as "both a framework or analytic model and a methodology" (p. 81) and offer their experiences using this method.

DATA ANALYSIS

*D*ata analysis relies on the statement of the subject, including the questions raised, the purpose, and the conceptual framework of the study. The themes developed by researchers direct data analysis. Researchers frame the findings according to research questions generated by the thesis. According to Spieseke (1953), the purpose of the study often directs the data analysis. If researchers want to teach a lesson, answer a question, or support an idea, they organize the selection of relevant data accordingly. How researchers analyze the material depends, in part, on the thematic organization of conceptual frameworks used in the study. Use of social, political, economic, or feminist theory will structure the data and enable researchers to concentrate on particular areas. Who the researcher is also influences the way data may be analyzed. "Each historian approaches the process from their own perspective, thus adding to the larger picture" (Lewenson & Herrmann, 2008a, b, p. 10).

In data analysis, researchers must deal with the tension between the conflicting truths so that they may find interpretations or understandings regarding the subject. In some way, researchers must strike a "balance between conflict" (Tholfsen, 1977, p. 246). They need to ask questions such as, Is the content found in the primary and secondary sources congruent with each other, or are there conflicting stories? If a conflict does exist, is there supporting evidence to explain either side of the argument?

Another important aspect of analysis is researcher bias about the subject and the influence of that bias on data interpretation. Awareness of personal bias improves the researcher's ability to provide an accurate interpretation of events. Self-awareness promotes a researcher's honesty in finding the truth and decreases the influence of bias on data interpretation (Austin, 1958; Barzun & Graff, 1985).

Through data analysis, researchers should develop new material and new ideas based on supporting evidence rather than just rehash ideas (Matejski, 1986). Researchers seek to discover new truths from the assembled facts. However, given the same data, individuals will analyze the data differently and thus contribute to the tentative nature of interpretation (Austin, 1958). To interpret the findings and get at a truth, historians must be conscious of the role ideology plays in analysis. Researchers must question how ideology, or any set of ideas, influences the analysis of a particular event. For example, a paternalistic ideological view of the nurse's role in the health care system may starkly contrast with an interpretation of the same data using a feminist lens. Awareness of ideological influence enhances researchers' abilities to study the full effect that ideas have on events and to avoid accepting ideas on face value. Tholfsen (1977) argues that history will suffer if taught from any one ideological stance; instead, its aim should be the "commitment to the disinterested pursuit of truth, accompanied by an openness to continuing debate and discussion" (p. 255). With this understanding, researchers examine and analyze data to try to find alternative truths supported in the available evidence.

Analysis occurs throughout the process of data collection. Historians look for evidence to explain events or ideas. By interpreting primary and secondary documents, researchers form a picture of historical antecedents. However, these documents become part of history only when "they have been subjected to historiography that bridges the gap between lived occurrences and records" (Matejski, 1986, p. 180).

In the search for true meanings and in the attempt to bridge identified gaps, researchers must be aware not only of their own bias and the effect of ideology but also of bias found in the sources themselves that may impede interpretation. For example, in biographical research, the use of both informants through interviews and materials found in archival collections may raise issues regarding the accuracy and validity of the data. Historians doing a biographical study need to be cautious of interviews that often present a biased or one-sided view of the individual being studied. Researchers may also suspect bias in archival holdings of an individual's papers because the individual may have determined what to include in the collection (Brown et al., 1991). Olson's (2000) concern that nurse historians have maintained a "uniform reliance on a narrative approach" and excluded using quantifiable data in their analysis of historical events highlights another type of potential bias in interpreting historical data.

ETHICAL CONSIDERATIONS

An ethical concern regarding the use of an institution or individual's private papers is the right to privacy versus the right to know. Although discussion of this concern is beyond the scope of this chapter, it is important for historical researchers to be aware of this dilemma. Researchers must have a clear idea of the kinds of information they need to obtain from data. If they find the source in an archive, then the archivist is responsible for seeing that "policy, regulations, and rules—governing his action do exist and are effective" (Rosenthal, 1982, p. 4). However, scholars are ultimately responsible for using data appropriately. If historians have as a goal to further the understanding of social, political, or economic relationships among individuals, institutions, events, or ideas, they must question what purpose is served if they expose exploitative or embarrassing details. Historians who misuse data and generate sensationalism by "[presenting] conclusions regarding motives and behavior that transcend the evidence . . . [and] turn an ordinary book into a best seller" (Graebner, 1982, p. 23) are discouraging future access and preservation of primary sources. If this type of misuse involves the people or events in the past, then only a historical reputation is damaged; however, if it involves people who are still living or their immediate ancestors, then it places at risk the right to access future contributions of papers from families or institutions. When determining how to use data, Graebner suggests that "decisions, events, and activities which affect the public welfare or embrace qualities of major human interest—and thus add legitimately to the richness of the historical record—set the acceptable boundaries of historical search and analysis" (p. 23).

The confidentiality of source material has become more of an ethical concern for historians as researchers have placed greater emphasis on the lives of ordinary people (Lusk, 1997). Several professional organizations, such as the American Historical Association (1987), the American Association for the History of Medicine (1991), and the Oral History Association (2000), have developed ethical guidelines for historical research. Nurse historians Birnbach, Brown, and Hiestand (1993a, 1993b), members of the American Association for the History of Nursing, have published ethical guidelines as well as professional standards for doing historical inquiry in nursing. Birnbach (2008) recently republished these guidelines and the use of these guidelines can be found in the case studies that are presented by Lewenson and Herrmann (2008c).

INTERPRETATION OF FINDINGS

*T*he historical narrative is the final stage in the historical research process. During this stage, researchers tell the story that interprets the data and engages readers in the historical debate. Synthesis occurs, and findings are connected, supported, and molded "into a related whole" (Austin, 1958, p. 9). Decisions regarding what to include and what to emphasize become important. Hallett (2008) considers how historians approach the "truth" in their interpretation of the archival data. "Once the sources have been collated and read carefully, most historians will find that an interpretation begins to emerge . . . it is important, however, to avoid the assumption that this is a purely intuitive process" (Hallett, 2008, p. 154). The combination of the ideas generated in the source material integrated with the historians' own value laden thoughts create the necessity to stop and consider what the truth is in the interpretation of the material.

In historical exposition, researchers explain not only what happened but how and why it happened. They explore relationships among events, ideas, people, organizations, and institutions and interpret them within the context of the period being studied. The political, social, and economic factors set a stage or backdrop from which to compare and contrast collected historical data. Historical judgments, based on historical evidence, must pass through the filter of "human understanding of human experience" (Cramer, 1992, p. 7). To accomplish this task, researchers must be sensitive to the material; must show genuine engagement in the subject; and must balance the forces of self, societal, and historical interest. Along with these attributes, researchers need creativity to achieve a coherent, convincing, and meaningful account (Ashley, 1978; Spieseke, 1953). Historians need to be mindful of what they learn from the source material and interact with that material as they interpret the findings (Hallett, 2008). Hallet explains that "strong history writing is marked by the care and openness with which the historian engages their source. It is, furthermore, characterized by a consciousness about the way in which those sources are used to support interpretation" (Hallett, 2008, p. 156).

When writing the narrative, researchers are charged with creatively rendering the events, explaining the findings, and supporting the ideas. Researchers must possess discipline, organization, and imagination to accomplish this Herculean task. Historians must set aside time to write daily, finding a quiet place to concentrate and contemplate the data. They will use a detailed outline to direct the writing of the manuscript, plan the story using a thematic framework established early in the study, and use time and place as landmarks to give balance and direct the flow of the story while critically interpreting the findings (Austin, 1958).

Historians weave historical facts, research findings, and interpretations influenced by the conceptual framework into a coherent story. To guide them in the writing process, researchers may divide the narrative into chronologic periods. Or, they may use geographic places such as regional areas in the United States, thematic relationships, research questions, or political, social, cultural, or economic issues to organize the narrative. These ad hoc inventions are determined by individual researchers and as such are subject to researcher interest, bias, and understanding of the historical method (Cramer, 1992; Fondiller, 1978).

Writers of history who want readers to hear the words spoken during the period studied may use direct quotations. Direct quotations provide corroboration of and credibility to a researcher's interpretation. However, although authentic quotes are a useful narrative tool, researchers must avoid using too many direct quotations. It is better to paraphrase and use limited direct quotes to give the narrative the flavor of a person.

A well-written historical research study illustrates the investigator's creativity and imagination as the story unfolds. Creativity connects thoughts, quotes, and events into a readable story and gives birth to new ideas (Christy, 1978). The interpretations and responses to the themes and questions rely on historians' abilities to go beyond the known facts and develop new ideas and new meanings. No two historians who view the same data will respond in exactly the same way. The human filter through which all information passes will alter researchers' responses to the data and will provide the catalyst for the creation of new ideas (Barzun & Graff, 1985; Christy, 1978).

D'Antonia (2008) writes that while the goal of the narrative is to produce a "seamless and coherent argument" that in the end seems "innately intuitive," the process of writing is "fraught with almost endless choices and decisions about what to include or exclude, which points in the chronology deserve more or less attention, and will anyone even care" (p. 21). The other salient point that D'Antonio shares is that the historian must write. For it is in the writing of the narrative that the historian again considers the various elements in the study, such as the nature of the primary and secondary sources, the "meaning of one's variables and context, and the validity of one's interpretation" (p. 21). The historian writes and tells the story after interpreting and considering the data. The narrative holds the reader's attention and makes history understandable and meaningful.

SUMMARY

*T*he nursing profession needs the infusion of new ideas, new meanings, and new interpretations of its past to explain its place in history and its future direction. Ashley (1978) confirmed this connection when she wrote, "With creativity as our base, and with strong historical knowledge and awareness, nurses can become pioneers in developing new types of inquiry and turn inward toward self-knowledge and self-understanding" (p. 36). The historical method gives researchers tools to explore the past. Even though it is challenging to fully explain and perhaps understand historical methodology, as D'Antonio (2005) notes, it is important to continue to find ways to do so. Using certain guideposts along the way, historical researchers formulate ideas, collect data, validate the genuineness and authenticity of those data, and narrate the story. However, to make the research meaningful, historians must relate the research questions and the findings to the present. Connolly (2004) and other historians in the 21st century ask us to examine our nursing stories so that we can learn about what we do, how we do it, where we do it, and who has done nursing work before us. History, in this way, becomes what D'Antonio (2004) has proclaimed as a "new paradigm for nursing knowledge" (p. 1). It is imperative, therefore, to understand the historical method of inquiry as it is up to historians to make this new paradigm happen.

References

American Association for the History of Medicine. (1991). Report of the committee on ethical codes. *Bulletin of the History of Medicine, 65*(4), 565–570.

American Historical Association. (1987). Statement on standards of professional conduct. *History Teacher, 21*(1), 105–109.

Ashley, J. (1978). Foundations for scholarship: Historical research in nursing. *Advances in Nursing Science, 1*(1), 25–36.

Austin, A. (1958). The historical method. *Nursing Research, 7*(1), 4–10.

Barzun, J., & Graff, H. F. (1985). *The modern researcher* (4th ed.). San Diego, CA: Harcourt Brace Jovanovich.

Biedermann, N. (2001). The voices of days gone by: Advocating the use of oral history in nursing. *Nursing Inquiry, 8,* 61–62.

Birnbach, N. (2008). Ethical guidelines and standards of professional conduct. In S. B. Lewenson, & E. K. Herrmann (Eds.), *Capturing nursing history: A guide to historical research* (pp. 167–172). New York: Springer.

Birnbach, N., Brown, J., & Hiestand, W. (1993a). Ethical guidelines for the nurse historian. *American Association for the History of Nursing Bulletin, 38,* 4.

Birnbach, N., Brown, J., & Hiestand, W. (1993b). Standards of professional conduct for historical inquiry into nursing. *American Association for the History of Nursing Bulletin, 38,* 5.

Boschma, G., Scaia, M., Bonificio, N., & Roberts, E. (2008). Oral history research. In S. B. Lewenson, & E. K. Herrmann (Eds.), *Capturing nursing history: A guide to historical research* (pp. 79–98). New York: Springer.

Brown, J., D'Antonio, P., & Davis, S. (1991, April). *Report on the Fourth Invitational Nursing History Conference.* Unpublished manuscript.

Buck, J. (2008). Using frameworks in historical research. In S. B. Lewenson, & E. K. Herrmann (Eds.), *Capturing nursing history: A guide to historical research* (pp. 45–62). New York: Springer.

Chaney, J. A., & Folk, P. (1993). A profession in caricature: The changing attitudes towards nursing in the *American Medical News,* 1960–1989. *Nursing History Review, 1,* 181–201.

Christy, T. (1978). The hope of history. In M. L. Fitzpatrick (Ed.), *Historical studies in nursing* (pp. 3–11). New York: Teachers College Press.

Connolly, C. A. (2004). Beyond social history: New approaches to understanding the state of and the state in nursing history. *Nursing History Review, 12,* 5–24.

Cramer, S. (1992). The nature of history: Meditations on Clio's Craft. *Nursing Research, 41*(1), 4–7.

Cordeau, M. A. (2009). Method for historicizing lived experience. *Advances in Nursing Science: History of Nursing, 32*(1), 75–90.

D'Antonio, P. (1999). Rewriting and rethinking the rewriting of nursing history. *Bulletin of the History of Medicine, 73,* 268–290.

D'Antonio, P. (2004). Editor's note. *Nursing History Review, 12,* 1–3.

D'Antonio, P. (2005). Editor's note. *Nursing History Review, 13,* 1–3.

D'Antonio, P. (2008). Conceptual and methodological issues in historical research. In S. B. Lewenson, & E. K. Herrmann (Eds.), *Capturing nursing history: A guide to historical research* (pp. 11–23). New York: Springer.

Fitzpatrick, M. L. (2001). Historical research: The method. In P. L. Munhall (Ed.), *Nursing research: A qualitative perspective* (3rd ed., pp. 403–414). Boston: Jones and Bartlett.

Flynn, K. (2009). Beyond the glass wall: Black Canadian nurses, 1940–1970. *Nursing History Review, 17,* 129–152.

Fondiller, S. (1978). Writing the report. In M. L. Fitzpatrick (Ed.), *Historical studies in nursing* (pp. 25–27). New York: Teachers College Press.

Gaddis, J. L. (2002). *The landscape of history: How historians map the past.* New York: Oxford Press.

Graebner, N. A. (1982). History, society, and the right to privacy. In *The scholar's right to know versus the individual's right to privacy.* Proceedings of the first Rockefeller

Archive Center Conference, December 5, 1975 (pp. 20–24). Pocantico Hills, NY: Rockefeller Archive Center Publication.

Grypma, S. J. (2005). Critical issues in the use of biographic methods in nursing history. *Nursing History Review, 13,* 171–187.

Grypma, S. J. (2008). Critical issues in the use of biographic methods in nursing history. In S. B. Lewenson, & E. K. Herrmann (Eds.), *Capturing nursing history: A guide to historical research* (pp. 63–78). New York: Springer.

Hallett, C. (2008). "The truth about the past?": The art of working with archival materials. In S. B. Lewenson, & E. K. Herrmann (Eds.), *Capturing nursing history: A guide to historical research* (pp. 149–158). New York: Springer.

Hamilton, D. (1991, April). *Intellectual history.* Paper presented at the meeting of Fourth Invitational Conference on Nursing History: Critical Issues Affecting Research and Researchers, Philadelphia, PA.

Hamilton, D. B. (1993). The idea of history and the history of ideas. *Image, 25*(1), 45–50.

Hanson, K. S. (1989). The emergence of liberal education in nursing education, 1893 to 1923. *Journal of Professional Nursing, 5*(2), 83–91.

Herrmann, E. K. (2008). About artifacts. In S. B. Lewenson, & E. K. Herrmann (Eds.), *Capturing nursing history: A guide to historical research* (pp. 159–166). New York: Springer.

Hofstadter, R. (1959). History and the social sciences. In F. Stern (Ed.), *The varieties of history* (pp. 359–370). New York: Meridian.

Kirby, S. (1997/1998). The resurgence of oral history and the new issues it raises. *Nurse Researcher, 5*(2), 45–58.

Kerlinger, F. N. (1986). *Foundations of behavioral research* (3rd ed.). New York: Holt, Rinehart & Winston.

Kruman, M. (1985). Historical method: Implications for nursing research. In M. M. Leininger (Ed.), *Qualitative research methods in nursing* (pp. 109–118). Orlando, FL: Grune & Stratton.

Lewenson, S. B. (1990). The woman's nursing and suffrage movement, 1893–1920. In V. Bullough, B. Bullough, & M. Stanton (Eds.), *Florence Nightingale and her era: A collection of new scholarship* (pp. 117–118). New York: Garland.

Lewenson, S. B. (1996). *Taking charge: Nursing, suffrage and feminism, 1873–1920.* New York: NLN Press.

Lewenson, S. B. (2008). Doing historical research? In S. B. Lewenson, & E. K. Herrmann (Eds.), *Capturing nursing history: A guide to historical research* (pp. 25–43). New York: Springer.

Lewenson, S. B., & Herrmann, E. K. (2008a). *Capturing nursing history: A guide to historical research.* New York: Springer.

Lewenson, S. B., & Herrmann, E. K. (2008b). Why do historical research? In S. B. Lewenson, & E. K. Herrmann (Eds.), *Capturing nursing history: A guide to historical research* (pp. 1–10). New York: Springer.

Lewenson, S. B., & Herrmann, E. K. (2008c). Using ethical guidelines and standards of professional conduct. In S. B. Lewenson, & E. K. Herrmann (Eds.), *Capturing nursing history: A guide to historical research* (pp. 173–179). New York: Springer.

Lorentzon, M. (2004). Nursing record/British journal of nursing archives, 1888–1956. *British Journal of Nursing, 13*(5), 280–284.

Lusk, B. (1997). Historical methodology for nursing research. *Image, 29*(4), 355–359.

Lynaugh, J. (1996). Editorial. *Nursing History Review, 4,* 1.

Lynaugh, J., & Reverby, S. (1987). Thoughts on the nature of history. *Nursing Research, 36*(1), 4–69.

Mages, K. C., & Fairman, J. A. (2008). Working with primary sources: An overview. In S. B. Lewenson, & E. K. Herrmann (Eds.), *Capturing nursing history: A guide to historical research* (pp. 129–148). New York: Springer.

Matejski, M. (1986). Historical research: The method. In P. L. Munhall, & C. J. Oiler (Eds.), *Nursing research: A qualitative perspective* (pp. 175–193). Norwalk, CT: Appleton-Century-Crofts.

Melchior, F. (2004). Feminist approaches to nursing history. *Western Journal of Nursing Research, 26*(3), 340–355.

Morse, J. M., & Field, P. A. (1995). *Qualitative research methods for health professionals* (2nd ed.). Thousand Oaks, CA: Sage.

Newton, M. (1965). The case for historical research. *Nursing Research, 14*(1), 20–26.

Oral History Association. (2000). Oral history evaluation guidelines (Pamphlet No. 3) [On-line]. Available at: http://omega.dickinson.edu/organizations/oha/pub_eg.html.

Olson, T. (2000). Numbers, narratives, and nursing history. *Social Science Journal, 37*(1), 137–144.

Rafferty, A. M. (2004). Pre Conference. Paper presented at the meeting of the American Association for the History of Nursing, Charleston, SC.

Rines, A., & Kershner, F. (1979). *Information concerning historical studies.* Unpublished manuscript. New York: Teachers College, Columbia University, Department of Nursing.

Rosenthal, R. (1982). Who will be responsible for private papers of private people? Some considerations from the view of the private depository. In *The scholar's right to know versus the individual's right to privacy.* Proceedings of the first Rockefeller Archive Center Conference, December 5, 1975 (pp. 3–6). Pocantico Hills, NY: Rockefeller Archive Center Publication.

Sampson, D. A. (2009). Alliances of cooperation: Negotiating New Hampshire nurse practitioners' prescribing practice. *Nursing History Review, 17,* 153–178.

Spieseke, A. W. (1953). What is the historical method of research? *Nursing Research, 2*(1), 36–37.

Termine, J. (1992, March). A talk about archives. Paper presented at the State University of New York, Health Science Center at Brooklyn, College of Nursing, Brooklyn, NY.

Tholfsen, T. R. (1977). The ambiguous virtues of the study of history. *Teachers College Record, 79*(2), 245–257.

Ulrich, L. T. (1990). *A midwife's tale: The life of Martha Ballard based on her diary, 1785–1812.* New York: Vintage Books.

Yuginovich, T. (2000). More than time and place: Using historical comparative research as a tool for nursing. *International Journal of Nursing Practice, 6,* 70–75.

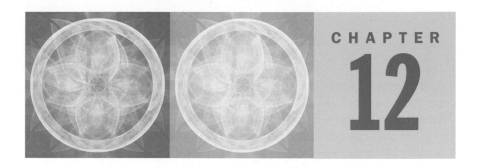

Historical Research in Practice, Education, and Administration

*U*sing historical research methods to study nursing practice, education, and administration allows us to understand relationships and to view the world from a broader perspective. It provides "us with a way of knowing what happened before, a way of understanding current issues, and offers a way to glean an insight into the future" (Lewenson & Herrmann, 2008, p. 2). *Nursing History Review* editor D'Antonio (2003) states that "history matters" (p. 1). History provides an "overarching conceptual framework that allows us to more fully understand the disparate meaning of nursing and the different experiences of nurses" (p. 1). Understanding how nurses practiced, how they educated future generations of nurses, and how they administered hospitals, community agencies, and schools of nursing lends itself to historical inquiry. Historical method provides a way to examine specific periods or events in time and place them within a broader context, giving the researcher insights that numbers alone cannot provide. Self-reflection, imagination, and an awareness of a world beyond oneself are essential tools for the historian to have when looking for relationships between the past and present (Lynaugh, 1996, p. 1). This chapter highlights how historical researchers study and interpret patterns of our past to gain a better understanding of the current and future world. Three critiques of historical research studies in the areas of practice, education, and administration are presented. Based on criteria developed from the material discussed in Chapter 11, guidelines were created for critiquing historical research (Box 12-1). A reprint of the

Box 12-1

Guidelines for Critiquing Historical Research

Data Generation

Title

1. How does it concisely reflect the purpose of the study?
2. How does it clearly tell readers what the study is about?
3. How does it delineate the time frame for the study?

Statement of the Subject

1. Is the subject easily researched?
2. What themes and theses are studied?
3. What are the research questions?

Literature Review

1. What are the main works written on the subject?
2. What time period does the literature review cover?
3. What are some of the problems that may arise when studying this subject?
4. What primary sources can be identified?
5. How was the subject narrowed during the literature review?
6. What research questions were raised during the literature review?

Data Treatment

Primary Sources

1. How were primary sources used?
2. Were they genuine and authentic?
3. How was external validity determined?
4. How was internal validity determined?
5. Were there inconsistencies between the external validity and internal validity?
6. Does the content accurately reflect the period of concern?
7. Do the facts conflict with historical dates, meanings of words, and social mores?
8. When did the primary author write the account?
9. Did a trained historian or an observer write the source?
10. Were facts suppressed, and if so, why?
11. Is there corroborating evidence?
12. Identify any disagreements between sources.

Secondary Sources

1. What were the secondary sources used?
2. How were secondary sources used?
3. Do they corroborate the primary source?
4. Can you identify any disagreements between sources?

Data Analysis

Organization

1. What conceptual frameworks were used in the study?
2. How would the study be classified; for example, intellectual, feminist, social, political, biographical?
3. Were the research questions answered?

Box 12-1   Continued

4. Was the purpose of the study accomplished?
5. If conflict exists within the findings, was there supporting evidence to justify either side of the argument?

Bias

1. Was the researcher's bias identified?
2. Was analysis influenced by a present-mindedness?
3. What were the ideological biases?
4. How did bias affect data analysis?

Ethical Issues

1. Was there any infringement on a historical reputation?
2. Was there a conflict between the right to privacy and the right to know?
3. Did the research show that decisions, events, and activities of an individual or organization affected the public welfare or embraced qualities of major human interest?

Interpreting the Findings

Narrative

1. Does the story describe what happened, including how and why it happened?
2. Were relationships among events, ideas, people, organizations, and institutions explained, interpreted, and placed within a contextual framework?
3. How were direct quotations used? (Too limited or too long?)
4. Was the narrative clear, concise, and interesting to read?
5. Was the significance to nursing explicit?

---

article "Alliances of Cooperation: Negotiating New Hampshire Nurse Practitioners' Prescribing Practice," appears at the end of the chapter to help readers understand the critiquing process. Table 12-1 offers a sampling of selected historical research publications.

CRITIQUE GUIDELINES

As noted in Chapter 11, D'Antonio (2005) reflects on how difficult it is to explain historical research methodology. This difficulty can potentially jeopardize our ability to pass this knowledge onto new historians. There is a certain "inexactness" which historians experience when trying to explain the process of historiography (D'Antonio, 2005). Readers must keep this in mind as they attempt to understand the process of historical research, which is often circuitous in nature. Guidelines are just that—guidelines. They serve as a way to "light the path" and keep the researcher "on track." Historians search for meaning in past events and face the ever-present concern that they will not be able to find data to tell "the whole story." Critique guidelines help the historian on this journey of discovery and also help consumers of historical research understand what should be expected from this

Table 12-1 • Selective Sampling of Historical Research Studies

Author	Date	Domain	Title	Findings
Abrams	2007	Education	The report of the conference on redesigning nursing education for public health	This study examines highlights of a conference organized by the Division of Nursing Bureau of Health Professions, Health Resources Administration, of the US Department of Health, Education and Welfare in May 1973. By exploring the "selected discussions" (Abrams, 2007, p. 198) reflecting trends, challenges, and inferences about public health nursing education, offers insight for public health nurse educators today. Several of the issues faced over 34 years ago continue to "remain salient lessons for contemporary readers" (p. 198).
Rima	2007	Practice	Much instruction needed here: The work of nurses in rural Wisconsin during the depression	This study examines the reports of Wisconsin public health nurses during the 1930s about the maternal child health care they provided to women in a rural community. It explores the relationship between these nurses and the local physician's with whom they worked. This study offers insights about gender relations and how the delivery of health care is shaped by contemporary health care policy, norms of medical practices, and patient circumstances.
Buck	2007	Practice	Reweaving a tapestry of care: Religion, nursing, and the meaning of hospice, 1945–1966	This article uses the development of the hospice movement in Britain and in the state of Connecticut as a case study. The case study serves to study the transition in community-based care for the dying before and after the beginning of the hospice movement in the United States. It allows the study of the "interplay among religion, nursing, and the modern conceptualization of hospice" (p. 114).

Fairman	2008	Education	Context and contingency in the history of post World War II nursing scholarship in the United States	This study examines the social, political, economic context in which nursing scholarship developed during the post World War II period in the United States. Three contextual strands are identified that influenced nursing scholarship: the use of experiential clinical knowledge to raise questions; the move toward higher education in nursing which in turn led to scholarly activity focused on reintegrating practice and education; and the scholars that emerged during this period and influenced the development and understanding of nursing knowledge.
Hobbs	2009	Practice	Defining nursing practice: The ANA social policy statement, 1980–1983	This study examines the development of the American Nurses Association (ANA) Social Policy Statement (SPS). The SPS reflects a "particular view of nursing practice" (p. 15). Academics devised the SPS based on what they viewed as important such as the separation of nursing and medical roles and nursing's reliance on theory rather than practical experience in their clinical decision-making. Implications for current practice requires one to consider who develops information tools like the SPS, and include those that practice, teach, and research in their development.
Wall	2009	Administration	Catholic sister nurses in Selma, Alabama, 1940–1972	This study examines the activities of religious sister nurses when faced with the racism in Selma, Alabama between 1940 and 1972. The effort these nurses took to reach out to the community of African Americans during the civil rights movement while obeying the hierarchical male leaders showed a level of political activism. Including the analysis of their activism is needed in order to fully understand the issue of race in nursing.

(*Continued*)

Table 12-1 • (Continued)

Author	Date	Domain	Title	Findings
Ament	2004	Education	The evolution of midwifery faculty practice: Impact and outcomes of care	Midwifery education has undergone changes, and this study examines some of the changes that occurred at the oldest programs of its kind. Yale School of Nursing Nurse-Midwifery program began in 1956 and has adapted more recently to the changes in student enrollment and availability of clinical sites. To understand how this school has adapted over time, this study examines the history of midwifery faculty practices. The outcomes of this historical inquiry are clearly stated and include the need for a "good business infrastructure."
Buck	2004	Administration	Home hospice versus home health: Cooperation, competition, and cooptation	This study examines attitudes about death and dying in the United States during the later half of the 20th century and how these attitudes influence both the care and cost related to death and dying. The sociopolitical development of hospice care and the changes in end-of-life care offer a historical perspective on a difficult and often considered "taboo" subject. The study presents the complexities required to negotiate the tensions between the "systems of care and cure" and then balancing this between "a philosophy of care and the realities of sustainability" (p. 41). The study presents the political issues surrounding control of end-of-life care, federal reimbursement for care, and the role nurses played in changing care for the dying. The study raises questions about future health care policy and reform and the need to continue studying in this area.

Author	Year	Type	Summary
D'Antonio	2004	Education	Women, nursing, and baccalaureate education in 20th-century America	The purpose of this study was to "analyze the social meaning of the American system of education for nursing practice" (p. 379). Historical analyses of the educational levels of various groups of American women were compared with current data on educational levels of nurses and women. D'Antonio raises questions about the social class and community status of nurses in relation to their educational levels. Findings revealed that raising the educational level of nurses provided an avenue for upward mobility into middle-class America. The data illustrated that more African American, Hispanic, and Asian American nurses hold baccalaureate degrees than their Caucasian counterparts. The study also reveals that during the 20th century, the level of education decreased among nurses in the United States in comparison to the educational level of all women in the United States. An increase in social and political support for raising the level of nursing education is needed to make changes in that direction. D'Antonio further suggests that the "language of class and community status" be linked with the language of "science, knowledge, and clinical excellence" (p. 384) to gain this support.
Evans	2004	Practice	Men nurses: A historical and feminist perspective	This study examines the history of men in nursing in Britain, Canada, and the United States using CINAHL, Pubmed, and Sociological Abstracts databases. The findings show that documentation of men's role in nursing has been sparse and incomplete.

(*Continued*)

famous" (p. 45). The reader is cautioned, however, not to assume that the person being studied is "undistinguished or unexceptional" (p. 45).

Marshall (2009) provides context in which to study the particular relationship between Margaret Shanks and Susan B. Anthony, including "time, place, and context" (p. 45). Shanks, Marshall explains, went to nursing school in 1897 during a period of reform in nursing and health care in the United States. Marshall provides the reader a brief history of this period when the leaders in nursing were organizing to provide standards for both nursing education and practice. The efforts by nurses to establish standard curriculum, nursing registration laws, specializations such as public health nursing, and the publication of a professional journal *The American Journal of Nursing*, provide a backdrop to understanding the context of the world in which Margaret Shanks lived. The connection between the dominantly women's profession of nursing, the political efforts of nurses to organize the profession, and the efforts toward achieving woman suffrage further enriches the time, place, and context in which Shanks and Anthony lived. Marshall explains the relationship that Anthony had with nursing at that time, identifying one of Anthony's speeches to the New York State Nurses Association in Rochester, New York in 1902. Anthony, Marshall states, was familiar with the issues nursing leaders experienced in their efforts to professionalize nursing. While many nurses supported women suffrage, several did not. Marshall believes that Shanks was among those nurses who may have been indifferent to efforts to achieve women suffrage being more focused on her own life and her work as a private duty nurse than the political issues of the day. According to Marshall, Anthony accepted Shanks limitations in regard to political activity and expected that she would focus on her own nursing needs. They maintained their complementary roles as patient and nurse and yet their legacies were to change as a result of this relationship.

The narrative provides an interesting story about the life of Margaret Shanks and her work as Susan B. Anthony's private duty nurse. Marshall (2009) enriches the narrative using primary source material that includes letters, school records, annual reports, editorials, and other documents. Books about the period and social history add to the list of secondary source material. Marshall does not explicitly list for the reader the primary and secondary sources; however, she addresses the need to examine all kinds of sources using the work of Ulrich (1990, 1994) as an example. Primary and secondary sources support the narrative throughout the study, and although Marshall does not pause in the narrative to distinguish between the two types, the introduction of direct quotes and other supporting evidence allows the reader to easily identify the two types of sources. Although, for a novice researcher, it may have been easier and clearer if the researcher had delineated the primary and secondary sources.

When addressing questions related to whether sources are genuine or authentic, each historian must determine this by drawing on where he or she found the documents and what he or she found within the material examined. Marshall (2009) does not reflect on the methodology used to determine the genuineness or authenticity of the sources. However, the documents that are identified in the references are found in archival collections, prestigious journals, and other sources where the nature of the material would have been verified already. However, even when using sources that appear reliable, the researcher must have an understanding of the time period studied. For example, when reading about the role of the nurse during the late 19th and early 20th centuries, the researcher must possess an understanding of the particular time period to determine whether the comment makes "sense." The researcher must also ask, "Do the documents accurately reflect the period?" This is an important question and one that Marshall, by virtue of the use of historical documents, seems to implicitly verify in terms of authenticity. For newcomers to historical research, this is a difficult determination to make and one that would be easier if Marshall had been more explicit.

Ethical concerns are not explicitly addressed in Marshall's study, yet using Birnbach, Brown, and Hiestands's (1993a, 1993b) and Birnbach's (2008) Ethical Guidelines and Standards of Professional Conduct, the reader can discern that no specific issues relating to ethical concerns seems to be present in this historical investigation. Birnbach (2008) explains that the historian addresses ethical issues and maintains professional standards throughout the research process and Marshall's work demonstrates that any concerns were addressed. Archives were used, the reputations of both Shanks and Anthony in the study were seemingly treated respectively, and direct quotes were used frequently adding to the "truthfulness" of the data presented. The reader may consider that ethical concerns were addressed and yet, when reviewing historical research, they may want to consider the guidelines and standards and make their own decisions about the work. For example, Lewenson and Herrmann (2008) present cases where the reader might consider various ways of reviewing the ethical decisions that were made in regard to the use of data.

Marshall presents an interesting examination of the life of one nurse as she cared for a noted suffragist in the 20th century. This glimpse of the work and life of Margaret Shanks juxtaposed against the extraordinary work and life of Susan B. Anthony allows for interesting reflection of that period. Marshall creatively weaves the evidence together and brings the reader along so that the interpretation of the events becomes part of the story. She uses direct quotes from Margaret Shanks that reflects who she was and the work she did. Marshall's historical study uncovers the life of an individual and places her within the broader context of the progressive period where women strove for suffrage and nursing strove to be professional. Marshall (2008) provides an excellent example of historical research sharing her thoughts and explanations about the process with the reader.

APPLICATION TO EDUCATION

Researchers interested in nursing education are concerned with varied aspects of this subject, such as the entry into practice dilemma (D'Antonio, 2004), the move of nursing education into the university (Bartal & Steiner-Freud, 2005; Lewenson, 2008), the development of nursing scholarship (Fairman, 2008a), or the biography of an important figure in nursing education (Hawkins & Watson, 2003). By using a historical approach, researchers are able to address topics in nursing education ranging from curriculum design to control of education. This approach not only provides background descriptive information but also answers relevant questions regarding issues that concern nursing today.

Currently, topics such as recruitment of adult learners, critical thinking, and culturally competent care concern nursing educators. However, historians may question whether the concept of recruitment of adult learners is a new idea in nursing education and may attempt to understand this topic by studying nursing students of the past. Historians may examine past records of nurse training schools or professional studies of nursing. For example, the 1923 Goldmark (1984) study *Nursing and Nursing Education in the United States* indicated that, in 1911, about 70% of the training schools required students to be 20 or 21 years old for admission; however, within 7 years, the age requirement had dropped to 18 or 19 years. Given this information, the historian might ask, Why did the admission age drop at that time, and why did training schools initially believe older women would be better training school candidates? What teaching strategies worked better with older women than with younger ones? Both questions address the past and yet relate to current, pertinent issues related to adult learners.

Another contemporary nursing education issue, critical thinking, has its roots in nursing's history. For example, in 1897, Superintendent of Bellevue Training School Agnes Brennan addressed the Superintendent's Society. She stated, "An uneducated woman may become a good nurse, but never an intelligent one; she can obey orders conscientiously and understand thoroughly a sick person's need, but should an emergency arise, where is she? She works through her feelings, and therefore lacks judgment" (Brennan, 1991, p. 23). Was Brennan referring to critical thinking when she reasoned that nurses needed to have the knowledge and theory regarding pathology to understand the appropriate care of sick people? Brennan suggested it was equally important for nurses to spend time in clinical practice learning the "character of the pulse in different patients or finding out just why some nurses can always see at a glance that this patient requires her pillow turned" (p. 24). She firmly believed that a trained nurse required both theoretical and practical knowledge and that, without both, something would be missing in the nursing care provided. As she pointed out, "Theory fortifies the practical, practice strengthens and retains the theoretical" (p. 25). Brennan clearly described her views on the theory–practice dichotomy that still challenges nursing educators today. Brennan firmly believed that nurses must be educated to think so that they can practice.

Historical researchers have addressed the contemporary issue of cultural diversity by studying racial tensions in nursing and in society and offering nurses a better understanding of the inherent conflicts. Questions that might be asked related to the topic include, Was there cultural diversity in nursing or any interest in providing culturally competent care before the current interest in the topic? From where did the nursing student at the beginning of the 19th century come? What socioeconomic–political background did the student bring to nursing? How does nursing interface with race and gender? In the book *Black Women in White: Racial Conflict and Cooperation in the Nursing Profession, 1890–1950*, Hine (1989) described the opening of nurse training schools for African Americans who had been excluded from most of the existing U.S. nurse training schools. Of the schools that did not racially discriminate, many admitted African Americans using quotas. The very origin of the National Association of Colored Graduate Nurses (NACGN) in 1908 speaks to the early exclusion of African Americans from the first two national nursing organizations: the American Society of Superintendents of Training Schools for Nurses (renamed the National League of Nursing Education in 1912) and the Associated Alumnae of the United States and Canada (renamed the American Nurses Association [ANA] in 1911). Young (2005) re-examines the 1925 Johns Report on African American nurses and adds to the ongoing discussion about how race affected the education and practice of nurses. Historians need to look at what was, as well as what was not, to better understand historic events. For example, How did nursing handle diversity? What was the reaction of nurses to institutional racism? When did the profession welcome people of a different race, color, and religion into the profession? Who were the advocates of an integrated profession? Who responded to political movements that advocated racial and gender equality?

Historians who search for answers may learn that nursing political activist Lavinia Dock spoke out against prejudicial treatment of any professional nurse. Dock (1910) cited the need for nursing to demonstrate practical ethics and ardently hoped that the nursing association (ANA) would not ever "get to the point where it draws the color line against our negro sister nurses" (p. 902). She believed that the nursing association was one place in the United States where color boundaries were not drawn. As the ANA expanded, however, Dock witnessed evidence that made her remark "that this cruel and unchristian and unethical prejudice might creep in here in our association" (p. 902). Dock said that under no circumstances should nurses emulate the cruel prejudices displayed by "men" and urged nurses to treat each nurse of color "as we would like to be treated ourselves" (p. 902). She supported politically active, black nursing leader Adah Thomas, who became president of the NACGN and who, in 1929, wrote the history of African American nurses in the book *The Pathfinders* (Davis, 1988).

Questions that arise from conflicting ideas in the existing data and the omission of information in published narrative suggest new areas for historic inquiry. An example is Mosley's (1996) historical study based on examining the influence of four black community health nurses on public health nursing in New York City between 1900 and 1930. Mosley included a discussion specifically addressing institutional racism as it existed in nursing during the first 30 years of the 20th century. To understand the prejudice experienced by African American nurses, Mosley focused on the lives and contributions of four leaders in public health nursing: Jessie Sleet Scales, Mabel Staupers, Elizabeth W. Tyler, and Edith M. Carter.

To really understand nursing education (and all aspects of nursing for that matter), historians need to use a more global perspective. Examining, for example, contextual factors such as gender, race, class, and economics internationally, allows us to place nursing education and the challenges it has faced within a larger (both local and global) setting. Boschma (2008) explains that:

> good international nursing history . . . is historical scholarship that contributes to the exploration of diversity in local contexts, helps to unsettle parochial assumptions about nursing and health care, and most of all, assists us in reaching a deeper understanding of what it means to be different. (p. 11)

Critique of a Study in Education

In "Beyond the Glass Wall: Black Canadian Nurses, 1940–1970," Karen Flynn (2009) examines the historical experience of some of the first black nurses to be educated in Canada and how they served as "trailblazers" for future black nurses. These trailblazers entered nursing education at a time when typically only white nurses were eligible to be educated and practice. Yet these women, aware of the racial bias and negative stereotypes that existed, focused on the work of nursing, became friends with other nursing students, continued their nursing education, and developed successful professional careers. This study examines these nurses' experiences during the years 1940 and 1970. The title of the study clearly informs the reader of the time frame for the study, as well as the subject. While readers may not be familiar with the meaning of "glass wall," and may at first glance surmise its meaning, Flynn eventually does explain where this term is derived. Flynn takes the term "beyond the glass wall" from a fictional work titled, "The Glass Wall," written in 1964 by Sheila Mackay Russell and published in the *Chetelaine*. In this story, Flynn explains the anxiety and racist attitudes that black Canadian nurses experienced. Flynn uses the fictional story to understand the context of nursing and the attitudes about race during this period of time in Canada.

Flynn (2009) opens the narrative with a direct quote from Agnes Scott Elesworth, one of the women she has interviewed for this study. From the start, Flynn informs the reader of the purpose of the study citing that it "explores the complex subjectivities of the first cohort of Black Canadian registered nurses embodied in Agnes Scott Elesworth's quote at the beginning" (p. 130). The reader also learns that this study is part of a larger one where Flynn is collecting oral histories of black Canadian and Caribbean nurses who were born between 1929 and 1950; who were educated either in Britain, in one of the Caribbean islands, or Canada; and who came from Ontario, Nova Scotia, and Manitoba. Flynn explains that this larger study needs to be done to address the lack of research in the experience of these nurses who were educated at a time when nursing education in Canada excluded, for the most part, black women. The nurses interviewed for the study blazed a trail, breaking down some of the racial barriers and became successful in their nursing careers. Their experiences are important to collect and document because, Flynn writes, they "provide a unique perspective on constructions of race and gender" (Flynn, 2009, p. 130.).

Flynn (2009) provides the reader with a contextual backdrop of life in Canada, attitudes about race, common practice in exclusion of black Canadians in nursing education and practice, and essentially prepares the reader to understand the experiences of the black Canadian nurses that are interviewed. The author specifically identifies the sources used in the study as oral histories, a fictional story published in a magazine, nursing and non-nursing texts. Looking at the references used throughout the study, additional source material includes personal letters, archival material, film, and journal articles. Flynn does not, however, delineate whether they are primary or secondary source and leaves this up to the reader to discern. Although this is not always necessary, it would help the reader to understand how the author selected the primary sources, including how the author collected the oral histories used. The author writes an interesting narrative that illustrates the history of the exclusionary practices in nursing education in Canada as well as the experiences of the nurses interviewed for the study. The use of oral histories as part of the evidence in this paper is nicely woven into the fabric of the study and provides most of the primary source data.

A separate literature review section is not clearly labeled as such in Flynn's (2009) article. This may not be necessary because the author tells the story by using the literature throughout the article. In other words, the use of various data sources provides the basis for the literature review and becomes part of the narrative. Flynn (2009) also does not clearly identify a framework for the study. The historian appears to use a social history framework because the study examines the contextual factors of race and gender by gathering the experiences of this group of women who entered nursing training.

Whether the author's bias is evident when the data are interpreted is not clear and is not addressed in the paper. Yet, Flynn (2009) clearly explains why the study was done, why this particular group of nurses was studied. The author voices her argument that these nurses "secured a place in an occupation that defined itself around Victorian ideals of 'true womanhood,' an archetype that excluded Black women . . . Black Canadian nurses nevertheless capitalized on opportunities nursing offered to carve out a satisfactory professional and personal life" (p. 130). The data presented and the interpretations of the findings are reported in such a way as to provide readers with the opportunity to question and/or accept the findings based on their own critique of the study and further exploration in this area of nursing education and practice.

The ethical issues related to historical studies when subjects are still alive and the history is more recent are not addressed in the study. However, there is no evidence suggesting unethical treatment of those interviewed. It is important to ask whether or not there was an infringement on the historical reputation of those interviewed. The oral histories spoke favorable about the experiences they had while in nursing training yet unveil sensitive issues about relationships between white and black Canadians. For example, one of the women interviewed shares some good memories about the other nurses she trained with at the Hotel Dieu. In that interview, it was recalled that "I think our method of training melded us together. One girl told me that she would not talk to Blacks until she met us . . . She was ripped of all the stereotypes and rumors. She had no real experience to compare; we became fast friends and remain friends today" (Flynn, 2009, p. 143). Flynn (2009) addresses difficult issues about race and nursing education that can be uncomfortable for some to discuss. Yet, the narrative carefully integrates the literature, documentation, and oral histories to present a story of how a group of women entered nursing education and forged a successful personal and professional life. While sharing stories about racial bias that may conflict with the perception that Canada did not experience these issues, the author presents various views of those involved without seemingly violating their right to privacy.

Flynn (2009) explores the legacy of struggle that blacks in Canada experienced as earlier ancestors struggled to find freedom from racism and violence found in the United States. They came to Canada in search of freedom, but found that here too, they had to struggle with acceptance, negative stereotypes, and segregation. The black Canadian nurses that entered nursing training in the 1940s found that like other black Canadians they also had to serve as trailblazers for others who wanted nursing as a career, breaking down some of the existing barriers. "It was this history, then, coupled with their belief that they had a right to train as nurses that provided Black Canadian nurses the necessary affirmation to begin their training in the postwar era and to blaze a sometimes arduous trail for the generation of Black Canadian and Caribbean nurses who followed" (Flynn, 2009, p. 148).

APPLICATION TO ADMINISTRATION

*B*y now, it should be clear to readers that doing historical research requires creativity. Researchers may select a topic of interest and study it using different approaches. The history of nursing organizations founded by nursing leaders is an excellent subject for a nursing history. As an example, Birnbach and Lewenson (1991) examined the early speeches presented at the National League for Nursing (NLN), an organization that epitomizes the efforts of nurse administrators to organize and control nursing education and practice. The NLN began in 1893 when a group of nursing superintendents in charge of nurse training schools met in Chicago at the Canada and Columbian Exposition. Superintendents throughout the United States met and founded the American Society of Superintendents of Training Schools for Nurses. In 1912, this organization became the National League of Nursing Education, and, in 1952, became the NLN. Superintendents started this organization so they could collectively address the issues confronting the developing profession. They advocated reforms such as improving educational standards, developing uniform training school curricula, decreasing working hours, and increasing the number of years of training. Through their efforts, the organization developed needed educational reforms in nursing and fostered the control of practice.

To study nursing administration, researchers might use biographies of nursing leaders. A biography offers insight into the characteristics of people as well as their roles. It some cases, it allows the "dots to be connected" and provides insight into broader historical studies. Biographies of leaders before the modern nursing movement, such as the one done by Griffon (1998) on Mary Seacole, give a different perspective on women who contributed to establishing independent practice and setting the stage for future nurses. A biography need not be limited to one person but may compare and contrast the relationships among a group of leaders, such as the study by Poslusny (1989): "Feminist Friendship: Isabel Hampton Robb, Lavinia Lloyd Dock, and Mary Adelaide Nutting." Grypma (2005) believes that biography enables researchers to ask the "newer" questions being asked by historians. Looking at the lives of ordinary nurses, for example, tells a different story than that of more famous nursing leaders who have been captured in biographical sketches. For example, in "Careful Nursing: A Model for Contemporary Nursing Practice," Meehan (2003) presents a "new" model for nursing care that was derived from a historical study of the nursing system developed in Ireland by Catherine McAuley, the founder of the Religious Sisters of Mercy, in the early 19th century.

Whelan's (2005) study that examines the change in employment of nurses from private duty to hospital-based practice highlights the dilemma nurses experience in meeting supply and demand needs caused by economic, social, and political factors. The lessons learned from the decline in the use of private duty nurses following World War II and the inevitable affect on employment practices reverberate today as administrators respond to the continuing concerns produced by the nursing shortage.

The following section presents a critique of Sampson's (2009) study that examines the issues surrounding the efforts to secure appropriate nursing legislation that supports the work of nurse practitioners'.

Critique of a Study in Nursing Administration

Sampson (2009) writes about the efforts of nurse practitioners to obtain the right to practice independently. The author does this by presenting an historical account of the legislative experience nurse practitioners underwent in the state of New Hampshire as a case study. The title, "Alliances of Cooperation: Negotiating New Hampshire Nurse Practitioners Prescribing Practice" offers the reader an understanding of what the study is about. Although no dates were given in the title that would have immediately clarified the time period, the title speaks about alliances and negotiation of nurse practitioners "prescribing" practice. It is a title that captures the imagination right away and briefly lays out what to expect.

The opening paragraph brings the reader directly into the time period under study. Beginning with, "in 1973, the New Hampshire Board of Nursing recognized a new category of nurses called 'advanced registered nurse practitioners' when the legislature passed an addendum to the nursing practice act formally recognizing this emerging group of nurses" (Sampson, 2009, p. 153). For four years following the passage of this addendum, New Hampshire nurse practitioners practiced independently assuming some of the responsibilities typically found in the medical domain such as ordering diagnostic tests, diagnosing patients, and prescribing and dispensing medications. This continued unchallenged by other health care providers and often with the support of the medical community. Yet, by 1977 the Commission on Pharmacy "formerly challenged" the New Hampshire nurses' expanded role into the prescribing and dispensing medication. The Commission on Pharmacy, responsible for inspecting pharmacies and the handling of prescriptions, observed a discrepancy in a physician's signature noting that the signature was signed differently on his prescriptions. It seemed that the physician's wife, a practicing nurse was signing his name, although she also said that she was a nurse practitioner.

The inspector contacted the New England Regional Office of the Federal Drug Enforcement Agency, and then informed the physician and the nurse practitioner that they were breaking the law (Sampson, 2009). The Commission on Pharmacy filed a formal complaint with the New Hampshire Board of Nursing and Nursing Registration asking for a "strict interpretation of the law" (p. 155). As a result of this action, New Hampshire nurse practitioners became embroiled in a political battle in which they sought to "legally define" their practice as well as amend the restrictive pharmacy laws that already existed.

While Sampson (2009) does not clearly state the purpose of the study, it is clearly explained in the narrative. Sampson (2009) explains that examining the efforts of nurses in one particular state can yield information about how nurses cooperate with others when seeking legislative change pertaining to their practice. Specifically, Sampson explores the actions of "two powerful bureaucrats" (p. 155) and their cooperative efforts. Marguerite Hastings, executive director of the New Hampshire Board of Nursing and Maynard Mires, the executive director of the New Hampshire Board of Medicine worked closely and in support of the political efforts of the nurse practitioners in their state. Their alliance, Sampson writes, demonstrates "the power of interprofessional relationships and respect to support change in spite of opposition from state professional organizations and boards" (p. 156).

Sampson (2009) provides the reader with a discussion about state professional boards and practice acts and uses New Hampshire's laws as an exemplar. The literature search for the study is also not separately identified in the narrative. Yet the narrative provides excellent documentation and explanation of the events that occurred during the 1970s in New Hampshire. This is typical of a well-written historical study, where the story flows without separately identifying the various sections in the critique. After reviewing the references one finds extensive use of primary sources including archival records from the State of New Hampshire, minutes of meetings of the various organizations and commissions, and oral histories of nurse practitioners and others embroiled in legislative actions in New Hampshire. Secondary sources used in the study include published research in this area. The "Notes" section is rich with additional information about the findings and explanations distinguishing nurse and nurse practitioner, for example. By using the Chicago Style Manual 15th edition as required by the journal in which this article appears, the author has an additional avenue in which to assist the reader understand various facets of the study as opposed to those who write historical studies using the American Psychological Association Publication Manual (APA). Without completely reading the "Notes" section of a published paper, important information and nuances of the story may be lost to the reader.

The authenticity and genuine nature of the primary sources also can be determined within the "Notes" section. By offering the reader explanations about the subject, such as "For excellent in-depth discussion of nursing and the contested terrain of medical boundaries see . . ." (p. 174). Sampson (2009) places the citation in context and thus implies its appropriateness to the study. Throughout the "Notes" section, Sampson explains the data adding to the readers understanding of the ideas presented. For example, Sampson clarifies the terms of nurse and nursing in the article writing that these terms "are used to denote all licensed nurses and their practice" (p. 173) and then explains that "nurse practitioners are one branch of nursing . . . while all nurse practitioners are nurses first, not all nurses are nurse practitioners" (p. 173). She frequently alerts the reader to various histories on the subject of collaborative practice, nurses work identity, and other areas that impact on the study. In the references, Sampson highlights disagreements among scholars about nursing and this too adds an important dimension to understanding Sampson's work. The presentation of various opinions, theses, and ideas about the subject illuminates possible inconsistencies between and among the sources, as well as offers corroboration of certain facts. The numerous articles published during the time frame of the study and used to corroborate facts gives the reader needed information to determine the authenticity and genuine nature of the sources. Sampson does an excellent job of letting the reader know about the sources and offers important evidence that supports the quality and strength of the sources used.

Sampson (2009) implicitly embraces a social and labor history framework to examine how nurses, specifically nurse practitioners, negotiated and developed alliances with others to garner legislation that supported their practice. Sampson explains that

> nursing history is the history of women (and men) workers in women's sphere in an industry (health care) dominated by powerful traditionally male professionals. It is the story of conflict and cooperation as women negotiate for credibility, economic legitimacy, autonomy, and power in the professional arena, while defining an occupational sphere (p. 171).

Another framework that Sampson seems to use is the biographical description of two of the important people engaged in the New Hampshire effort. We learn about Marguerite Hastings and Maynard H. Mires and how their ability to work together aided the nurse practitioner's cause. Framing the analysis through the lens of women's work, nurses' work, cooperation, and conflict enables the researcher and reader to begin to understand the possible consequences an independent nursing practice have on individual nurses and on the profession as a whole. The researcher's beliefs about the outcome of the New Hampshire's nurses' successful bid for independent practice were stated in the opening section; however, bias was not explicitly addressed, nor were any of the ethical issues that may have surrounded the topic presented. Nevertheless, the study represents an appropriate use of data, and no ethical concern about the people involved is evident.

The narrative in Sampson's (2009) study tells the story of a particular group of people sparring for control of practice in New Hampshire. She integrates social, economic, biographical, and political factors that influenced the "story." By weaving in the insights gained from the primary and secondary sources, Sampson makes connections, such as

> Hastings undoubtedly had a keen understanding that patients would suffer if nurse practitioners could no longer practice in their full role. She probably also understood that they would no longer

have the jobs for which they had recently been educated if they were unable to continue to provide comprehensive care that included prescribing and dispensing . . . perhaps caught between her roles as state bureaucrat and nursing advocate, Hastings encouraged the nurse practitioners to mobilize to change the nurse practice act to redefine the disputed tasks as sanctioned nurse practitioner practice. (p. 160)

By using direct quotes, the author adds richness to the narrative. The narrative clearly presents Sampson's ideas and theses. The significance of the study, identified in the beginning of the study, was again explicitly shared with the readers in the concluding section of the paper. The case study using the political efforts of nurse practitioners in New Hampshire serve as an exemplar for all nurse practitioners and nurses in each state. The narrative creatively weaves together the story, relates it to the broader issues of nurses' work, political activism, and cooperative alliances. Sampson (2009) ends her compelling narrative by connecting the events in one particular state to broader issues in nursing noting that this story "illustrates the significance of networks and intraprofessional and interprofessional relationships in supporting women's voice and power over their work and stimulating alliances with and across professional lines to influence legislative outcomes" (p. 172).

SUMMARY

Grypma (2005) describes the allure of historical research, citing the "thrill of discovery" (p. 171) upon handling papers and materials from noted leaders in the past. Yet Grypma notes that historical research methodology is undergoing changes that require the researcher to question the readership and audience of historical studies. Important information gleaned from the past must be critically examined for themes such as power, ethics, diversity, technology, political activism, and other compelling concerns that continue to affect nursing practice, education, and administration. Issues in nursing that are affected by gender, race, and ethnicity lend themselves to study through historical research. D'Antonio's (2005) statement about the lack of specificity surrounding historical research methods does not necessarily alter the quality, importance, or relevance of the historical studies. Nurse researchers must use the appropriate method to gain insights into their practice and explore the relevance of historical evidence to current and future practice issues in nursing. Lynaugh (2008) speaks of the importance of historical scholarship as well as the "integrity" of the historical research.

This chapter enables the audience of historical research to better understand the method and provides a guide for critiquing historical studies. The guide should not be considered the only way to understand the historical process, nor is it meant to fit all historians into a single mold. As in the case of the critiques presented in this chapter, the research often did not present their material in a lock-step manner as suggested by the criteria. Rather, the rich narratives of each of the three studies presented in this chapter offer connections and meaning to the data. What it is meant to provide is a framework that will allow nurses to assess historical research evidence affecting a particular nursing technique, an educational reform, or an administrative decision. The reader should ask, Does the study meet the guidelines, and if not, why? What is explicitly stated in the narrative, and what must the audience infer from the work? These questions may be more realistic than expecting historians to fit a proscribed set of criteria. Nursing history, as D'Antonio (2003) notes, "matters." For history to matter, it must first be understood. And we need to study history, as Lynaugh (2009) writes, "it is our history, our known and ordered past, that makes it possible to imagine new goals and envision a collective future for nursing" (p. ix).

References

Abrams, S. E. (2007). The report of the conference on redesigning nursing education for public health. *Public Health Nursing, 24* (2), 198–201.

Ament, L. A. (2004). The evolution of midwifery faculty practice: Impact and outcomes of care. *Nursing Outlook, 52*(4), 203–208.

Bartal, N., & Steiner-Freud, J. (2005). Nursing education moves into the university: The story of the Hadassah school of nursing in Jerusalem, 1918–1984. *Nursing History Review, 13,* 121–145.

Barzun, J., & Graff, H. F. (1985). *The modern researcher* (4th ed.). San Diego, CA: Harcourt Brace Jovanovich.

Birnbach, N. (2008). Ethical guidelines and standards of professional conduct. In S. B. Lewenson, & E. K. Herrmann (Eds.), *Capturing nursing history: A guide to historical research* (pp. 167–172). New York: Springer.

Birnbach, N., & Lewenson, S. (Eds.). (1991). *First words: Selected addresses from the National League for Nursing 1894–1933.* New York: National League for Nursing Press.

Birnbach, N., Brown, J., & Hiestand, W. (1993a). Ethical guidelines for the nurse historian. *American Association for the History of Nursing Bulletin, 38,* 4.

Birnbach, N., Brown, J., & Hiestand, W. (1993b). Standards of professional conduct for historical inquiry into nursing. *American Association for the History of Nursing Bulletin, 38,* 5.

Boschma, G. (2008). Writing international nursing history: What does it mean? *Nursing History Review, 16,* 9–11.

Brennan, A. (1991). Comparative value of theory and practice in nursing. In N. Birnbach, & S. Lewenson (Eds.), *First words: Selected addresses from the National League for Nursing 1894–1933* (pp. 23–25). New York: National League for Nursing Press. (Original speech presented in 1897.)

Bloch, M. (1964). *The historian's craft.* New York: Vantage Books.

Buck, J. (2004). Home hospice versus home health: Cooperation, competition, and cooptation. *Nursing History Review, 12,* 25–46.

Bullough, B. (1992). Alternative models for specialty nursing practice. *Nursing and Health Care, 13*(5), 254–259.

Connolly, C. A. (2004). Beyond social history: New approaches to understanding the state of and the state in nursing history. *Nursing History Review, 12*, 5–24.

D'Antonio, P. (2003). Editor's note. *Nursing History Review, 11*, 1.

D'Antonio, P. (2004). Women, nursing, and baccalaureate education in 20th century America. *Journal of Nursing Scholarship, 36*(4), 379–386.

D'Antonio, P. (2005). Editor's note. *Nursing History Review, 13*, 1–4.

Davis, A. T. (1988). Adah Belle Samuels Thomas. In V. Bullough, O. M. Church, & A. P. Stein (Eds.), *American nursing: A biographical dictionary* (pp. 313–316). New York: Garland.

Dock, L. (1910). Report of the thirteenth annual convention. *American Journal of Nursing, 10*(11), 902.

Fairman, J. (2008a). *Making room in the clinic: Nurse practitioners and the evolution of modern health care.* New Brunswick, NJ: Rutgers University Press.

Fairman, J. (2008b, First Quarter). Context and contingency in the history of post World War II nursing scholarship in the United States. *Journal of Nursing Scholarship,* 4–11.

Flynn, K. (2009). Beyond the glass wall: Black Canadian nurses, 1940–1970. *Nursing History Review, 17*, 129–152.

Goldmark, J. (1984). *Nursing and nursing education in the United States.* New York: Garland. (Original work published 1923.)

Griffon, D. P. (1998). A somewhat duskier skin: Mary Seacole in the Crimea. *Nursing History Review, 6*, 115–127.

Grypma, S. J. (2004). Neither angels of mercy nor foreign devils: Revisioning Canadian missionary nurses in China, 1935–1947. *Nursing History Review, 12*, 97–119.

Grypma, S. J. (2005). Critical issues in the use of biographic methods in nursing history. *Nursing History Review, 13*, 171–187.

Hallett, C. (2008). The truth about the past?: The art of working with archival materials. In S. B. Lewenson, & E. K. Herrmann (Eds.), *Capturing nursing history: A guide to historical research* (pp. 149–158). New York: Springer.

Hawkins, J. W., & Watson, J. C. (2003). Public health nursing pioneer: Jane Elizabeth Hitchcock 1863–1939. *Public Health Nursing, 20*(3), 167–176.

Hine, D. C. (1989). *Black women in white: Racial conflict and cooperation in the nursing profession, 1890–1950.* Bloomington, IN: Indiana University Press.

Hobbs, J. L. (2009). Defining nursing practice: The ANA social policy statement, 1980–1983. *Advances in Nursing Science, 32*(1), 3–18.

Houweling, L. (2004). Image, function, and style: A history of the nursing uniform. *American Journal of Nursing, 104*(4), 40–48.

Lewenson, S. B. (2008, September). *Transforming Nursing Education: History of the Phasing Out of Bellevue and Mills School of Nursing and the Expansion of Hunter College Department of Nursing, 1967.* Paper presented at the 25th Annual Meeting of the AAHN hosted by the University of Pennsylvania in Philadelphia, PA.

Lewenson, S. B., & Herrmann, E. K. (2008). Why do historical research? In S. B. Lewenson, & E. K. Herrmann (Eds.), *Capturing nursing history: A guide to historical research* (pp. 1–10). New York: Springer.

Lorentzon, M. (2004). Nursing Record/British Journal of Nursing archives, 1888–1956. *British Journal of Nursing, 13*(5), 280–284.

Lusk, B. (1997). Historical methodology for nursing research. *Journal of Nursing Scholarship, 29*(4), 355–400. (Retrieved from Gale Group Information Integrity, pp. 1–5.)

Lynaugh, J. E. (1996). Editorial. *Nursing History Review, 4,* 1.

Lynaugh, J. E. (2008). Foreword. In S. B. Lewenson, & E. K. Herrmann (Eds.), *Capturing nursing history: A guide to historical research* (p. xi). New York: Springer.

Mages, K. C., & Fairman, J. A. (2008). Working with primary sources: An overview. In S. B. Lewenson, & E. K. Herrmann (Eds.), *Capturing nursing history: A guide to historical research* (pp. 129–148). New York: Springer.

Meehan, T. C. (2003). Careful nursing: A model for contemporary nursing practice. *Journal of Advanced Nursing, 44*(1), 99–107.

Mosley, M. O. P. (1996). Satisfied to carry the bag: Three black community health nurses' contributions to health care reform, 1900–1937. *Nursing History Review, 4,* 65–82.

Poslusny, S. (1989). Feminist friendship: Isabel Hampton Robb, Lavinia Lloyd Dock, and Mary Adelaide Nutting. *Image, 21*(2), 64–68.

Reedy, E. A. (2003). From weakling to fighter: Changing the image of premature infants. *Nursing History Review, 11,* 109–127.

Sampson, D. A. (2009). Alliances of cooperation: Negotiating New Hampshire nurse practitioners' prescribing practice. *Nursing History Review, 17,* 153–178.

Spieseke, A. W. (1953). What is the historical method of research? *Nursing Research, 2*(1), 36–37.

Thomas, K. K. (2004). A law unto themselves: Black women as patients and practitioners in North Carolina's campaign to reduce maternal and infant mortality, 1935–1953. *Nursing History Review, 12,* 47–66.

Ulrich, L. T. (1990). *A midwife's tale: The life of Martha Ballard based on her diary, 1785–1812.* New York: Vintage Books.

Ulrich, L. T. (1994). About Laurel Thatcher Ulrich's work on A Midwife's Tale: Interviews with Laurel Thatcher Ulrich. Available at http://dohistory.org/book/100_interview.html. Accessed August 22, 2009.

Wall, B. M. (2003). Science and ritual: The hospital as medical and sacred space, 1865–1920. *Nursing History Review, 11,* 51–68.

Whelan, J. (2005). A necessity in the nursing world: The Chicago Nurses Professional Registry, 1913–1950. *Nursing History Review, 13,* 49–75.

Wolf, A. (1991). How can general duty be made more attractive to graduate nurses? In N. Birnbach, & S. Lewenson (Eds.), *First words: Selected addresses from the National League for Nursing, 1894–1933* (pp. 138–147). New York: National League for Nursing Press. (Original speech presented 1928.)

Young, J. (2005). Revisiting the 1925 Johns Report on African-American nurses. *Nursing History Review, 13,* 77–99.

Research Article

Alliances of Cooperation: Negotiating New Hampshire Nurse Practitioners' Prescribing Practice

Deborah A. Sampson, *University of Michigan School of Nursing*

ABSTRACT

Nurse practitioner legislation varies among states, particularly in relation to practice without physician oversight, altering the legal environment within which nurse practitioners can use knowledge and skills to meet patient needs. Using New Hampshire as a case study, this historical analysis of nurse practitioners' negotiations over time for independent practice, defined in state practice acts, illuminates the complex social and economic factors affecting nurses' struggle to gain legal rights over their own professional practice without supervision and intervention from another profession. In New Hampshire, not only did organized medicine oppose nurses' rights to practice, but pharmacists demanded the right to control all aspects of medication management, including who could prescribe and under what circumstances prescribing could occur. Shifting social and political terrain as well as changes in legislative and state professional board leadership affected the environment and negotiations of a small group of nurses who were ultimately successful in obtaining the right to define their own professional practice.

In 1973, the New Hampshire Board of Nursing recognized a new category of nurses called "advanced registered nurse practitioners" when the legislature passed an addendum to the nursing practice act formally recognizing this emerging group of nurses.[1] Following a growing national trend, these nurse practitioners had obtained additional education that enabled them to diagnose disease, order diagnostic tests, and prescribe and dispense medications to patients, activities that had been traditionally designated as only within the realm of medicine. For the next four years, New Hampshire nurse practitioners worked in this expanded role diagnosing disease, dispensing contraceptives and drug samples, and prescribing medications by using physician presigned prescriptions or under physician auspices by telephoning prescriptions to community pharmacies under a physician's name. Most often the nurse practitioners were making their own clinical decisions about the drug, prescribing or dispensing without directly consulting doctors. Physicians, who were not always on

From Sampson DA. *Nursing History Review*. vol. 17, pp. 153–178. Copyright © 2009 by Springer Publishing Company. Reprinted with kind permission of the American Association for the History of Nursing (AAHN).

premises when nurse practitioners examined patients, diagnosed illness, and prescribed or dispensed drugs (and may not even have worked in the same practice as the nurse practitioner), were fully aware and sanctioned this practice.[2] The nurse practitioners reasoned that since the New Hampshire Nurse Practice Act was broadly written and allowed nurses to practice consistent with their education, they were fully within their rights to diagnose and prescribe in the manner that they were doing, even though the practice act did not specifically address diagnosis or prescribing. The nurse practitioners, after all, were educated to perform these functions, and they were bound by state nursing statutes rather than by pharmacy or medical practice acts. The physicians supported these nurse practitioners' actions because, they believed, the Medical Practice Act allowed them to "delegate" with impunity any function they wished to another health care provider, and the physicians with whom the nurse practitioners worked were fully supportive of the practices. Both groups believed they were meeting patient needs without breaking the law.[3]

This practice had been going on for several years without question from any state regulatory office. Community pharmacists, another party to the discussion, occasionally complained to the Commission on Pharmacy, but these rare complaints brought forth no action other than an occasional brief notation in Commission on Pharmacy Board meeting minutes.[4] Both physicians and nurse practitioners were unaware that they were breaking a state pharmacy law that permitted only physicians, dentists, and veterinarians to prescribe and dispense. For almost five years, neither physicians, pharmacists, nor any other professional group seemed interested in ending the nurse practitioners' practices, despite state pharmacy law to the contrary.

But at the end of 1977, the Commission on Pharmacy formally challenged nurse practitioners' diagnosing, prescribing, and dispensing medications. The Commission was under pressure from the New England Regional Drug Enforcement Agency office in Boston and the New Hampshire State Police Drug Investigation Unit to tighten the filling of potentially specious prescriptions for controlled substances through pharmacies in New Hampshire.[5] The Pharmacy Commission, which was charged with inspecting community pharmacies' handling of prescriptions, put pharmacists on notice that prescriptions would be meticulously reviewed at each inspection, a practice that had previously been done in a more random and haphazard way.

During one such inspection in June 1977, a Commission on Pharmacy inspection pharmacist found several prescriptions for controlled substances that, while bearing one physician's name, had markedly different signature styles. Upon visiting the physician's office, the Commission on Pharmacy inspector found that the physician was unavailable. The physician's wife, who worked in the office, claimed to be a nurse practitioner and admitted to signing her husband's name to some prescriptions. She insisted that she had been taught at a prestigious Boston university–based nurse practitioner program that what she was doing was legal. The inspector, in front of the nurse practitioner, called the New England Regional Office of the Federal Drug Enforcement Agency, where an agent informed them both that the nurse was indeed breaking the law, and that she and the physician could be prosecuted under federal statutes.[6]

In July 1977, after discussing the issue at scheduled meetings, the Commission on Pharmacy filed a formal letter of complaint with the New Hampshire Board of Nursing Education and Nursing Registration against the nurse practitioner's practice.

The substance of the complaint was that nurse practitioners were prescribing and dispensing drugs, a practice nurses were specifically prohibited to perform by state-mandated Pharmacy Board rules and regulations, and physicians could not abrogate their responsibilities by delegating this task to any person who was not a physician. The Commission moved to pursue a strict interpretation of the law but did not name the nurse practitioner or physician or move to have the nurse practitioner disciplined.[7] Subsequently, New Hampshire nurse practitioners became involved in a lengthy and often contentious legislative process to legally define not only their own practice act rights, but to enlist changes in pharmacy laws.

An examination of the legislative process in a particular state, New Hampshire, can give us information on how nurses cooperate to define their work through legislative negotiations around state practice acts. These negotiations encompass the highly gendered work roles of nursing, medicine, and pharmacy in the health care arena.[8] New Hampshire nurse practitioners' pursuit of prescribing legislation, which began in 1977, demonstrates the power of cooperation that transcends differences in nursing education and experience. Nurses at the New Hampshire state nursing board, most of whom were from academia, provided unqualified support of the nurse practitioners' endeavors. Perhaps most imperative, the cooperative actions of two powerful bureaucrats (Marguerite Hastings, executive director of the New Hampshire Board of Nursing, and Maynard Mires, executive secretary of the New Hampshire Board of Medicine, a leader in the New Hampshire Medical Society and director of New Hampshire Public Health) to support nurse practitioners' prescribing authority demonstrate the power of interprofessional relationships and respect to support change in spite of opposition from state professional organizations and boards.

State Professional Boards and Practice Acts

Professional licensing and oversight by state-mandated boards are an extension of the state's social contract with citizens. The intent of state laws and governing boards is to monitor and regulate professional activity as defined by state regulation. State professional regulation is designed ostensibly to protect the citizens of the state, but also to limit competition so that some groups or organizations are protected.[9] Each state has boards or commissions that oversee regulations for the practice of nursing, medicine, and pharmacy. The names of these boards and their structure, function, power, and laws vary significantly from state to state. Regardless of differences, however, these boards are responsible for administering and enforcing the state practice act. Although many board activities under the act may be mandated, funds may be insufficient to carry out their duties in a comprehensive way, and boards may have to prioritize activities, including oversight of professionals and maintaining boundary infringement by other professionals.

Board members are usually unpaid, overwhelmingly drawn from the professional practitioners the board is charged with overseeing, and often members of the professional organizations involved, a priori, in any legislative activity affecting professional boundaries and practice. A professional group often believes that only those within that profession should have jurisdiction of their practice. Physicians believe that only the medical board and the medical practice act have authority over medical practice. Nurses correspondingly believe that the nursing board and corresponding practice act have sole jurisdiction over nursing. But, in truth, in

New Hampshire as elsewhere, the Pharmacy Practice Act also affects all health practitioners' management of drugs requiring a prescription. The boundaries of professional practice are thus not solely defined by one practice act but may extend through those of several professions. Practice acts may delineate the boundaries for each profession, but interpretation of such acts is evidenced by how the laws are clarified through rules and regulations, and board interpretations may conflict with the interests, responsibilities, or rules of other professional boards. In New Hampshire, the Boards of Nursing, Medicine, and Pharmacy all influence legal aspects of medication prescribing and dispensing.

In many states, New Hampshire being no exception, it is common for professional organizations to submit nominations for empty board seats to the governor, and often the nominee is appointed without question. Under this system, the agenda of the professional board may conflict with patient needs. Physician Maynard Mires, director of the New Hampshire Public Health Department and an influential member of both the New Hampshire Medical Society and Board of Medicine in the 1970s and early 1980s, recalled that in New Hampshire in the 1970s,

> members of the Board of Registration and Medicine really came from the Medical Society. So they were together in all of their ideas. I think that the Division of Public Health Services sort of resented time that I would spend with the board or with the Medical Society . . . and I almost got into some binds because the Medical Society [and therefore the Board of Medicine membership] would like me to take part in something, which I felt would not be in the best interests of the Division of Public Health.[10]

The ethics of such arrangements, where members of boards charged with protecting the public are intimately involved with promoting the interests of the professions, contains obvious ethical conundrums, but is nonetheless a common occurrence. The actions of regulatory boards, whose formal function is to protect the public, often echo the interests of the profession, particularly when the goals of public safety and protection of the profession conflict.[11] In New Hampshire the practice acts, organizations, configurations, and titles of the boards have changed over time based on legislative mandates. Moreover, state practice acts rarely keep up with "role evolution."[12] Nurse practitioners needed to prescribe before states implemented legal regulations and nurse practitioners found ways to do so.

Cooperation, Coalitions, and Alliances

On July 28, 1977, after receiving the Commission on Pharmacy letter demanding that nurse practitioners no longer prescribe drugs, even under the instructions of a physician, Marguerite Hastings, executive director of the New Hampshire Board of Nursing, sent a letter to the leaders of the New Hampshire Nurse Practitioners Association detailing the Commission on Pharmacy complaint. Hastings informed the leaders that under current statue it was illegal for nurse practitioners to prescribe or dispense medications, practices nurse practitioners had been performing without challenge, sometimes alongside physicians, but also alone in geographically isolated areas or to low-income, underserved patients throughout the state.[13] The nurse practitioner leaders realized that they needed to mobilize their membership quickly to plan a strategy. The law needed not only to be revised but to be crafted and passed in a form that would assure New Hampshire nurse practitioners the legal right to prescribe and dispense under their own names.[14] Nurse practitioner leadership first gathered in October 1977 to discuss the situation.

The New Hampshire nurse practitioner and physician alliance that had worked well, and presumably safely, for both patients and providers was suddenly under threat from the formerly disinterested Commission on Pharmacy, which used state law to halt a practice all stakeholders had tacitly agreed to honor. New Hampshire nurse practitioners found themselves in the middle of a political battle for their livelihood and practice prerogatives. Assumed practice boundaries, within the usual "contested terrain" of medicine and nursing, were suddenly open to interpretation by pharmacists.[15] The nurse practitioners quickly learned not only how to maneuver the difficult, often ambiguous, lengthy, and gritty political process of moving a bill from initial draft into final law, but also how to use intra-, inter-, and extraprofessional networks to negotiate legislation that assured the nurse practitioners prescribing authority without physician oversight. They also had to continue practicing so that patient care would continue without difficulty for patients, physicians, or nurse practitioners.

Hastings was a native of Massachusetts and a 1937 graduate of Newton-Wellesley Hospital School of Nursing. While working as a nursing instructor and nursing administrator in several Massachusetts hospitals and serving as president of the Massachusetts Nurses Association, she earned a Bachelor of Science degree in nursing education from Boston University. After earning a graduate degree in education from Northeastern University in 1966, she moved to New Hampshire to become executive director of the New Hampshire State Board of Nursing, a position she held for 22 years. During her tenure, she also assumed leadership positions in the National Association of Parliamentarians and as chair of the National Council of State Boards of Nursing.[16] Hastings's leadership skills, which she honed through her leadership positions in national and international organizations, earned overwhelming respect and admiration from New Hampshire legislators, the nursing community, and leadership of other state professional boards.[17]

Hastings was never called anything but "Miss Hastings" except by her closest friends and, although she was diminutive, she was known to be intelligent, gracious, and poised. Because she frequently visited schools of nursing and hospitals in New Hampshire, meeting with administrators and staff nurses alike, virtually all nurses in the state knew and respected her. The level of respect she engendered translated into significant personal and professional power when negotiating change for New Hampshire nurses. Moreover, Hastings was a shrewd and meticulous planner when developing strategies for change or shaping nursing practice that could cross medical boundaries. She often asked for input from others within and outside the Board of Nursing to assure that she understood all aspects of an issue and had a reputation for always being well-prepared at meetings and when testifying before the legislature.[18] Under Hastings, the Board of Nursing, unlike the Board of Medicine and Commission on Pharmacy, decisively disciplined nurses who violated nurse practice act mandates, particularly those that involved threats to patient safety or nurse substance abuse. Although she was a staunch advocate for nurses, Hastings took seriously the Board of Nursing charge to protect the public. Board of Nursing adjudication often involved license suspensions and revocation, Board actions that rarely happened to physicians or pharmacists.[19]

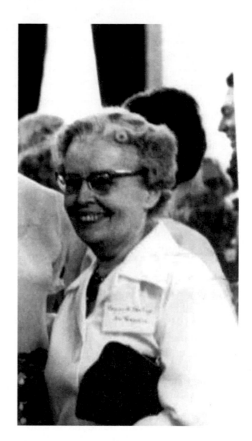

Figure 1: **Marguerite Hastings, MS, RN, former Executive Director of the New Hampshire Board of Nursing. Reprinted courtesy of the New Hampshire Historical Society, Tuck Library.**

Hastings worked, often successfully in terms of nurses' position, to negotiate nursing-medical boundaries at fairly regular and amicable Board of Medicine and Board of Nursing joint meetings. For example, in March 1973 the two boards agreed to issue a joint statement that nurses should not be responsible for pronouncing death; that a properly trained nurse was not practicing medicine by inserting a vaginal speculum to perform a pelvic exam; that nurses should not take physician assistants' orders (a practice nurses and the Board of Nursing vehemently opposed); and that nurse midwives were practicing nursing, not medicine, and were exempted from Medical Practice Act, with the Board of Nursing solely responsible for their oversight. The two boards agreed that the issue of a nurse "hanging out a shingle" to give foot care to the elderly should be referred to the Board of Podiatry (nominally under the Board of Medicine), and further that, "If she hangs out a shingle, she could be in trouble."[20] The Board of Medicine often described negotiations with Hastings as "felt meeting was good and were able to discuss and solve problems," and the Board of Nursing, with Hastings's leadership, was able to "win" all the nursing positions.[21]

Hastings undoubtedly had a keen understanding that patients would suffer if nurse practitioners could no longer practice in their full role. She probably also understood that they would no longer have the jobs for which they had recently been educated if they were unable to continue to provide comprehensive care that included prescribing and dispensing. The best interests of the residents of New Hampshire would not be served if these nurses could not continue to dispense and prescribe. Perhaps caught between her roles as state bureaucrat and nursing advocate, Hastings encouraged the nurse practitioners to mobilize to change the nurse practice act to redefine the disputed tasks as sanctioned nurse practitioner practice.

Shortly after meeting with the nurse practitioners, Hastings met with Mires. Their close professional relationship, as noted above, not only facilitated boundary negotiations but also prompted their alliance to promote nurse practitioner practice, even when opposed by pharmacists or the medical society. Mires, appointed director of public health in December 1973, held a position of significant state power. He had an extensive public health background and family ties to New Hampshire, although he was a native of upstate New York. Before coming to New Hampshire, he had served as a public health physician in the U.S. Navy and subsequently attended Harvard University School of Public Health in the early 1950s. Dr. Alfred Frechette, a former Harvard faculty member and Massachusetts commissioner of public health, encouraged Mires to apply to the New Hampshire Health Department. Undoubtedly Mires's military service influenced his subsequent leadership decisions in New Hampshire. During World War II and after, he worked with military nurses of equal and higher rank who were in leadership positions. Yet he also may have recognized the ambiguities of upholding military regulations while providing health services to individuals and populations.

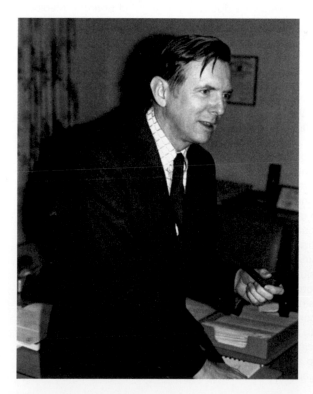

Figure 2: **Maynard H. Mires, MD, MPH, former Executive Secretary of the New Hampshire Board of Medicine, leader in the New Hampshire Medical Society, and Director of New Hampshire Public Health. Photograph courtesy of Maynard H. Mires and used with permission.**

Mires believed in loyalty to his superiors, in this case the governor, who had administrative oversight of all state boards, but he also believed in "doing his duty" to support unpopular decisions in the best interests of patients, even when this meant defying his colleagues or the governor. Like Hastings, he had the respect of his colleagues, the governor, and legislators. He maintained close personal friendships with politicians, the New Hampshire attorney general, other Board of Medicine members, and the chair of the Commission on Pharmacy, Kenneth Fortier. Mires also had great admiration for Hastings, acknowledging that "Marguerite and I saw eye-to-eye. I worked very closely with her."[22] Whatever the two negotiated jointly, the Board of Nursing and Board of Medicine seemed to approve. Mires affirmed, "The two boards trusted Marguerite and me to the effect they thought, 'You just go ahead and take care of it.'"[23] The Board of Medicine was apparently content to abdicate all nurse practitioner practice issues to Mires and Hastings.

The Hastings/Mires alliance worked well to negotiate, often under the radar, all manner of Board of Medicine and Board of Nursing joint issues. For example, when the Commission on Pharmacy objected to nurse practitioners dispensing contraceptive medications in family planning clinics and private medical offices, Mires and Hastings, with the attorney general's sanction, collaborated to change the Board of Nursing rules and regulations to permit the dispensing.[24] Under the Hastings and Mires alliance, the Board of Nursing led the Joint Practice Committee, comprising the Board of Medicine, Board of Nursing, and New Hampshire Nurses Association, to interpret and implement the amendment to the nurse practice act that defined nurse practitioner status.[25] Mires and Hastings jointly developed protocols for nurse-run immunization clinics, which the Board of Nursing and Board of Medicine approved without fuss. Given that all other Board of Medicine members were practicing physicians with private practices, it is probable that the Joint Health Council medical representation consisted solely of Mires. When Mires, the Board of Medicine, and the New Hampshire Medical Society expressed strong concern that diploma schools of nursing were closing in New Hampshire and community college academic programs were replacing hospital-based training schools, there was little disruption in the cordial relationships between the Board of Nursing and Board of Medicine.[26] Undoubtedly the Mires/Hastings relationship could surmount interboard discord.[27]

When the Commission on Pharmacy complained about nurse practitioner prescribing it also objected to nurse practitioners dispensing medications and contraceptives. Nurse practitioners dispensing medications in public clinics, especially contraceptives at family planning clinics, was critical to meeting patient needs, and physicians would rarely be onsite to oversee the dispensing. Hastings and Mires recognized that patients would suffer needlessly. Therefore, they initiated a process available to state administrative department heads in New Hampshire to facilitate nurse practitioner dispensing of medications without involving the lengthy legislative process or the recalcitrant Commission on Pharmacy. After consulting with Attorney General David Souter, Hastings and Mires quickly changed administrative rules of the Board of Nursing and the Board of Medicine practice acts to permit nurse practitioners to dispense medications and contraceptives legally under protocols jointly developed with a collaborating physician. The attorney general agreed that physicians could delegate the legal right to dispense, and that defining a process and mechanism to accomplish this only required Boards of Medicine and Nursing agreement about administrative rules.[28] The Commission on Pharmacy, not included in this process, spent the next four years trying to convince the attorney general's office that the rule change should be deemed illegal. The Commission was not successful and New Hampshire nurse practitioners' legal practice boundary was explicitly expanded without the legislative initiative that can often take years in New Hampshire's complex citizen legislature.[29]

What is particularly interesting is that the expansion of nurse practitioner practice was accomplished quickly through the collaboration and cooperation of a physician and a nurse, both state bureaucrats. Mires, a close friend of Attorney General Souter, also believed that the rural center patients needed nurse practitioners to have more freedom in treating and prescribing without physician supervision.[30] Hastings was able to develop a rule that met the needs of clinics and patients as well as legal rulemaking requirements, and was acceptable to Mires. They presented the rule to their respective Boards (incidentally indicating that they had modeled it together), and after approval by Souter it was enacted into law. The Commission on Pharmacy was dismayed and filed a futile formal complaint with the attorney general's office.

The Commission on Pharmacy strongly opposed allowing nonphysician health care professionals, including nurse practitioners, to prescribe or dispense medication.[31] The crux of the opposition was twofold. First, the Commission argued that only physicians had the requisite education for safe medication prescribing. Medications were potentially dangerous, and "patient safety" could be compromised if nonphysicians were allowed to prescribe. Moreover, under current state statutes, prescribing to patients was a legal prerogative limited to physicians and dentists. Any other professional group that prescribed was breaking the law.

Prescribing Medications—Whose Privilege?

The issue of prescriptive privilege for nurse practitioners required a major legislative initiative. Furthermore, New Hampshire Nurse Practitioner Association members had no experience or knowledge about this process. So when Hastings informed the New Hampshire Nurse Practitioner Association leadership that nurse practitioners could no longer prescribe, nurse practitioner leaders Betty Mitchell and Donna White, who worked together at a women's health practice and lived in the same small New Hampshire town, took action. They met with their state representative, George Roberts, Jr., to ask for his guidance for changing the nurse practitioner laws. Roberts, who was not only Donna White's neighbor and high school friend but also speaker of the New Hampshire House of Representatives and former House majority leader, enlisted the help of the legislative attorney to draft a plan for the nurse practitioners to use to change the law.[32] When asked why he bothered to take time to help the nurse practitioners, Roberts said, "My wife was Donna's patient and loved her. I'd have never heard the end of it. I think the local doctors' wives went to her too."[33] Through incredibly valuable community and family networks, these two nurse practitioners were able to enlist the help of a seasoned and powerful legislator and premier legislative attorney to make a solid start in the change process.

In the meantime, the New Hampshire Nurse Practitioner Association leadership continued to hold planning and information meetings for all New Hampshire nurse practitioners and began sending letters to keep them informed and to mobilize political action. The letters urged all nurse practitioners that "this is your chance to participate and whatever happens will affect your nursing practice . . . think about New Hampshire Nurse Practitioner Association's future . . . be prepared to [mobilize] to get through a special [legislative] session" if necessary.[34] This professional network was tapped for practical and financial reasons. Cynthia Cote, former Association treasurer, recalls that members sat around a conference table at the meetings and emptied purses onto the table for postage money to mail the letters. Cote recalls, "I think often a lot of us just paid for the mailings and for any of the supplies and whatever we had to do. We were a very low-budget operation."[35]

The very small group of 20 regular New Hampshire Nurse Practitioner Association meeting attendees had a sparse financial base, but that would not be an obstacle. They had no central office from which to work, so, as women have often done, they met in public spaces such as restaurants and conference rooms in hospitals and clinics, and ran their campaign from their homes, often paying for telephone bills, stationery, and travel out of pocket.[36] The political was indeed both personal and professional, and the boundaries between personal and professional lives were often blurred.

New Hampshire Nurse Practitioner Association leaders immediately formed a Prescription Task Force led by Christine Kuhlman to implement the legislative action plan facilitated by Roberts. Kuhlman and Donna Cassidy, another task force member, worked at the progressive private Concord Clinic with physicians who supported independent prescribing for nurse practitioners. The clinic was often used for strategy meetings; clinic telephones, stationery, copy machines, and other office services were openly used without cost by Task Force leadership with full clinic physician support.[37]

Prescription Task Force members worked hard to organize a successful legislative initiative. They sent frequent information and strategy letters to all New Hampshire nurse practitioners outlining the legislative process, where negotiations and actions stood, names and towns of residence of key state committee legislators, sample letters to send to legislators, and dates of public hearings. The letters stressed that nurse practitioners should let their patients know that their help was needed to assure successful passage of the law. Nurse practitioners also intensively lobbied legislators. Paula Weeman, a member of the Task Force, recalled:

> It seems like, anybody in the legislative process that we needed to talk to . . . well, if we needed to talk in the halls [of the State House], we'd talk in the halls. If we needed to take a senator to lunch, we'd go to lunch; we'd invited the senator to lunch, or a representative. Or we'd go to representatives' breakfasts. We just became much more present, all the while, while we're working, raising families. But we were doing it.[38]

Prescription Task Force members enlisted other tactics as well. They made a presentation to the Commission on Pharmacy, which still actively opposed nurse practitioner prescribing. Hoping to bring the commission into the legislation change support group, the Task Force hoped to increase commission members' understanding about nurse practitioners' practice and the realities of New Hampshire patient care, and convince them that nurse practitioners' education was adequate to assure safe prescribing. Nurse practitioners had been educated to prescribe, and their prescribing practice was safe according to the physicians with whom they worked. Chris Kuhlman recalls "feeling very frustrated because we were taught prescriptive information in school for sure."[39] The Task Force presented details of pharmaceutical education and subsequent practice. Although there were little survey data for nurse practitioner prescribing safety (nor for physicians, for that matter), the Pharmacy Commission may have been mollified. After the presentation, for reasons as yet unclear, the commission neither publicly supported nor actively opposed the legislation during legislative hearings.[40]

The nurse practitioners continued to work with Marguerite Hastings and the Board of Nursing, who in turn continued to work with Maynard Mires and the Board of Medicine. In an interesting contrast to actions in many states, where those groups were opposing camps, in these early years the Board of Medicine and Board of Nursing often presented a united front in support of nurse practitioners against the Commission on Pharmacy. Nurse practitioner leaders used their cooperative networks with patients, physicians, colleagues, and neighbors to coalesce support, develop strategies, and mobilize action, while state leaders Mires and Hastings maintained their support for nurse practitioners' prescribing legislation.

Partial Success

The nurse practitioner practice prescribing legislation passed the House in spring 1979 without difficulty in spite of strong opposition from several powerful and vocal physician and pharmacist representatives from the heavily populated, nurse practitioner-scarce southern tier of the state. But the corresponding Senate bill was defeated on June 6, 1979, delaying hope for legislation until the next legislative session, several years hence.[41] Hamilton Putnam, administrative director of the New Hampshire Medical Society, later took credit for the defeat, insisting that his testimony stressing the need for "safeguards" missing in the bill had influenced the Senate vote.[42] Although Putnam may have had some influence on the outcome, other factors may also have been at play. George Roberts stresses that legislation on new ideas, no matter what the issue, might pass the House but is almost always defeated on the first "go 'round" in the Senate. "In the world of pragmatism [in New Hampshire politics] . . . the kill is in the Senate."[43]

Laurie Harding, community health nurse, former lobbyist for the New Hampshire Nurses Association and the New Hampshire Nurse Practitioners Association, and current House representative and member of the Health and Welfare Committee, had insight into why the New Hampshire Senate is traditionally a difficult place to pass a bill.

> The House will study an issue very diligently, because you're only assigned to one committee as opposed to being a Senator and assigned to four committees. They [the Senate] get a hair across their tail end and they make a lot of arbitrary decisions sometimes and they're heavily influenced by outside forces, depending on who is able to influence them at what times, and there have been times when nurses have been able to influence them in a positive way for nursing and for health care. Sometimes it has to do with the numbers, and it's a very individual thing and you really just can't tell sometimes about that Senate. It's highly unpredictable as to what the Senate will do.[44]

The nurse practitioners had been naïve. They had never attempted legislative action and perhaps relied too heavily on the belief that, since what they were trying to do was in the best interests of patients and they were filling a need supported by their collaboration, there would be no question of success. They believed that the backing of Hastings and Mires, representing a medical-nursing alliance, and the support of several legislators who were friends and neighbors, would also guarantee support. They clearly underestimated the possibility of opposition and were unaware of the power of behind-the-scenes political shenanigans that could blindside their attempts. Finally, as nurses often do, they tried to do everything themselves: organizing, testimony, lobbying, strategizing, fund-raising, educating, coalition building, and negotiating in a complex and sometimes covert world, the state legislature, where they had no experience. The term *babes in the woods* comes to mind. They needed more professional assistance than even George Roberts and legislator friends could give, but they did not even know enough on this first go-around to know what they didn't know. They would not be so naïve in the future.

When the bill failed the Senate, the nurse practitioners were discouraged but not defeated. At the next New Hampshire Nurse Practitioner Association meeting, they decided to try again. They discussed what they had learned from the years of strategizing, the lessons in the defeat, and how they could be more successful for their next attempt.[45] They would continue to use cooperation to attempt legislative change to assure their right to cross the medical (and in this case, pharmacy) boundaries for prescribing medications. They would continue to work toward prescribing rights legislation for as long as it took to pass the requisite laws. Unfortunately, they would have to do so without the powerful support of Hastings and Mires.

Hastings was required by state age limitation laws to retire at age 70, effective October 6, 1980. Although she continued to attend Board of Nursing meetings (as can any member of the public), she was no longer in an official leadership position and was unable to participate in a formal way. Mires, who had a close rapport with previous governor Meldrim Thomson, had a less than cordial relationship with Hugh Gallen, elected in 1980. An incident with Gallen changed leadership at the Department of Public Health. Mires evoked the incident, illustrating his own sense of fairness, belief in bipartisan cooperation, and integrity, that led to his leaving New Hampshire:

> The next administration [after Thomson] . . . really caused me to have to leave.
> I'd never been in a political situation like this before, where Republicans and
> Democrats really went at it hammer and tongs. I guess I was naïve enough to
> think they should get along. Anyway, they started saying something that was
> very untrue about the previous administration, that Governor Thomson had
> approved the dumping of hazardous materials some place. I believe that's
> what it was about. I knew that was definitely not true. I called Peter Thomson,
> his son. We met for lunch, and I said, "Peter, they're trying to blacken your
> father's name, and I don't think it's right." So somehow that word got back to
> the governor, Hugh Gallen. . . . I was told that I would have to leave.[46]

When Mires left New Hampshire in early 1981, there was little left of the strong interpersonal linkage and mutual support between the Board of Nursing and Board of Medicine. Stephen Tzianabos, a surgeon in private practice with no personal or professional relationships with nurse practitioners, or physician assistants for that matter, was appointed to the Board of Medicine along with other physicians who were less than friendly to nursing autonomy. Although neither Tzianabos nor other Board physicians were disposed to an alliance with the Commission on Pharmacy, the Board of Medicine became a vocal opponent of nurse practitioner prescribing. Times and leadership in boards and state had changed, and the relationship between the boards would continue to deteriorate.[47] The nurse practitioners needed new strategies.

Perhaps the nurse practitioners did not realize that the Hasting/Mires alliance was a source of power, and that its loss would make the second legislative attempt all the more difficult. Or perhaps they still believed in pursuing the support of the House of Representatives rather than initiating the bill with the more contentious but powerful Senate. Only 2 of the 24 senators attended the Senate Health and Welfare Committee hearings in May; one was Vesta Roy, Senate president. The minimal attendance may have signaled that the Senate decision had already been determined. At the hearing, House health and welfare chair Roma Spaulding unexpectedly introduced an amendment, undoubtedly originating from the New Hampshire Medical Society or Board of Medicine, adding physician assistants to the prescribing bill and requiring both physician assistants and nurse practitioners to be overseen by the Board of Medicine.

The nurse practitioner leaders were blindsided and were not sure how to proceed. If they opposed this arrangement, their hard work could continue to another session. If they agreed, they would possibly be subjected to the supervision of a now-hostile medical board, an abhorrent thought to all. They voted unanimously to oppose any bill that included Board of Medicine supervision of nurse practitioners. This proved to be a moot issue, since on June 12 the prescribing bill was once again "killed in the Senate," when Roy and the Senate Health and Welfare Committee recommended that the bill "ought not pass."[48] Once again, the House had passed the bill only to have it fail in the Senate. The exact reasons for the Senate defeat are unclear. Perhaps influenced by the Board of Medicine,

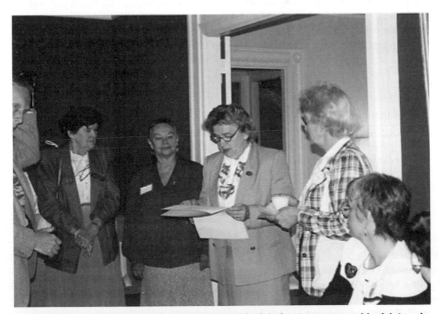

Figure 3: **Senator Ruth Griffin, RN, reading recent legislation to nurses and legislators in the New Hampshire State House (approximately 1980). Photograph used with permission of the New Hampshire Historical Society, Tuck Library.**

powerful legislators were content to play politics rather than support the nurse practitioners and the health care needs of the citizens. The nurse practitioners had underestimated the importance of winning over Roy and Spaulding, both powerful women legislators.

Still determined, the nurse practitioners were finally successful on the third try, in the 1984 legislative session. In large part the third attempt was successful because they enlisted initial sponsorship from the dynamic and powerful (and nurse practitioner-friendly) Senator Susan McLane, who was also chair of the Senate Health and Welfare Committee, which would hear the nurse practitioner prescribing bill.[49] Success was undoubtedly also due to the tenacity, cohesiveness, and determination of the nurse practitioners, and their awareness that starting a bill in the Senate, with powerful Senate backing, would be more likely to engender success.

Even though the final bill allowed nurse practitioners to prescribe, the Board of Medicine and Commission on Pharmacy insisted on oversight requirements for ongoing approval of a prescribing formulary. The formulary would define, and therefore limit, the drugs nurse practitioners would be able to prescribe. This was more oversight than the nurse practitioners or the Board of Nursing had hoped, but half a loaf was better than none.[50] Cynthia Cote recalls:

> It was a compromise. I think it was win-win. If you want this, you got to have that. And it was kind of like the safety net. . . . I think it was some of those back-room kind of deals, and maybe the Board of Pharmacy said as well. "OK, if you say that you, nurse practitioners, are skilled and educated and this is the only way that they really can deliver health care to those that are in need, then we'll go there so long as we have some safeties to protect the citizens from any malpractice on the part of nurse practitioners." And I remember those discussions so heatedly at our meetings, where there were some factions of our group. "We've been through this, didn't make it. Let's come up with a compromise so that we can move." It was a win-win for everybody, and their concerns are being addressed and we can get what we want too, which was to have the ability to write prescriptions legally.[51]

Even though they disagreed in private meetings, the nurse practitioners decided to go along with the compromise and present a united front in public. They had not entirely gained independence over their own practice, but they had made strides toward breaking down medical boundaries over prescribing. The victory they had won would quickly be followed by other major changes, including the legal right to receive direct insurance reimbursement for medical care services in New Hampshire regardless of collaboration with a physician.

Conclusion

For the most part, specialist nurses, particularly advanced practice nurses, have sought to gain independence from oversight by other health professions. Nurse practitioners seek the legal right to apply *medical* knowledge and practice independent of physician oversight, and have endeavored, state by state, for the right to define their own practice as professionals. The crux of this struggle seems to lie in questions such as what is nursing and what is medicine, who controls the practice of each, how control is implemented, who gets paid, and who gets control of health care access.[52] Nurse practitioners and physicians may not practice in the same physical space, and often do not collaborate to share knowledge. Negotiation was complex and sometimes painful but was a process between intricately related individuals and groups.[53] Although organized medicine has generally sought to maintain control and oversight over nurse practitioners, many other physicians were, and to some degree always have been, supporters of autonomous advanced practice nursing.[54]

New Hampshire nurse practitioners were breaking new ground both politically and in practice. They were pioneering to define new state sanctions for a nursing practice role while negotiating legislative change against some formidable opposition. They were political novices who "really learned a lot through trial and error," becoming more cohesive as a faction and "empowered and assertive and outspoken."[55] A small group, they were determined to have "a big voice," and they "weren't going to go away."[56] Leaders relied on politicians and physicians, other nursing organizations, patients and other community members, state bureaucrats, and each other for political alliances, and these alliances of cooperation shifted and changed over time. Community and professional networks mattered. The nurses formed an identity based on a shared belief about what they, as nurse practitioners, could do to provide care for people in the community, and this care included prescribing medications. Alliances between state bureaucrats of different professional backgrounds, based on respect and common goals, facilitated rules changes supportive of the nurses' goals. The nurse practitioners, with the support of Hastings, Mires, and influential politicians, were ultimately successful in passing the legislation defining new professional responsibilities for nurses.

Nursing history is the history of women (and men) workers in women's sphere in an industry (health care) dominated by powerful traditionally male professionals. It is the story of conflict and cooperation as women negotiate for credibility, economic legitimacy, autonomy, and power in the professional arena, while defining an occupational sphere.[57] It is a tale of women's efforts for professional status in an industry bound in male paradigms of occupational practices, particularly within the parameters of state practice acts. Advanced registered nurse practitioners challenge these male paradigms since they are, first and foremost, nurses, but also have knowledge and skills traditionally identified as reserved for the male physician's sphere.

While nurses have always challenged medical boundaries, the original intent that nurse practitioners could fill medical needs when physicians were not available meant that these nurses would openly diagnose disease and prescribe medications in publicly sanctioned ways. Yet the road to fulfilling their role, particularly around prescribing medications as defined in state practice act law, has been difficult in all states. Advanced registered nurse practitioners have faced opposition by medical and pharmacy organizations and boards, and they have had varying success overcoming this resistance. Current state nurse practice acts vary widely with regard to nurse practitioners prescribing as a nursing activity without state-required physician oversight.[58]

The history of New Hampshire nurse practitioner political activism during a time of significant legislative activity illustrates the concepts of nursing as gendered work, including how women's alliances and cooperation informs negotiations for occupational place in the hierarchy of health professions. This story illustrates the significance of networks and intraprofessional and interprofessional relationships in supporting women's voice and power over their work and stimulating alliances within and across professional lines to influence legislative outcomes.

DEBORAH A. SAMPSON, PHD, ARNP
Assistant Professor
University of Michigan School of Nursing
400 North Ingalls
Ann Arbor, MI 48109
734–647–0146
sampsond@umich.edu

Acknowledgments

Funding support for this research was provided by National Institute for Nursing Research/National Institutes for Health predoctoral research training award F31-NR008302–01A1: Doctoral Student Research Award, The American Association for the History of Nursing; Sigma Theta Tau, Xi Chapter.

Signed informed consents and releases of all oral histories are on file in the author's records or at the Tuck Library of the New Hampshire Historical Society.

Notes

1. The New Hampshire 1973 legal designation "advanced registered nurse practitioners" included nurse practitioners, nurse midwives, and psychiatric clinical nurse specialists, adding nurse anesthetists in 1991. Perhaps because there have been few clinical nurse specialists in New Hampshire other than those in psychiatry, they have never been designated advanced practice nurses. For documents related to the 1973 designation, see Box 1–1, folders marked "Legislation 1970," "Charters," "Minutes 1970s," New Hampshire Nurse Practitioners Association (hereafter NHNPA) Papers, archived in the Tuck Library of the New Hampshire Historical Society, Concord, New Hampshire. See also *Registered Nurses and Practical Nurses,* RSA 326-B: 1–22, Laws of the State of New Hampshire (January 1, 1973), Concord, New Hampshire.

2. For documentation of prescribing practices see oral history transcripts of Donna White recorded December 28, 2004 (cited as White), lines 390–408, 445–62; Jeanne Charest recorded May 15, 2005 (cited as Charest), lines 437–72; Joyce Cappiello recorded August 2, 2005 (cited as Cappiello), lines 229–77; Mary Bidgood-Wilson recorded May 27, 2005 (cited as Bidgood-Wilson), lines 535–45, 574–615; Nancy Dirubbo recorded February 23, 2005 (cited as Dirubbo), lines 240–61; Paula Weeman recorded January 24, 2005 (cited as Weeman), lines 294–381. Transcripts and tapes cited are archived in the Tuck Library of the New Hampshire Historical Society unless otherwise noted.

3. Oral histories from practicing nurse practitioners at this time document the nurse practitioners' prescribing practices and the physician complicity. See, for example, Weeman, Dirubbo, and Charest, also oral history transcript of John Argue, May 3, 2005 (cited as Argue), lines 493–513, 626–49; Maynard Mires recorded April 6, 2005 (cited as Mires), lines 883–944; letter dated July 20, 1977 from Thomas Nadeau, MD, to Commission on Pharmacy, attached to Commission on Pharmacy meeting minutes, July 20, 1977. All Commission on Pharmacy minutes cited are found in the Office of Paul Boisseau, Board of Pharmacy, Concord, New Hampshire. Board of Medicine minutes, December 5, 1977, January 5, 1978. All Board of Medicine minutes cited are found in the conference room, Board of Medicine, Concord.

4. See Commission on Pharmacy minutes, January 17, 1973, December 18, 1974, November 19, 1975.

5. See Commission on Pharmacy minutes, June 10, 1972, all minutes of 1974 and 1975, July 20, 1977, December 13, 1978; Board of Medicine minutes, February 16, 1971, February 19, 1972, December 3, 1973, January 4, 1979; *New Hampshire Medical Society News 28,* no. 4 (October 1977), 1. All *New Hampshire Medical Society Newsletters* cited are found in the Office of the New Hampshire Medical Society, Concord.

6. See a complete discussion of the Pharmacy Commission investigator's report incident in the Commission on Pharmacy minutes, July 22, 1977.

7. An interesting footnote is that the so-called nurse practitioner in question was not licensed in New Hampshire as a registered nurse or nurse practitioner, although she became licensed in both categories. Moreover, the prestigious university she claimed to have attended had no nurse practitioner program at that time. Yet her individual actions, sanctioned by the physician with whom she worked (who also happened to be her husband, a physician well known to the State Drug Investigation Unit), set in motion a lengthy struggle for all New Hampshire nurse practitioners to gain prescriptive authority. It was also at this time that the Board of Nursing was making considerable efforts to address the significant problem of unlicensed nurses working in physicians' offices. According to Board of Nursing minutes, this was a common problem well known to the Board of Medicine. It was not necessarily unusual for an office "nurse practitioner" not to be licensed. See Board of Medicine minutes, May 5, 1977; "Doctor, Is Your Nurse Licensed?" *New Hampshire Medical Society News* 31, no. 1 (February 1979): 2; Board of Nursing minutes, October 1, 1979, May 15, 1980; *Board of Nursing Newsletter* 15, no. 1 (May 1980), 3 . All Board of Nursing minutes and newsletters cited are found in the conference room, Board of Nursing office, Concord.

8. For the purposes of this article, the terms *nurse* and *nursing* are used to denote all licensed registered nurses and their practice. Nurse practitioners are one branch of nursing. They are educated to work in capacities that include concepts of nursing care and also provide some components of medical care traditionally performed by physicians, such as diagnosing and treating disease, prescribing medications, and even performing surgery and invasive procedures. While all nurse practitioners are nurses first, not all nurses are nurse practitioners. Therefore, the concepts and contexts of nursing history are applicable, for the most part, to nurse practitioner history. The converse, however, may not be entirely true.

9. Julie Fairman, "Delegated by Default or Negotiated by Need? Physicians, Nurse Practitioners, and the Process of Critical Thinking," *Medical Humanities Review* 13, no. 1 (1999), 38–58. State regulation is often shared with federal legislation, but states, even in the same geographic region such as New England, can vary widely in their ideology about regulation of citizens.

10. Interview with Maynard Mires, Georgetown, Delaware, April 6, 2005 (cited as Mires 2005), lines 173–82; Ronald L. Akers, "The Professional Association and the Regulation of Practice," *Law & Society Review* 2, no. 3 (1968), 463–482.

11. It is not unusual for professional organizations to form coalitions to combat other competing professional groups, particularly when negotiating mutually amenable legislation. Conversely, professions may introduce or support legislation that is actually detrimental to the public interest. The Commission on Pharmacy introduced legislation in 1975 to prevent outpatient clinics and physicians' offices from dispensing more than a 24-hour supply of medications, including contraceptives from family planning clinics. Patients would be forced to take a prescription to a pharmacy instead. Limiting access to often free or low-cost contraceptives would most certainly be detrimental to patients. Fortunately for many women of New Hampshire, this Commission on Pharmacy initiative failed. Commission on Pharmacy minutes, April 2, 1975, book marked "NH Commission of Pharmacy Minutes January 1975–December 1978."

12. Bobbie Schwaninger Hughes, "Role Evolution vs. Legislation," *Nurse Practitioner* 8, no. 3 (1983), 9, 12.

13. Letter dated July 28, 1977 from Marguerite Hastings, Executive Director of New Hampshire Board of Nursing, to Gloria Klein, President NHNPA, folder "Legislation 1970s."

14. Letter dated November 29, 1977 from Betty H. Mitchell and Donna White to "Dear Fellow Practitioners" sent to all New Hampshire nurse practitioners; letter dated January 24, 1978 from Debbie Clark, RN PNP, Recording Secretary NHNPA, to "Dear Practitioner," folder "Legislation 1970s."

15. For excellent in-depth discussions of nursing and the contested terrain of medical boundaries, see Julie Fairman, "Playing Doctor? Nurse Practitioners, Physicians and the Dilemma of Shared Practice," *Journal of the Massachusetts School of Law* 4, no. 4 (1999); Arlene Keeling, *Nursing and the Privilege of Prescription, 1893–2000* (Columbus: Ohio State University Press, 2007), 27–35.

16. See Obituaries, *Berkshire Eagle* (Pittsfield, Massachusetts), July 7, 1998, Marguerite Hastings, http://oa.newsbank.com.oa-search/we/Archives (accessed December 13, 2005).

17. Hastings was also New Hampshire representative to the National Council of State Boards of Nursing and consulted to the Caribbean Nurses Association. After her retirement from nursing, she was New Hampshire director of the New Hampshire Association of Retired Persons, an active member of the Boston University Alumni Association, and volunteered every winter to help elderly people prepare their federal income taxes. Carolyn Andrews recorded May 16, 2005 (cited as Andrews), lines 480–599.

18. The admiration Hastings engendered is consistently repeated in oral histories collected for this research. For information on Hastings's power, stature, and relationships see, for example, transcripts of Charest, lines 832–937; Andrews, lines 240–309, 971–1020; Christine Kuhlman recorded November 19, 2004 (cited as Kuhlman), lines 314–32, 882–88; Stanley Plodzik recorded March 4, 2005 (cited as Plodzik), lines 465–529. Also personal communication June 6, 2005 with Doris Nuttelman, former executive director of the New Hampshire Board of Nursing; transcript may be obtained from the author.

19. See, for example, adjudication discussions in minutes of each meeting of Board of Nursing and the Commission on Pharmacy through 1986. Nurses routinely had licenses suspended or revoked for actions including mishandling medications, IRS fraud, or substance abuse. Pharmacists routinely had licenses suspended for similar actions, but often had the majority of the suspension period "stayed" or forgiven. The Board of Medicine, however, rarely suspended or revoked licenses even after Drug Investigation Unit investigations (see Board of Medicine minutes, January 5, 1978). One physician who was found guilty of Medicare and Medicaid fraud had no action (Board of Medicine minutes, December 11, 1978). One who was found guilty of breaking prescription narcotic laws was allowed to "retire with dignity," as were others (Board of Medicine minutes, August 15, 1972, July 7, 1977). Another physician, while spending the night at a patient's hospital bedside, injected himself with massive amounts of Demerol, a potent morphinelike narcotic, while the patient died. Although the physician was subsequently found to exhibit bizarre and unstable behavior and to have a drug and alcohol abuse problem, the Board of Medicine left his license intact for many months (Board of Medicine minutes, July 6, 1978, October 5, 1978, December 11, 1978). These examples are a few of many during the years of study. Mires indicated that there were many "problem" physicians but due to the threat of being sued for an adjudicatory decision, the Board of Medicine was reluctant to take action against physicians (Mires, lines 121–55). Physicians did, however, have licenses revoked if their relicensing fee checks were returned to the Board of Medicine for insufficient funds (Board of Medicine minutes August 7, 1980).

20. Minutes of Special Joint Meeting, Board of Registration in Medicine, Board of Registration in Nursing, Thursday, March 8, 1973, Board of Medicine minutes files, 2.

21. Minutes, March 8, 1973, 3.

22. Hastings died suddenly in 1985, several years after she retired from the Board of Nursing. Although she remained active in the New Hampshire Nursing Association, she

spent her time as an H&R Block consultant helping elderly people prepare their federal income tax reports and renovating the house she bought at her retirement (the first she had ever owned). Hastings never married (see Andrews, lines 808–50).

23. Mires was a close personal friend of New Hampshire Attorney General David Souter, who had a hand in backing several rulings supporting nurse practitioners' dispensing in defiance of the Commission on Pharmacy (Mires 2005, lines 18–81, 98–101, 202–25, 380–430, 668–86, 728–840, 1036–40, 1224–29).

24. Letter dated January 9, 1978 from Marguerite Hastings, Executive Director, New Hampshire Board of Nursing, to Deborah F. Clark, RN, PNP, Secretary NHNPA, folder "Legislation 1970s"; letter dated July 5, 1979 from Andrew R. Grainger, New Hampshire Assistant Attorney General, to Maynard Mires, MD, MPH, Executive Secretary, State Board of Registration in Medicine and Miss Marguerite Hastings, Director, Board of Nursing Education and Registration, folder "Joint Regulation Board of Medicine 1979"; letter dated September 13, 1982 from Assistant Attorney General James Townsend to Paul G. Boisseau, Secretary, Commission on Pharmacy, in reply to Subject; "Who Can Dispense," folder "Legislation 1980s." See also *Registered Nurses and Practical Nurses,* RSA 326-B: 4, Powers and Duties of the Board Laws of the State of New Hampshire (January 1, 1974), Concord, New Hampshire, and Commission on Pharmacy minutes, September 19, 1979.

25. See Board of Nursing minutes, January 14, 1974.

26. For comments by Mires and others on the impending closure of the last hospital-based nursing schools, see *New Hampshire Medical Society News* 32, no. 2 (March 1980), 4.

27. See Board of Nursing minutes, February 21, 1974. Selma Deitch, MD, another formidable woman with a national reputation in pediatric health and a significant statewide power base, was director of the New Hampshire Division of Maternal and Child Health services at the New Hampshire Department of Public Health, and reported directly to Mires. Deitch believed strongly in the need for, and abilities of, nurse practitioner care within the public health system, even meeting with Hastings and the Board of Nursing to explore sponsoring a nurse practitioner training program in New Hampshire. Although this idea never reached fruition, Deitch was responsible for facilitating nurse practitioner training for several New Hampshire public health nurses and also for assuring that nurse practitioners held significant positions of power in New Hampshire pediatric programs, public health department administration, and public clinic patient care. It is probable that Mires, when faced with negotiating nurse practitioner practice boundaries on behalf of the Board of Medicine and physicians, was keenly aware that Hastings and Deitch, with whom he had close and often daily working relationships, supported nurses and patients rather than focusing on protecting physician boundaries. Susan McKeown relates how Deitch was responsible for the state supporting education of pediatric nurse practitioners, including Susan herself, to staff federally funded public pediatric clinics in Manchester in the 1970s. McKeown also discusses the remarkable dedication Deitch had to multidisciplinary care for all children in New Hampshire. Transcript of oral history Susan McKeown recorded March 22, 2005 (cited as McKeown), lines 85–626. Kathleen Hoerbinger, former state coordinator and case manager for home care of children with spina bifida, relates that Deitch was "a character. She was dauntless and wouldn't take 'no' for an answer" (personal communication with Hoerbinger, August 22, 2005). Both nurses had great respect and admiration for Deitch.

28. Letter dated January 9, 1978 from Marguerite Hastings, Executive Director, New Hampshire "Legislation 1970s"; see "Joint Regulation of Board of Registration in Medicine & Board of Nursing Education and Nurse Registration relative to definition of professional nursing" discussing the rule for dispensing, attached to letter dated July 5, 1979 from Andrew R. Grainger, New Hampshire Assistant Attorney General to Maynard Mires, MD, MPH, Executive Secretary, State Board of Registration in Medicine, and Miss Marguerite Hastings, Director, Board of Nursing Education and Registration, folder "Joint Regulation Board of Medicine 1979"; letter dated September 13, 1982 from Assistant Attorney

General James Townsend to Paul G. Boisseau, Secretary, Commission on Pharmacy, in reply to Subject; "Who Can Dispense," folder "Legislation 1980s." In an interesting coincidence, in June 1978, while Hastings and Mires were negotiating the process to allow nurse practitioners to dispense, the Commission on Pharmacy refused to relicense the State Public Health Department Laboratory (which held pharmaceuticals over which the Commission on Pharmacy had jurisdiction) and required Mires, who oversaw the lab, to close the lab, move the facility, and install expensive and extensive environmental, architectural, and procedural controls prior to reopening. At this same time Mires was also in difficult and contentious negotiations with the Commission on Pharmacy to allow paramedics and emergency medical technicians to administer medications in emergencies, and the Commission on Pharmacy and Board of Medicine (of which Mires was a member) were disputing Board of Medicine handling of physicians referred for Board adjudication by the Drug Investigation Unit and Commission on Pharmacy, Commission on Pharmacy minutes, April 19, May 10, June 21, July 26, November 8, 1978.

29. Letter dated November 17, 1977 from Attorney General David Souter to Commission on Pharmacy, attached to Commission on Pharmacy minutes, December 14, 1977; Commission on Pharmacy minutes, September 19, 1979, August 13, 1980, May 26, 1982.

30. See Mires 2005, lines 675–91.

31. The Commission on Pharmacy also opposed dispensing, prescribing, or possessing medications by nurses in college health clinics, and by optometrists, chiropractors, paramedics, and emergency medical technicians. Commission on Pharmacy minutes, December 18, 1974, April 19, 1978, July 26, 1978, June 18, 1980, May 7, 1986.

32. See White, lines 909–31; letter dated November 12, 1977 from Betty H. Mitchell and Donna White to "Dear Fellow Practitioners," folder "Legislation 1970s."

33. Personal communication with George Roberts, February 8, 2005. See also transcript of oral history with George Roberts, January 22, 2005 (cited as Roberts), lines 105–50, 415–20, 681–88.

34. Letter dated January 24, 1978 from Debbie Clark, RN PNP, Recording Secretary, NHNPA, to "Dear Practitioner," folder "Legislation 1970s."

35. See transcript of oral history, Cynthia Cote recorded February 11, 2005 (cited as Cote), lines 860–63.

36. Cote, also lines 1353–86.

37. Kuhlman, lines 118–25, 1037–51; Interview with Donna Cassioly, March, 3, 2005, lines 403–24. All NHNPA meetings from January 1977 through September 1983, with the exception of a few dinner meetings at area restaurants, were held after hours or on Saturdays at the Concord Clinic in Concord, where Kuhlman and Cassidy worked with Kuhlman's husband, obstetrician Gerry Hamilton. See NHNPA minutes, January 11, 1977–September 18, 1983. Letters sent to nurse practitioners through January 1980, when NHNPA had its own letterhead printed, were sent on Concord Clinic letterhead.

38. See Weeman, lines 934–41; Cote, lines 617–716; Charest, lines 1060–70, 1500– 1580; Dirubbo, lines 440–57, 815–29, 844–80; letter dated January 24, 1978 from Debbie Clark, RN PNP, Recording Secretary, NHNPA, to "Dear Practitioner"; letter dated January 29, 1979 from Kathy Higgins Cahill, President, NHNPA, and Prescription Task Force members Chris Kuhlman, Gloria Klein, and Paula Weeman, to "Dear Nurse Practitioner," folder "Legislation 1970s"; NHNPA minutes May 1, 1979, folder "Minutes 1970–1980."

39. Kuhlman, lines 215–16.

40. See NHNPA minutes September 11, 1978, folder "Legislation 1970s."

41. NHNPA minutes June 5, 1979, folder "Minutes 1970–1980."

42. Reginald W,. Rhein, Jr, "Nurses Colleagues or Competitors," *Medical World News,* 1979, 20–65, 69–71, 73.

43. Roberts 2005, lines 552–54.

44. Interview with Laurie Harding, White River Junction, Vermont, June 14, 2005 (cited as Harding), lines 683–716.

45. NHNPA minutes, January 12, 1980, NHNPA Papers, Box 1–1, folder "Legislation and Minutes 1980."

46. Mires 2005, lines 239–81.

47. Board of Medicine minutes, October 1979, New Hampshire Board of Medicine Minutes, July 6, 1978–December 16, 1979.

48. NHNPA minutes, June 12, 1981, folder "Legislation and Minutes 1981."

49. The June 2, 1981 NHNPA minutes discusses the second legislative attempt and failure. See May 1980 minutes, folder "Minutes 1980s"; minutes, January 1, February 2, September 16, 1983, folder "Minutes & Correspondence 1980–1983."

50. NHNPA minutes June 5, September 11, 1979, folder "Legislation & Minutes 1978 & 1979."

51. Cote, lines 1120–65.

52. Medical-nursing boundaries are further discussed in Fairman, "Delegated by Default or Negotiated by Need?"; Keeling, *Nursing and the Privilege of Prescription.*

53. Julie Fairman, "The Roots of Collaborative Practice: Nurse Practitioner Pioneers' Stories," *Nursing History Review* 10 (2002), 159–194.

54. Susan M. Reverby, "The Sorcerer's Apprentice," in *Prognosis Negative: Crisis in the Health Care System,* ed. David Kotelchuck (New York: Vintage Books, 1976) , 170–183. Other scholars disagree with Reverby's analysis in this early work. For example, in more recent scholarly work, Fairman, "Delegated by Default" (1999) has found that nursing academics' dismay at the idea of nurse practitioners was more an aspect of "insecurity" and a "prevailing fear of a middle man between nursing and medicine taking away nurses' power," while physicians were supportive of and encouraged nurses crossing medical boundaries. See also O'Reilly, *Health Care Practitioners: An Ontario Case Study on Policy Making.* (Toronto: University of Toronto Press, 2000).

55. Weeman, lines 1165–74.

56. Cote, lines 1336–86.

57. Nursing history is, of course, more varied and nuanced. For a comprehensive discussion of nurses' work identity intermingled with personal, cultural, and community identity, see Patricia D'Antonio, "Revisiting and Rethinking the Rewriting of Nursing's History," *Bulletin of the History of Medicine 73 (1999): 268–90,* at 270.

58. Nancy Rudner Lugo, Eileen T. O'Grady, Donna R. Hodnicki, and Charlene M. Hanson, "Ranking State NP Regulation: Practice Environment and Consumer Healthcare Choice," *American Journal for Nurse Practitioners* 11, no. 4 (2007), 8–9, 14–18, 23–24.

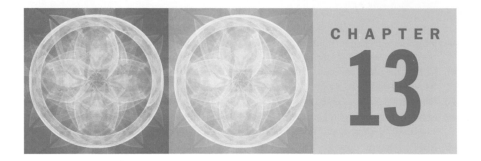

Action Research Method

"*T*he theory of action research grew out of the practice of problem solving in groups and organizations. The theory of participatory research grew out of the practical efforts at conscientization and empowerment of the marginalized" (Brown & Tandon, 2008, p. 227). Problem solving in groups and organizations and empowerment of the marginalized are two very significant activities which are a part of nursing's history. The characteristics of action research provide nurse researchers with a framework for exposing group knowledge and planning *with* those most involved rather than imposing expert knowledge and planning. The essential characteristics of action research require that the researcher work within the group to understand or improve a situation identified by the group using systematic, analytical, and reflective techniques to gather data that lead to the development of an action plan for solving the problem based on the information gathered *and* in collaboration with those *in* the group (Hinchey, 2008).

Nurses in recent years have been challenged to provide documentation to support how what they do makes a difference in peoples' lives. Although it would seem obvious that improving outcomes based on nursing practice would necessarily involve those who are the recipients of care in an active way, this is not often the case. Traditional research methods value objectivity. Consequently, much of nursing research focuses on measuring the effect of what we do to our patients rather than working with them to discover what creates the overall best outcomes. Action research offers nurse researchers the opportunity to work *with* their patients to discover what make the greatest difference in their lives. Letts (2003) states that "participants are involved in planning and evaluating actions to address issues of importance to them, so that knowledge is gained through the process of acting to improve or address issues" (p. 78). Action research method is participatory. It is based on democratic principles. According to Stringer (2007),

> The desire to give voice to people is derived not from an abstract ideological or theoretical imperative but from the pragmatic focus of action research. Its intent is to provide a place for the perspectives of people who have previously been marginalized from opportunities to develop and operate policies, programs, and services—perspectives often concealed by the products of a typical research process. (pp. 206, 207)

Action research seeks to empower those who are part of the process to act on their own behalf to solve *real world problems*.

Nurses conducting research in the United States have been slow to embrace action research. This is despite the fact that it is a research method that has demonstrated great success in the areas of social research. It is particularly interesting, given federal support for this type of research. Minkler, Blackwell, Thompson, and Tamir (2003) report the Centers for Disease Control and Prevention (CDC) has

> funded 25 community-based prevention research grants totaling $13 million; these 3-year grants are intended to fund multidisciplinary, multilevel, participatory research with the goal of enhancing capacity of communities and population groups to address health promotion and prevention of disease, disability, and injury. (p. 1211)

It is the intent of this chapter to help the reader understand the collaborative, emancipatory process that is known as action research. The goal will be to share important insights about action research development, its fundamental roots, characteristics of the method, and information on how to generate, analyze, and utilize the findings of an action research study. Once knowledge of the method is acquired, it is hoped that it will be incorporated more often by nurse researchers because of its significant utility in offering an action-based, emancipatory approach to problem solving for nurses and those they serve.

ACTION RESEARCH DEFINED

*A*ction research is known by various names, including *cooperative inquiry, action inquiry, participatory action research, community-based action research, collaborative research,* and *participative inquiry* (Reason & Bradbury, 2008; Stringer, 2007; Tetley & Hanson, 2001). The various terms make using one definition difficult, although the definition of this approach may not be as important as its assumptions. It is the assumptions of the action research process that can better assist the nurse researcher in deciding whether action research is a useful research approach for the problem to be studied.

Hinchey (2008) defines action as "a process of systematic inquiry, usually cyclical conducted by those inside a community rather than by outside experts; its goal is to identify action that will generate some improvement the researcher believes important" (p. 4). According to Winter and Munn-Giddings (2001), action research "is a form of social research which involves people in a process of change, which is based on professional, organizational or community action" (p. 5). "Action research is first and foremost a group activity" (Bennett, 2000, p. 1). Reason and Bradbury (2008) offer a particularly inclusive definition of action research:

> a participatory process concerned with developing practical knowing in pursuit of worthwhile human purposes. It seeks to bring together action and reflection, theory and practice, in participation with others, in the pursuit of practical solutions to issues of pressing concern to people, and more generally the flourishing of individual persons and their communities. (p. 4)

Some action researchers have suggested that rather than offering a single definition, action research should be seen as a continuum of methods, with the ends of the continuum being both insider and outsider models (Badger, 2000; Rolfe, 1996; Tichen & Binnie, 1993).

> At the outsider end [is] the sociological approach of testing out theory in a real situation and Lewin's (1946) traditional approach of the researcher as professional expert entering the situation to facilitate and evaluate change. At the continuum's other end, termed endogenous research by DePoy & Gitlin (1994), lie those approaches where practitioner and researcher collaborate loosely, or are even the same person. (Badger, 2000, p. 202)

Coghlan and Casey (2001) share that the insider is sometimes the nurse working in his or her own situation: "Rarely is there much consideration of action by the permanent insider" (p. 675).

To assist in understanding the action research method, four specific approaches will be described. These are cooperative inquiry, community-based action research, participatory action research, and action science or action inquiry.

Cooperative inquiry is a type of action research that values above all else the notion that the individual is self-determining, and as such, cannot be researched without full participation. John Heron first advanced the ideas related to cooperative inquiry (Brown, 2001; Reason, 1998). According to Heron and Reason (2008) "cooperative inquiry is a form of second-person action research in which all participants work together in an inquiry group as co-researches and co-subjects" (p. 366).

> One can only do research on persons in the full and proper sense of the term only if one addresses them as self-determining, which means that what they do and what they experience as part of the

research must be to some significant degree determined by them. (Reason, 1998, p. 264)

Therefore, the implementation of cooperative inquiry requires that both researchers and informants cooperate to derive new knowledge.

As suggested earlier, the definitions/descriptions of the approaches presented here are not fundamentally different. The emphases in all action research studies are the reciprocity between researchers and informants and empowerment of those who have not traditionally had a voice. Participatory action research (PAR), as described by William Foote Whyte (1984), is a type of action research that is best known because of its interdisciplinary focus. Also, it is recognized for its political aspects (Reason, 1998). In more recent years, researchers have sought to remove the strong political overtones that characterize the method. According to Tetley and Hanson (2001), "it is these issues of knowledge creation, control and power that makes participatory research distinctly different from other types of social research" (p. 71). In PAR, the emphasis is on relinquishing control, learning through mutual interactions between researchers and participants, and giving voice to those who would otherwise not be heard.

Community-based action research represents the ideas advanced by Stringer (2007). Like PAR, community-based action research has faced some difficult times because of its association with radical political activism.

it has reemerged in response to both pragmatic and philosophical pressures and is now more broadly understood as "disciplined inquiry (research) which seeks focused efforts to improve the quality of people's organizational, community and family lives" (Calhoun, 1993, p. 62). Community-based action research is also allied to recent emergence of practitioner research (e.g., Anderson et al., 1994), new paradigm research (Reason, 1988), and teacher-as-researcher (Kincheloe, 1991). (Stringer, 2007, p. 10)

As a research method, its most frequent application has been in problem solving by practitioners such as educators, occupational therapists, social workers, nurses, organizational leaders, and human service workers. According to Stringer (2007), "community-based action research works on the assumption . . . that all stakeholders—those whose lives are affected by the problem under study—should be engaged in the process of investigation" (p. 11). The method can be used to improve work activities, resolve problems or crises, and develop special projects. The overall goal is to deal with the problems that practitioners face in their everyday lives.

Action science or action inquiry is described by Reason (1998) as "forms of inquiry into practice" (p. 273) with the greatest emphasis being on developing action that will lead to systemic change within organizations, ultimately leading to "greater effectiveness and greater justice" (p. 273). The emphasis is on identifying theories of action that guide behavior (Reason, 1998). According to Argyris, Putnam, and Smith as cited in Reason (1998), theories-in-use are rendered explicit by reflection on action. Therefore, action science concerns "itself with situations of uniqueness, uncertainty, and instability which do not lend themselves to the mode of technical rationality. It would aim at the development of themes from which . . . practitioners may construct theories and methods of their own" (Schon, 1983, p. 319). Friedman and Rogers (2008) offer four key features of action science: creating communities of inquiry, developing theories of action, framing as a process for making sense of the problem, and designing for change. These four features guide the research. Ultimately, the researchers are focused on gaining a fuller understanding of the problem and how theory can guide practice.

Holter and Schwartz-Barcott (1993) offer three classifications of action research. These are technical collaboration, mutual collaboration, and enhancement. In the technical collaboration approach, the researcher has a predetermined agenda that often involves intervention or theory testing; in the mutual collaboration approach, the researcher and participants identify the focus of the research together and decide together how to study and ultimately manage the problem; finally, in the enhancement approach, the researcher and participants work together but move beyond the collaborative approach to engage in critical dialogue to raise group consciousness (Sturt, 1999, p. 1059). According to Holter and Schwartz-Barcott (1993) and Kendall and Sturt (1996), most reported nursing action research studies use the technical collaboration approach.

Given a basic understanding of the multiple definitions and descriptions of action research, it is important to examine the historical roots of this important research methodology. It is only through understanding of the method that nurse researchers will have an appropriate framework to determine its applicability to problems faced in practice.

ACTION RESEARCH ROOTS

Action research is a method that might well be described as a research approach that has gone through several phases. The early work is attributed to Kurt Lewin. Lewin, a social psychologist, is cited frequently as the first person who coined the term *action research*. Most nurses know Lewin as the person who described change theory. Lewin's theoretical ideas about change were very basic. Simplistically, Lewin said that for a change to occur, individuals would need to unfreeze—give up their ideas about something or give up the dominant structure. They would then need to change. The change would require the acceptance of new ideas or a new structure. Finally, once the new ideas were formally in place, the individuals involved in the change would refreeze, or hold the new ideas or structure as permanent. Lewin's change theory remains an influential model for social change up to the present (Greenwood & Levin, 1998).

Lewin, based on his ideas about change, saw action research as a process by which a researcher could achieve a goal by constructing a social experiment (Greenwood & Levin, 1998). "This research approach . . . fell very much within the bounds of conventional applied social science with its patterns of authoritarian control, but it was aimed at producing a specific, desired social outcome" (p. 17). As action research has developed, there is less emphasis on the stagnant manner of change than on being a process with a definitive ending point. Current action researchers believe the process is open with ongoing dialogue and that the refreezing described by Lewin is not a permanent condition.

A group of individuals who worked on the ideas of action research in its early development is the Tavistock group. This group advanced Lewin's ideas in the post–World War II period. Following the war, when the English were rebuilding their industrial base, they found that traditional methods were not effective (Greenwood & Levin, 1998). To help with the understanding of why prewar strategies no longer worked, the British government called on the Tavistock Institute of Human Relations to study the problem. "Tavistock brought Lewin's work on the concept of natural experiments and [action research] (Gustavsen, 1992) back to the United States, and committed itself to doing direct experiments in work life" (Greenwood & Levin, 1998, p. 20). The works of Tavistock led to additional exploration of the work environment and change process in Norway. The Norwegian Industrial Democracy Project used the ideas of Lewin and further developed by Tavistock to advance understanding of the work environment. For a complete description of this period, the reader is directed to Greenwood and Levin (1998).

The expansions of Lewin's work in Norway led to yet other modification in Sweden. The term used to describe the application of action research in the work environment is *sociotechnical thinking* (Greenwood & Levin, 1998). This type of organizational thinking and action spread to the United States. Trist (1981) identified the new paradigm of sociotechnical design for organizations as follows: person was complementary to machine, people were resources to be developed, people should have broad skills and be grouped by tasks, people were internally motivated, organizations should be flat and represent participative models of functioning, activity should be collaborative and collegial, people in the organization should be supported in their commitment to the organization, and individuals should be rewarded for innovation. Ultimately, it was discovered that if individuals were part of identifying and creating their work environments, then based on the interaction among all concerned parties, positive action and direction for the organization would be achieved.

Hinchey (2008) provides a broader view of the history of action research. In addition to Lewin, she includes the works of John Dewey and John Collier as part of the foundation of this research approach. "While others imagine teachers as uncritical recipients of what expert researchers deemed best practices, Dewey argued that research findings need to be tested and adjusted by teachers in the field" (p. 8). Collier, not an educator was the Commissioner of Indian Affairs. His work was based on the idea that the American Indians could not all be treated by the US government as one group. Similar to Dewey, Collier argued that research needed to be done in the field with those who were most affected by US policy. Hinchey shares that based on Lewin's work, Stephen Corey, a dean at Teachers College, Columbia University promoted action research in education. More recently, she cites as significant contributors to the development of action research by Lawrence Stenhouse in England and Paulo Freire in Brazil. All of these researchers wrote extensively about the necessity of including those most affected by change in the process. The original works of these investigators are available for those interested in learning more about how action research has developed.

Brown (2001) states that Argyris and Schon represent the present-day transformation based on their conceptualization of action research as action science. Both Argyris and Schon are most interested in theory in action as described earlier in this section.

It should be obvious that action research has experienced a number of permutations. With the ongoing development, the fundamental principles of the design remain the same: its focus on emancipation of others and the collaborative nature of the research process. In the next section, the fundamental characteristics of the method will be explored.

FUNDAMENTAL CHARACTERISTICS OF THE METHOD

Similar to the definitions of action research, there is no one method of doing action research. According to Whitehead, Taket, and Smith (2003), "action research is methodologically flexible to the point that it encourages methodological triangulation/pluralism approaches" (p. 8). Despite the flexibility of the approach, there are some fundamental characteristics about the method and the way that it is executed. Common to all descriptions is the fact that the research is context bound. Second, the process seeks to have full engagement by researchers and participants. The process is truly collaborative. Third, those involved remain aware of the process and how it affects the lives of others. Fourth, an action or change is the focal point of the process. And finally, the decision to implement the action or change is in the hands of the stakeholders.

Like other types of qualitative research, the purpose is to produce not a generalizable study but rather one that is locally important. When initiating an action research study, the researcher would ideally become engaged in the process after a local group found a problem that it wanted to solve and when the group sought the insights of an individual with research expertise. Because the problem is local and the planned change is practical, the findings will most likely be local. This is not to suggest that a local problem may not develop ideas or theories that can be applied in other situations but rather to state that the purpose of an action research study is to create a real change for the stakeholders involved in the situation.

The collaboration that is identified as fundamental is at the root of this emancipatory research process. Those engaged must be *equal* members of the research team. The use of a truly democratic process to create new knowledge is potentially liberating for those involved (Greenwood & Levin, 1998).

> The logic of inquiry is linked to the inquiry process itself; in the struggle to make an indeterminate situation into a more positively controlled one through an inquiry process where action and reflection are directly linked. The outside researcher inevitably becomes a participant in collaboration with the insiders. (p. 78)

For example, if a group of disabled individuals who require power chairs to participate in activities of daily living discover that the chairs do not give them the flexibility to function independently in their homes, they might enlist the help of local health care providers or researchers to help them determine the best way to influence the health care system to meet their needs. To do so, it would be necessary to bring all the stakeholders (therapists, insurers, manufacturers) to the table to examine the problem rather than just the power chair user's group to decide the best way to handle the situation. If all stakeholders work together to develop a practical solution to the problem, then the needs of all should be met. The researcher facilitates the process but does not control it. "The emphasis [in action research] is on a critical approach to social problems and practices which arise from and are embedded in social context" (Bellman, Bywood, & Dale, 2003, p. 187).

Those involved in the research process must be aware of the impact participation in the process will have on their lives. Those involved must agree to be constantly aware of the differences in beliefs, values, needs, and objectives of those involved to support an effective process. Using the example above, if the most powerful stakeholders come to the table with preconceived ideas based on their beliefs, cultural values, and class and are not attentive to those who require the power chair to live independently, then the process will not yield an outcome that is in the best interest of all concerned. Similarly, if those needing the power chairs are unwilling to collaborate with the researcher, therapists, manufacturers, and insurers because of preconceived notions about power, class, and existing systems, then again what is best for all concerned will not emerge. Once there is commitment on the part of all concerned to stay attuned to the needs of each person, then the process can proceed, ultimately leading to an effective change.

Implementation of an action or change is the fourth fundamental characteristic of the action research process. The purpose of the process is not to describe an existing situation but rather to construct new knowledge, a new way to deal with a practical problem (Winter & Munn-Giddings, 2001).

"Participants are empowered to define their world in the service of what they see as worthwhile interests, and as a consequence they change their world in significant ways, through action" (Reason, 1998, p. 279). The action is developed based on what is discovered through the process of dismantling the problem. For example, in work completed by Jones et al. (2008), the researchers were interested in changing stroke services. As such those who had utilized stroke services were one group of informants who participated.

The last characteristic of action research is that the power to act is always in the hands of the stakeholders. If the process works as it should, the action determined through collaboration results in an outcome that is acceptable and can be implemented by those involved. The action is part of the continuing process of emancipation and democracy. No one outsider or no one insider can determine the action that needs to be taken. The conclusion and subsequent action must reflect the collective thinking of the group.

SELECTION OF ACTION RESEARCH AS METHOD

Nurses who choose to use action research as an approach to solve a particular practice problem should have a clear understanding of what the purpose of their research is. As described earlier, action research is specifically designed as a research method whose outcome is the implementation of an action or change. The types of action that can be considered include bringing about a change in behavior, developing a plan of action to deal with resistance to change, implementing new nursing practices, or empowering providers or those for whom they care (Hart & Bond, 1996; Jenks, 1999). In addition to dedication to action or change, the nurse interested in using action research must be committed to the development of local theory. The outcomes of an action research study will not be generalizable and will usually not have broad reaching application outside of the context in which the study occurs.

Second, the nurse researcher must be committed to collaboration. The collaboration in action research is different from that which generally occurs among researchers in a typical nursing research study. In action research, the collaboration is not between colleagues with equivalent knowledge and power but rather among individuals who may have little or no understanding of research and be seen as having little or no power to affect change. The participants usually are members of groups who come from backgrounds that are different from the researcher's. For example, the women living in a low-income housing development may be interested in improving the quality of care provided to their children in a neighborhood clinic. In this case, the women interested in solving the problem most likely come from a different socioeconomic background than the nurse. As a result, the nurse researcher will need to take his or her lead from what the women living in the community think the problem is, rather than the nurse researcher determining what the problem is and moving forward to solve it. There may be any number of differences between the participants and researchers. What is most important in the collaboration is that nurse researchers *must* view those with whom they engage in the research process as *equal* partners. Without this commitment, another method of inquiry will be most helpful.

Another important consideration in the selection of action research is the value placed on empowerment and voice. Nurse researchers interested in engaging in action research must be comfortable with self-reflection relative to the issues of process, power, and control. "The process of reflection is used to understand the power relationships and imbalances in the experiences of the participants" (Koch, Selim, & Kralik, 2002, p. 111). Lee (2009) contends that the researcher must go beyond reflection to reflexivity. She states that reflexivity includes being attentive to "preconceptions, values or beliefs about the research topic and the processes of data collection and analysis, as a mean of quality assurance, or to enhance the credibility and rigour of the research" (p. 31). An important characteristic of action research is the empowerment of others. True empowerment can only occur when the researcher regularly attends to the issues of power and control in the research process and the setting in which the research takes place. For instance, if the nurse researcher is interested in studying student nurses who are intimidated in the clinical education setting, then the researcher must be ready to listen carefully to what is said, help the participants find their voice, and assist them in the development of a process that will empower them to take action.

The final consideration in choosing action research is the realization that in action research, the power to act resides exclusively with those who engaged in the process. "Change may come in the form of individual or group empowerment, greater community capacity to solve shared problems, or transformed organizational structures" (Cockburn & Trentham, 2002, pp. 21–22). No amount of external pressure can force the participants to carry out the change or action that becomes apparent during the conduct of the study. The nurse researcher who chooses action research has to be comfortable with "others" making the decision about what is best for them. Corbett, Francis, and Chapman (2007) share that the experience participating in action research is validating in that it is the first time the co-researchers have ever been heard. Consequently, it may also be the first time they have ever been given a public opportunity to create the change they desire.

Once the nurse researcher is comfortable with the fundamental characteristics, understands the outcome of the method, and is willing to share the power and control, which is ordinarily the purview of the principal investigator, then and only then should action research be selected. Action research has the potential to dramatically change the life experiences of many individuals. However, the study must be conducted with attention to the fundamental issues of empowerment and action.

ELEMENTS AND INTERPRETATIONS OF THE METHOD

*A*ction researchers have many interpretations of method. This can be seen from the information provided earlier regarding the many terms and descriptions given to the process. There are, however, some basic elements to which most researchers engaged in action research subscribe. These will be shared in the hope that they give the nurse researcher who is interested in the methodology enough information to determine whether the approach will be useful in dealing with a specific problem. Once the decision is made to conduct an action research study, the researcher is encouraged to read primary sources on the method and engage a research mentor.

Data Generation

Data generation begins as soon as the problem becomes apparent. Ideally, this occurs when a community recognizes it has a problem and enlists the consultation of trained researchers to help its members deal with it. The initial discussions about the problem will become an important part of data analysis, as will all of the other information collected in the course of the study.

Defining the Problem

"An initial and large aspect of the process of participatory action research involves the careful documentation of the concrete and specific ways that people view a problem affecting their lives" (Taylor, Braveman, & Hammel, 2004, p. 75). For example, a group of young women who are pressured by some of their peers in the community to become gang members might discuss this with the nurse practitioner who runs the local clinic. Using the knowledge and skills of the nurse practitioner, these young women can work to understand the dynamics of their environment and move to change the variables within their social group that value gang membership over employment or academic success. Generally, this is not how action research problems in nursing are identified. More often, nurses see a problem in practice or a problem in the lives of those with whom they work and propose an action research approach to study and act on the problem. Regardless of who identifies the problem, it is likely that the stakeholders in an action research study will be more committed to an action or a change if they believe that the situation is important to them and that they can bring about a change in the situation.

It is important to recognize that there are two perspectives in any action research study. These are the insider, or emic, view and the outsider, or etic, view. This dichotomy exists because the insiders are living the problem and have a unique understanding of it. The outsider, the researcher, is the person who comes to the situation with the intention to assist those involved but who usually is unable to internalize the situation because he or she does not live it. It is also important to remember that insiders are the ones who will implement the change and thus have to live with the outcome. As can be seen, the insider's stake is much higher than the outsider's. Collaboration is essential. Thus, there may be two views on the problem. Both views are equally valuable because of the partnership that should develop while coming to fully understand the problem and create the change.

To fully define the problem and begin to understand it, the insiders will need to bring their personal knowledge of the problem to the researcher. The researcher will bring theoretical and practical information relative to the change process, and the ability to act as a liaison between those in power and those who have been marginalized. Together, the participants and the researcher will work to identify the problem. Ideally, the problem can be identified clearly. From a practical standpoint, clearly defining the problem will be an evolving process. It will require time and development of trusting relationships.

Planning

One of the important initial stages of an action research study is to identify all the stakeholders. It is essential to bring as many of the stakeholders as possible forward for initial conversations about the existing problem. All who may be affected in any way by the problem or the desired change need to be part of the early conversations.

Once the stakeholders are identified, it is important to determine how the investigation will proceed. Taylor et al. (2004) suggest that choosing an action-oriented solution and designing research methods and assessment procedures that will be used to solve the problem are important steps. To move these processes forward, a model advocated by Greenwood and Levin (1998), called the Cogenerative Action Research Model, might be useful. In the description of the model, Greenwood and Levin recommend that communication arenas be developed. Communication arenas are spaces where participants and researchers can come together for mutual learning. Developing these spaces will be one of the most important aspects of engaging all the stakeholders. "Arenas must be designed to match the needs of the issue" (p. 117). Therefore, there may be a need for large group, small group, and one-on-one meetings. There may be a need for specific meetings for explicit purposes, such as information sharing or team building. There also will be the need to develop spaces for reflection. Ground rules for participation are important. It is also essential that all parties clearly understand how the feedback loop for communication will work. As an example, the researcher or a member of the community group may record minutes. When the minutes become available, an appropriate forum should be created to discuss the recording.

As part of designing the study, the researcher should decide how information will be collected. Will interviews, observations, focus groups, and printed material comprise the major data collection strategies, or will survey and questionnaires be the tactics of choice? Who will be responsible for collecting data? These decisions must be made by all members of the research team. It will be the responsibility of the trained researchers to bring as much information as possible forward so that the members of the team who are not skilled in the strategies for data collection or the research process are provided with the opportunity to learn about the various data collection strategies and the method so that they can make informed decisions about how to proceed.

Reason and Bradbury (2008) describe the importance of being attuned to how individuals/researchers interact with community partners throughout the research activity. These action researchers discuss the importance of understanding the researcher as instrument, specifically how essential it is to consider how the researcher's ideas influence the framing and implementation of the study. One of the ways for the researcher to remain attuned to his or her actions throughout the study is to consider using some form of reflection. One of the better ways to encourage reflection is to include journaling or keeping a diary as one of the data collection strategies. Using a self-reflective mechanism can help sort out some of the important issues that may arise throughout the study. It is equally important that time and space be created for all members of the research team to reflect on their planning and implementation strategies. The opportunity for group members to consider their actions in a more formal reflection helps to manage differences in opinions about the way the research progresses.

Different from some other qualitative methods, the participants in an action research study are not separate from the research process. Those who are the stakeholders are often the ones who can most effectively inform the study. However, there will be times when data need to be collected to reflect the experience of members of affected groups who are not intimately involved with the study. For example, using the teen gang scenario presented earlier, all of the teens being pressured to join gangs in the community may not be part of the research team, but from time to time, it will be essential to collect information from as many of those teens as possible to fully understand the problem. When individuals are deliberately selected to inform the study, the sampling is called purposive. Depending on which data collection strategies are used, a decision will be made regarding who will conduct the interviews, do the observations, or collect survey or questionnaire data. It is important to consider whether data collectors should be from within or outside the group. Using outsiders to collect these data may provide a potentially more open-minded and detached view of the situation. However, using insiders may reduce potential barriers that arise when data collectors are not part of the group. There can be very intentional reasons for choosing insiders or outsiders to collect data. As long as the research team agrees on who the data collectors are and why they have been selected, data collection will move forward in a productive manner.

Jenks (1999) recommends that at least three strategies of data collection be utilized to ensure that there is cross-validation of information. All strategies will not need to be identified before the study begins. Because the question may not be clearly defined, data collection strategies not originally identified may need to be added in light of evolving data. For instance, using the example of teenagers and gang membership, a survey may be used as one of the data collection strategies. However, as the study progresses, it is discovered that there is information that the survey is not capturing. Focus group interviews or other data collection strategies can be added to explore information found in the survey.

The preparations that have been described represent the planning phase of the action research study. "Careful planning enables research participants, including the facilitator, to discover the makeup of the setting and establish a presence" (Stringer, 2007, p. 42). This is critical. Ownership by all involved is a condition of the action research process (p. 43).

Once the decisions are made regarding how best to collect data, data collection should commence. As stated earlier, the process of planning, collecting data, and analyzing data does not proceed in a linear manner. The process is dynamic and as such needs to respond to the changing needs of all involved.

Data Treatment and Analysis

As data are collected, they will be analyzed using the appropriate methodology for the strategy selected. For instance, if interviews were used, analysis can proceed using the constant comparative method. Jenks (1999) states that this method is useful in analysis of action research data. For a complete description of the constant comparative method, the reader is directed to Chapter 7.

The analysis phase of the study should include all stakeholders. Interpretations and explanations should not be offered unless the context is fully understood. The participants in the study will be the individuals who can most accurately determine whether the findings are appropriate. Conducting analysis as a joint activity, between researcher and participants, the entire research team can bring its perspectives to the discussion, providing the opportunity for dialogue and debate about the findings and their respective meanings. As stated earlier, it is appropriate to use a group reflection activity to make clear the possible influences on the interpretations.

Beyond preliminary analysis, the research team will likely begin to theorize about the findings. According to Hinchey (2008), theorizing provides the opportunity to interpret the findings and begin to discover what they really mean (p. 94). The type of theory that develops from action research studies is a local theory and it is based on the findings within the context in which they arise. Therefore, most theories developed will not be generalizable.

Action

Unlike some of the other types of qualitative research, action research does not end with documentation of the findings. When data analysis is completed, the team decides on an action or a change that they want to occur. The change is a result of and based on the findings. The outsiders take no active role in the change. They may remain part of the team by contributing to guiding the process or assisting with reflection, but they have no formal role in the change (Jenks, 1999).

In some instances, the action research process may start with the action or change, in which case the study is conducted to assess the change as it is implemented. When the study is implemented in this way, it is conducted as an evaluation study, with all members of the research team contributing. Modifications in implementation of the change can take place as the research team deems appropriate.

An important part of the change or action phase of the research process is reflection. Reflection is used in this stage of the process as a way of gaining insights about the change and its impact on those who are part of it. Reflection can be conducted as a one-on-one activity, in a group, or in a personal diary. "Data recorded during reflection are important contributions to the theory that emerges from the action research study" (Jenks, 1999, p. 260). Winter and Munn-Giddings (2001) speak to the cycle of action and reflection that is based on the work of Lewin. This spiral cycle includes planning, action, and fact finding. The cycle repeats itself to more effectively understand some aspect of the research process.

According to Jenks (1999), reflective critique can be used to facilitate reflection.

> Reflective critique is based on an understanding that all statements made during data generation—including participants' and researchers' written and verbal language—are subject to reflexivity. Reflexivity describes the belief that the language individuals use to describe an experience reflects that particular experience and also all other experiences in each individual's life. Knowing that observations and interpretations are reflexive creates two assumptions for action researchers: (1) a rejection of the idea of a single or ultimate explanation for an event and (2) the belief that offering various explanations for an experience explicitly increases understanding of the experiences. (p. 260)

Another process that can be used to assist in reflection is dialectical critique. In contrast to reflective critique, dialectical critique "probes data to make explicit their internal contradictions rather than complementary explanations" (Jenks, 1999, p. 261). The ultimate goals of each process are to ask important questions and reveal biases about data as they are revealed.

Evaluation

Evaluation of the action research process takes place throughout the study and at its end. A timeline for evaluation should be established during the planning phase. The timeline gives specific direction to keep evaluation in front of all members of the team. During evaluation, the process is assessed, and questions such as these can be asked: Are we using the correct instruments? Are we getting the data we need? Who else do we need to interview? Is the process working? These questions and others developed by the research team will keep the project focused.

Researchers have the responsibility to guide the evaluation process. This should not be done without consultation or the consent of the entire research team (Jenks, 1999). The evaluation process will be most effective if co-facilitated by members of the community and the trained researchers.

Writing the Report

The report that results from the study will be a document prepared by the team. Information to be included and excluded should be agreed on by all members of the team. The report is not necessarily the end of the action or change, but it does represent the end of the formal study. Hopefully, if the action is effective, the change will be evaluated for its long-term impact on the individuals involved and be part of the formal report.

One important feature of the report is the recommendations section. The recommendations are meant to be helpful and give direction for long-term implementation of the change. The recommendations should be determined collaboratively and should be based on a solid understanding of the problem, careful data collection, and analysis and review of appropriate literature. Review of the literature is an activity that takes place throughout the study. It should be part of informing the planned change or action in concert with the data that are collected. Conducting the literature review at the end of the study can place the findings in the context of what is already known. Because action research focuses on local problems, the literature review most likely will not yield directly applicable information. However, the researcher may find conceptual connections that can help make sense of the action or provide support for the local theory.

As part of the study process, the team should decide before initiation of data collection with whom the study report will be shared. This can be a very emotional conversation; therefore, the earlier the discussion takes place, the better. It is important to know who the primary recipient of the report will be for it to be written in a meaningful style for the intended audience. For example, writing the report for a city council will take a very different format than writing the report for the community at large.

Rigor

All research should be evaluated for its rigor. Action research is no exception. Stringer (2007) suggests that action researchers establish the rigor of their research by utilizing the trustworthiness criteria recommended by Lincoln and Guba (1985). These include credibility, transferability, dependability, and confirmability.

According to Stringer (1999),

> credibility is established by *prolonged engagement* with participants; *triangulation* of information from multiple data sources; *member checking* procedures that allow participants to check and verify the accuracy of the information recorded; and *peer debriefing* processes that enable research facilitators to articulate and reflect on research procedures with a colleague or informed associate. (p. 176)

Transferability is established by creating thick descriptions that, when read by another researcher, can be applied in other contexts. Generally, the results of an action research study are not generalizable. However, the possibility does exist that information gained can be used in other contexts. The ability to use the discovered information "lies in the detailed description of the context(s), activities and events that are reported as part of the outcomes of the study" (Stringer, 2007, p. 59).

Dependability and confirmability are established through an audit trail. The researcher is responsible for providing enough information so that another researcher reading the study would reach similar conclusions.

Waterman (1998) recommends that action researchers focus on the validity of their research. She offers three types of validity: dialectical, critical, and reflexive.

Dialectical validity "refers to the constant analysis and report of movement between theory, research and practice in examining the tensions, contradictions and complexities of the situation" (Badger, 2000, p. 204).

Critical validity involves analyzing the process of change. "The measure of validity is not the change effected but rather the analysis of intentions and actions, their ethical implications and consequences" (Badger, 2000, p. 204). "Action researchers tend to demonstrate a sense of timing or sensitivity to the situation which has been cultivated through an intimate understanding of the context and the people involved" (Waterman, 1998, p. 103).

Reflexive validity is the attempt by the researcher to constantly be examining the biases, suppositions, and presuppositions of the research. It is only through constant attention to the researcher's view that a true understanding can result. The researcher must be certain that in the end he or she has told the story of the insider.

The very real concern in any qualitative research study is that the story that emerges is the story of the people. Action research is no exception. Action research is useful because of its fundamental characteristics. It would be inadvisable to apply criteria for rigor that subtract from the value of the fundamental characteristics. The rigor of an action research study should be measured by how well the researcher has attended to the fundamental characteristics of the method.

Ethical Considerations

Action research studies have inherent ethical dilemmas that may not be seen in most other types of research. For example, one of the characteristics of an action research study is the focus on cooperation and collaborative decision making among stakeholders with the goal of carrying out a change or action project. Individuals from the marginalized group may become involved in the study without being aware of the potential tensions inherent in group process. For instance, individuals who share contrasting opinions from those in the dominant membership may find that although a consent form clearly stated the option to withdraw from the study at any time, pressure from within the group may be such that this is difficult or impossible to do so. The action researcher should try to identify as many of these tensions as possible. It may not be possible, however, to identify them all. The best that the researcher may be able to guarantee is a regular review of what the participants have agreed to. Munhall (2001) refers to this as process consent. Process consent is a procedure that allows the researcher and participants to renegotiate aspects of informed consent based on the changing nature of the inquiry.

Kelly and Simpson (2001) offer another ethical dilemma that may occur—the feelings of vulnerability felt by those who are invested in making a change. There are always those who are invested in maintaining the status quo who will work relentlessly to maintain their position. To limit the potential for oppression, Kelly and Simpson recommend that action researchers seek as much consultation as necessary with relevant authorities and provide for close inclusion of all participants throughout the process.

Williamson and Prosser (2002) speak specifically about the ethical dilemmas that may arise as part of conducting an action research study within one's own organization. Some of the areas of concern include difficulty guaranteeing confidentiality and anonymity, complexity of obtaining informed consent, and difficulty protecting subjects from harm. As these authors share, when involved in a study in one's own organization, it may be impossible not to be in a position of conflict with one's supervisors, particularly if the recommended action requires an organizational change. Similarly, when an organization grants permission for a study to be conducted, it is unlikely that those in power would not be aware of who the participants are. This compromises the participant's anonymity. Finally, it is very difficult to completely protect research participants from harm should they engage in debates with institutional administrators about how the organization functions or needs to be changed. Although these may appear to be insurmountable problems when conducting research in the parent organization, Williamson and Prosser suggest that using a steering group to convey information to the administration may be one way of limiting the ethical concerns raised here. If the steering group shares the problems and proposed actions, as well as assumes responsibility for conducting face-to-face confrontation, then those who are in less powerful positions in the organization may experience less of the anxiety and distress that may be an outcome of an organizational change.

Ethical issues can arise despite the most meticulous planning. Action researchers need to be cognizant of all the potential problems that may arise and inform their coresearchers of as many of them as can be identified before and during the study.

SUMMARY

Action research is a dynamic approach to inquiry. The researcher who opts to adopt the approach as a way to study a problem and assist in making a change in the lives of those who live in a particular situation must be willing to accept the important characteristics of this method. An attitude of collaboration, a commitment to cooperation, and an obligation to democracy and empowerment will be essential for the researcher who chooses the method. If the nurse researcher understands the possibilities that exist when adopting the method and is willing to participate in research that is locally meaningful, then action research can be an invigorating process that can create *real* change. According to Jenks (1999), "when used appropriately, action research can result in lasting change that creates a more meaningful nursing practice" (p. 263).

References

Anderson, G., Herr, K., & Nihlen, A. (1994). *Studying your own school: An educator's guide to qualitative practitioner research.* Thousand Oaks, CA: Corwin.

Badger, T. G. (2000). Action research, change and methodological rigor. *Journal of Nursing Management, 8,* 201–207.

Bellman, L., Bywood, C., & Dale, S. (2003). Advancing working and learning through critical action research: Creativity and constraints. *Nursing Education in Practice, 3*(4), 186–194.

Bennett, O. M. (2000). Action research: Reflective practice in occupational therapy education. *Education: Special Interest Section Quarterly, 19*(4), 1–2.

Bradbury, H., & Reason, P. (2003). Action research: An opportunity for revitalizing research purposes and practices. *Qualitative Social Work, 2*(2), 155–175.

Brown, C. L. (2001). Action research: The method. In C. L. Munhall (Ed.), *Nursing research: A qualitative perspective* (3rd ed., pp. 503–522). Sudbury, MA: Jones and Bartlett.

Brown, L. D., & Tandon, R. (2008). Action research, partnerships and social impacts: The institutional collaboration of PRIA and IDR. In P. Reason, & H. Bradbury (Eds.), *The Sage handbook of action research: Participative inquiry and practice* (2nd ed., pp. 227–234). Los Angeles: Sage.

Calhoun, E. (1993). Action research: Three approaches. *Educational Leadership, 51*(2), 62–65.

Cockburn, L., & Trentham, B. (2002). Participatory action research: Integrating community occupational therapy practice and research. *Canadian Journal of Occupational Therapy, 69*(1), 20–30.

Coghlan, D., & Casey, M. (2001). Action research from the inside: Issues and challenges in doing action research in your own hospital. *Journal of Advanced Nursing, 35*(5), 674–682.

Corbett, A. M., Francis, K., & Chapman, Y. (2007). Feminist-informed participatory action research: A methodology of choice for examining critical nursing issues. *International Journal of Nursing Practice, 13*, 81–88.

DePoy, E., & Gitlin, L. N. (1994). *Introduction to research: Multiple strategies for health and human services.* St. Louis, MO: Mosby.

Friedman, V.J. & Rogers, T. (2008). Action science: Linking causal theory and meaning making in action research. In P. Reason & H Bradbury (Eds.), *The Sage Handbook of Action Research: Participative Inquiry and Practice.* Thousand Oaks, CA: Sage.

Greenwood, D. J., & Levin, M. (1998). *Introduction to action research: Social research for social change.* London: Sage.

Gustavsen, B. (1992). *Dialogue and development.* Assen-Maastricht: Van Gorcum.

Hart, E., & Bond, M. (1996). Making sense of action research through the use of a typology. *Journal of Advanced Nursing, 23*, 152–159.

Heron, J., & Reason, P. (2008). Extending epistemology within a co-operative inquiry. In P. Reason, & H. Bradbury (Eds.), *The Sage handbook of action research: Participative inquiry and practice* (2nd ed., pp. 366–380). Los Angeles: Sage.

Hinchey, P. H. (2008). *Action research primer.* New York, NY: Peter Lang.

Holter, I. M., & Schwartz-Barcott, D. (1993). Action research: What is it? How has it been used and how can it be used in nursing? *Journal of Advanced Nursing, 18*, 298–304.

Jenks, J. (1999). Action research method. In H. J. Streubert, & D. R. Carpenter (Eds.), *Qualitative research in nursing: Advancing the humanistic imperative* (2nd ed., pp. 251–264). Philadelphia, PA: Lippincott Williams & Wilkins.

Jones, S. P., Auto, M. F., Burton, C. R., & Watkins, C. L. (2008). Engaging service users in the development of stroke services: An action research study. *Journal of Clinical Nursing, 17*, 1270–1279.

Kelly, K., & Simpson, S. (2001). Action research in action: Reflections on a project to introduce clinical practice facilitators to an acute hospital setting. *Journal of Advanced Nursing, 33*(5), 652–659.

Kendall, S. A., & Sturt, J. A. (1996). Negotiation access into primary health care: Insights from critical theory. *Social Sciences in Health, 2*(2), 107–120.

Kincheloe, J. (1991). *Teachers are researchers: Qualitative inquiry as a path to empowerment.* London: Falmer.

Koch, T., Selim, P., & Kralik, D. (2002). Enhancing lives through the development of community-based action research programme. *Journal of Clinical Nursing, 11*, 109–117.

Lee, N. (2009). Using group reflection in an action research study. *Nurse Researcher, 16*(2), 30–42.

Letts, L. (2003). Occupational therapy and participatory research: A partnership worth pursuing. *American Journal of Occupational Therapy, 57*(1), 77–87.

Lewin, K. (1946). Action research and minority problems. *Journal of Social Issues, 2*, 34–46.

Lincoln, Y. S., & Guba, E. G. (1985). *Naturalistic inquiry.* Beverly Hills, CA: Sage.

Minkler, M., Blackwell, A. G., Thompson, M., & Tamir, H. (2003). Community-based participatory research: Implications for public health funding. *American Journal of Public Health, 93*(8), 1210–1214.

Munhall, P. L. (2001). *Nursing research: A qualitative perspective* (3rd ed.). Sudbury, MA: Jones and Barlett.

Reason, P. (1988). *Human inquiry in action: Developments in new paradigm research.* New York, NY: Wiley.

Reason, P. (1998). Three approaches to participative inquiry. In N. K. Denzin, & Y. S. Lincoln (Eds.), *Strategies of qualitative inquiry* (pp. 261–291). Thousand Oaks, CA: Sage.

Reason, P., & Bradbury, H. (2008). *The Sage handbook of action research: Participative inquiry and practice* (2nd ed.). Los Angeles, CA: Sage.

Rolfe, G. (1996). Going to extremes: Action research, grounded practice and the theory-practice gap in nursing. *Journal of Advanced Nursing, 24,* 1315–1320.

Schon, D. (1983). *The reflective practitioner: How professionals think in action.* New York, NY: Basic Books.

Stringer, E. T. (1999). *Action research* (2nd ed.). Thousand Oaks, CA: Sage.

Stringer, E. T. (2007). *Action research* (3rd ed.). Los Angeles, CA: Sage.

Sturt, J. (1999). Placing empowerment research with an action research typology. *Journal of Advanced Nursing, 30*(5), 1057–1063.

Taylor, R. R., Braveman, B., & Hammel, J. (2004). Developing and evaluating community-based services through participatory action research: Two case examples. *American Journal of Occupational Therapy, 58*(1), 73–82.

Tetley, J., & Hanson, L. (2001). Participatory research. *Nurse Researcher, 8*(1), 69–88.

Tichen, A., & Binnie, A. (1993). Research partnerships: Collaborative action research in nursing. *Journal of Advanced Nursing, 18,* 858–865.

Trist, E. (1981). *The evolution of socio-technical systems* (Occasional Paper No. 2). Toronto: Ontario Quality of Work Life Council.

Waterman, H. (1998). Embracing ambiguities and valuing ourselves: Issues of validity in action research. *Journal of Advanced Nursing, 28*(1), 101–105.

Whitehead, D., Taket, A., & Smith, P. (2003). Action research in health promotion. *Health Education Journal, 62*(1), 5–22.

Whyte, W. F. (1984). *Learning from the field: A guide from experience.* Beverly Hills, CA: Sage.

Williamson, G., & Prosser, S. (2002). Illustrating the ethical dimensions of action research. *Nurse Researcher, 10*(2), 38–49.

Winter, R., & Munn-Giddings, C. (2001). *A handbook for action research in health and social care.* London: Routledge.

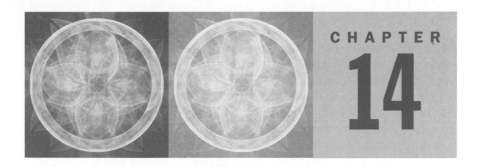

CHAPTER

14

Action Research in Practice, Education, and Administration

Action research is an exciting research methodology that "empowers people to bring [about] change by generating knowledge through reflection on their personal experiences and situations" (Glasson, Chang, & Bidewell, 2008, p. 34). As an approach to research, action research provides more than the opportunity for discovery; it has the potential to bring about long-term change. Nurses are uniquely positioned to support a research method that makes available new insight and creates new ways of advancing health care. The ability to use community engagement to enhance health care, particularly health care of underrepresented groups offers tremendous potential. Outside experts' perspectives have not been effective and more importantly are not well suited to address health needs of individuals from different ethnic or racial groups or those who experience health disparities (Minkler & Wallerstein, 2008). In light of the fact that nurses frequently find themselves caring for individuals from diverse backgrounds who have unmet health needs, working in a systematic way *with* individuals who have been marginalized by the current health care system can lead to improved outcomes. Action research can also be used to create change in nursing education and nursing administration. This chapter presents examples of nurse researchers who have used the method to solve local problems. More importantly, it demonstrates how collaborative research can empower individuals to make effective changes that improve their lives and be sustainable.

Table 14-1 offers a summary of recent action research studies to educate the reader about the ways action research has been used to solve nursing practice, education, and administration problems. In addition, a critical review of three studies is shared to give the reader a perspective on what is important in reporting action research. Box 14-1 provides a list of questions that is used for reviewing the articles presented in Table 14-1. The intent is to provide direction for critical review of action research studies and specifically to determine the merits of the study and the overall utility and practical application of the findings. A reprint of Gallagher, Truglio-Londrigan, and Levin's (2009) article is offered at the end of the chapter to facilitate the reader's understanding of the critique process.

APPLICATION TO PRACTICE

*T*he number of elderly in the world continues to grow. It is predicted that the population age 85 and over could grow from 5.3 million in 2006 to nearly 21 million by 2050 (US Census Bureau, 2008). In addition, it has been estimated that 10 million seniors live alone. As seniors continue to live out their lives without the support of family within their residences, questions arise as to who or what services will be or are available to fill the gaps. As community health professionals have learned, solving the problem as an outsider does not lead to long-term, sustainable change. For nurse researchers interested in learning about the unique challenges faced by seniors aging in place and to help find solutions to these challenges, it will be critical to commit to solving the problem by empowering others; understanding the situation through the eyes of the stakeholders; sharing power, information, and resources; and cocreating an action plan for change.

One group of nurse researchers interested in learning more about the impact community support had on the elderly used an action research approach to gain increased understanding of the problems faced by them. This group also helped to build a plan to maximize their ability to remain independent. Gallagher et al. (2009) published "Partnership for Healthy Living: An Action Research Project" that illustrates the use of this methodology to improve the lives of community-dwelling elders. The report is critiqued using the criteria given in Box 14-1. A complete reprint of this study can be found at the end of this chapter.

Gallagher et al. (2009) sought to develop, implement, and evaluate a nurse-managed model for supporting community-dwelling senior. The researchers selected action research because they wanted to use a collaborative model to identify the problems faced by aging seniors and empower them to act on their own behalf. The researchers reported that there was limited research on community support and its impact on community-dwelling seniors. Since the researchers were interested in more than just identifying the problem but also empowering the community-dwelling seniors to act on their behalf, action research is an appropriate research methodology.

Table 14-1 • Selective Sampling of Action Research Studies

Author(s)	Domain	Purpose	Coresearchers	Data Generation	Findings
Adams and Cancini (2008)	Education	To promote active involvement of BSN students in working with community partners to implement a community-based education program.	Community leaders, faculty, and BSN students	Survey, stakeholder meeting	The community had learning needs related to personal disaster management. BSN students were effective in providing education to meet this need. Further collaboration is planned.
Davidson et al. (2008)		To describe development of a nurse-directed cardiac rehabilitation program for women following an acute cardiac event.	Program participants, consumer representatives, clinical staff	Participant observation, reflective journaling, interviews, questionnaires, group interviews	Tailoring a cardiac rehabilitation program to meet the needs of women is feasible. The intervention to improved health-related outcomes will be tested in a randomized, controlled study.
Dickinson, Welch, & Ager (2007)	Practice	To improve mealtime experiences for older adults in the hospital through clinical practice changes.	Staff nurses, patients	Observations, focus groups, interviews	Staff changed nursing practices that led to improved patient mealtime experiences.
Gallagher, Truglio-Londrigan, & Levin (2009)	Practice	To develop, implement, and evaluate a nurse-managed program in a community center as a form of community support.	Recipients of service, senior center professional staff, primary political leaders	Focus groups, journals, semi-structured interviews	Educational programs and the "The Nurse is in" case-management model have been created as a method of community support for elders who live independently.

(Continued)

323

Table 14-1 • (Continued)

Author(s)	Domain	Purpose	Coresearchers	Data Generation	Findings
Jones, Auton, Rurton, & Watkins (2008)	Practice	To develop stroke services.	Patients, caregivers	Semistructured interviews, focus groups	Priorities for care of stroke patients and carers include information provision, preparation for transfer, integration of social and leisure activities.
Melrose (2006)	Education	To explore learners' ideas about seeking help when engaged in an online course.	Graduate students	Program satisfaction survey, focus groups, interviews	Strategies that facilitate help-seeking include reward for participation, introductions, creation of small group and private e-mail, identification of noncontributing students.
Phillips, Davidson, Jackson, & Kristjanson (2008)	Administration	To describe residential aged care nurses' and care assistants' perceptions of palliative care and identify actions to improve care.	Nursing directors, registered nurses, care assistants	Focus group	Increased understanding of palliative care concepts, enhanced competency, and desire to adopt a multidisciplinary approach to care planning.
Taylor et al. (2008)	Administration	Raise awareness of practice problems in palliative care specifically during times of pressure.	Registered nurses	Group meetings	Nurses gained insights into best practices during times of crisis. As a result, an action plan was developed.

Box 14-1

Critiquing Guidelines for Action Research

Planning

1. Does the researcher justify the use of action research?
2. Does the study begin with an analysis of the situation, or does it begin with implementation of the action?
3. Who initiated the study? The community? The researcher?
4. Does the research team demonstrate a commitment to mutual goal setting, sharing resources, and action?
5. Analysis of the situation
   a. Is the setting described in sufficient detail?
   b. What methods of data generation are used to describe the practice situation? Are qualitative and quantitative techniques used appropriately?
   c. Are procedures for selecting participants described? Are they the appropriate participants?
   d. What is the extent of collaboration between researchers and participants during the analysis of phase of the study?
   e. Is protection of human subjects documented?
   f. Are strategies for data analysis described? Are they used appropriately?
   g. Are participants involved in the interpretation?
   h. Does the description reflect understanding of the situation?
6. Action planning
   a. Is the planned change described in detail?
   b. Are methods of implementing the planned change described?
   c. Are methods for evaluating the planned change described?
   d. Are participants included in action planning?

Acting

1. Is the planned change implemented in the setting where the problem occurred?
2. Is the period for implementation specified?

Reflecting

1. Are methods for facilitating reflection specified?
2. Are the results of reflection described?

Evaluating

1. Are strategies for evaluating the change described?
2. Are the processes for implementing the change and the outcomes of the change evaluated?
3. Are data evaluation methods appropriate to factors evaluated?
   a. Are qualitative and quantitative techniques used appropriately?
4. Are participants included in the evaluation?
5. Are appropriate methods used to analyze evaluation data?
6. Does the research address validity and reliability of quantitative findings and trustworthiness of qualitative findings?

(Continued)

> **Box 14-1** *(Continued)*
>
> **Conclusions, Implications, and Recommendations**
> 1. Do the conclusions reflect the findings?
> 2. Is a local theory formulated from the findings?
> 3. Are implications described in sufficient detail?
> 4. Has the researcher discussed ethical and moral implications of the study?
> 5. Are recommendations for research and/or practice included?
> 6. Does the researcher describe the benefits participants gained from the study?

The first step of the four-step plan for action research is planning. The researchers need to make clear that the plan for action was a collaborative process.

This study was initiated by the nurse researchers. The stakeholders included the recipients of service, senior citizen community center professionals, and primary community political leaders. True to the method, the researchers stated clearly that the stakeholders needed to demonstrate a sense of ownership if the real change was to occur.

The setting for this study was a community center in a town north of New York City. The researchers collected demographic information. In addition, the investigators maintained a journal of semistructured interviews with center professionals and community leadership. Once data collection began, the senior center participants requested focus groups throughout the study. The focus groups initially were held every other week, but as time went by, they were reduced to monthly. The researchers spent 2.5 years in the site.

There is no documentation of informed consent. This is a good example of when "process consent" would be used to assure that the participants have the opportunity to reconsider their participation from time to time given the length of the study. There were initially eight members of the focus groups. For varying reasons by the end of the 2.5 years, only one informant remained.

Content analysis was used to analyze focus group information. Three major themes emerged from the analysis: "negotiating the health insurance bureaucracy, trials and tribulations of transport, and medication madness" (Gallagher et al., 2009, p. 17). The findings were reviewed with the members of the focus groups to assure accuracy. The researchers reported that as a result, the researchers and participants developed a plan for providing services to meet the needs identified. The action plan included two approaches to dealing with the problems identified. The first approach was to continue the focus groups. Participants enjoyed the group and stated that it gave them a forum to raise issues. As a result, educational programs and community projects were initiated. The second approach was a program titled, *The Nurse is in.* This program was focused on providing case-management services to the community center members a few hours a week. To illustrate the trust that developed between the researchers and informants, the nurse researchers were asked to be the case managers. This presented a number of issues for the nurse researchers; however, they believed that the good that would result outweighed the challenges that providing care presented.

It is clear from the report provided that the plan for change was codeveloped.

The second step of the action research process is acting. There are two main questions that need to be asked about the acting stage: (1) Does that change take place in the setting where problems exist? (2) Over what period of time is the action plan implemented?

In this study, the researchers report that the educational programs were implemented in the center. The topics were identified by the participants and the implementation of the programs was a cooperative activity. There were several community projects that were implemented. These included a health insurance program that was offered by a community group called Medicare Minute. The purpose of the group is to educate senior citizens on Medicare facts and issues. It is unclear from the report whether study participants actually became members of the Medicare Minute group.

The second community project was engaging local pharmacies in discussions regarding home delivery of medication. As a result of the conversations, one of the town pharmacies agreed to provide home delivery for a small charge.

The third project was related to availability of community seating outside of businesses regularly frequented by seniors. The researchers worked with the participants (seniors and center professionals) to inform store owners of the need for public seating in areas close to bus or train routes. This presented some unique challenges because store owners saw the seating areas as potential hangouts for teenagers and other groups that might detract from their business. Through the discussions, some seating was made available.

"The Nurse is in" program helped center participants to deal with individuals' difficulties. Seniors shared insurance, medication, and other common problems with the nurses working in the office.

The third step in action research is reflecting. The researchers tell the readers that they kept a journal. It is not clear from the report the role that the journal played in the overall study.

The final step is evaluation. The investigators report that during this stage, outcomes and their effectiveness were reviewed; client satisfaction was assessed as was the feasibility of implementing the project in a larger community. To accomplish this work, interviews were held with the participants. An outside evaluator was selected to conduct the interviews to provide for the integrity of the process. It was clear from the report that participants were part of the process. Unfortunately, only two individuals remained from the group who initially established the plan.

It is clear from the study that the purpose of the research was achieved. The center participants were able to develop health-related support in a community setting. By the investigators own admission, the number of individuals who remained after 2.5 years was too small to clearly determine the long-term impact of the plan. However, much personal and community learning occurred. The researchers planned to use what they learned to continue the education of town leaders about the unique needs of elderly within their community. Further, the investigators reported that the one remaining participant in the focus groups has developed advocacy skills.

APPLICATION TO EDUCATION

*T*here has been much literature lately on high-impact educational practices, those that make a significant difference in student learning. Several of these demonstrate similar principles to those required in action research. For example, the use of collaborative assignments, experiential or community-based learning, and the implementation of learning communities all require that students work together and with others to achieve specific outcomes. In this section, an action research study by Adams and Canclini (2008) titled "Disaster Readiness: A Community-University Partnership" illustrates the impact an experiential learning experience can have on the students and community members. The report is reviewed using the critiquing criteria found in Box 14-1.

In the article by Adams and Canclini (2008), the authors report on a participatory action research study that included students from Texas Lutheran University (TLU) and community members in the area. The study's genesis is a result of conversations with community members after hurricanes Rita and Katrina. Community members felt underprepared to meet the needs of evacuees and asked the faculty at TLU to involve nursing students in the education of community members on disaster response. Faculty who were knowledgeable about disaster response recognized the need for personal preparedness as a prelude to disaster response and sought to educate the community about this requisite. The researchers report that the aim of the study was to engage baccalaureate students with community members to plan, implement, and evaluate a health education program to respond to an identified community need. The focus on collaboration and action planning made this an appropriate research approach.

The researchers report that the study was approved by the TLC Institutional Review Board (IRB). Initially, they brought students and key community leaders together for a 1-day stakeholders meeting to build relationships. The "engaging" experience was a seminar on the basic concepts of disaster. The meeting was held as a result of a verbalized need on the part of the community.

Participation in the seminar resulted in the initiation of relationships between and among key community stakeholders and the students.

In the report, the researchers talk about the activities the students developed. However, there is less discussion of the role community stakeholders played in development of the activities. Initially, the faculty planned the 1-day seminar. As part of the all day event, students engaged participants in quantitative data collection. A survey was distributed to collect information on the participant's knowledge of personal disaster planning. Based on the findings, a poster session was planned to educate the community members. There is no description of how the community participants were engaged in developing this strategy or why the community perceived this to be an effective way to deliver the information. Adams and Canclini (2008) do report that the reason for the poster was its portability and the ability to communicate information on the major areas of concern reported by community stakeholders in the survey. Further, there is no indication that the stakeholders reviewed the findings and agreed that those were the topics that should be addressed. It is apparent that the faculty are aware of the importance of personal disaster preparation.

The plan for addressing the problem is clear. The duration of the plan is also included in the report. There is no indication that the community stakeholders collaborated in making the decision about the time frame for implementation.

Faculty and students of TLU engaged in the reflection process. As a result of this reflection, the faculty planned subsequent activities in the community on the basis of what they learned from the poster activity and community members' repeated requests for information. The study does not report whether the requests for additional information occurred as part of ongoing partnerships. As a result, the reader is unable to gauge whether there was a change and whether it has been sustainable.

Unlike many of the studies reviewed for this chapter, complete description of the process of engagement including the planning, acting, reflecting, evaluating is limitedly reported in this study. The researchers do provide a good description of the results of the survey, but it is hard to judge whether there was a strong partnership that developed with community members as part of the action research study. The benefits to the students and community are articulated in generalities. The specifics of how the community gained is inferred by references to continued community members' requests for additional information.

The conclusions, implications, and recommendations are focused on what students and faculty plan to continue to address. The aim of the project—to promote active involvement of baccalaureate students in working with community partners to plan, implement, and evaluate a community-based health education project (Adams & Canclini, 2008)—is to focus on the collaboration of the students with the community members. To fully meet the tenets of the action research methodology, collaboration with the community should be paramount.

APPLICATION TO ADMINISTRATION

The roots of action research are in organizational change.

Issues of organizational concern such as quality patient care, systems improvement, organizational learning and the management of change are suitable subjects for action research, as (a) they are real events, which must be managed in real time, (b) they provide opportunities for both effective action and learning and (c) can contribute to the development of theory of what really goes on in hospitals and to the development of nursing knowledge. (Coghlan & Casey, 2001, p. 676)

In this section, a publication by Phillips, Davidson, Jackson, and Kristjanson (2008) titled "Multi-faceted Palliative Care Intervention: Aged Care Nurses' and Care Assistants' Perceptions and Experiences" is critiqued using the criteria found in Box 14-1. This article gives the reader an understanding of how action research can be used to develop a new approach to patient care.

Phillips and associates (2008) engaged in the Residential-Palliative Approach Competency Project in Western Australia. The overall aim of the project was to improve care to clients requiring palliative care. This aim was selected based on changes that were occurring in the policy arena.

Action research was selected as the research approach because the authors believed that without adequate involvement of the stakeholders, no sustained change would be possible. This understanding demonstrates consistency of the research method with the intended outcome. Clearly, the researchers are interested in more than just discovery. They are interested in using what they discover to develop a plan for change.

Before beginning the study, IRB approval was gained. The researchers identify that the first step in their action research process is the completion of a needs assessment. In this stage, the researchers defined the scope of the problem. As a result of defining the problem, priorities for action were determined. These included: chart audits, focus groups with care providers, and a survey. The main caregivers for palliative care patients in institutions are registered nurses and care assistants. Twenty-eight individuals participated in the focus groups. They represented nine residential facilities in Australia. The study was conducted over a 3-year period. The researchers offer that focus groups continued until no new data were generated. This is consistent with the concept of data saturation.

It is not clear from the report how the actions that appear to have been developed were derived. Working from the assumption that educational programming, team building, and new data collection methods were the action steps in this action research study, the reader is left without a clear view of how these became the actions of choice. Additionally, there are no statements reflecting the involvement of stakeholders.

It is also unclear, what role the care providers had in the development of the strategies for data analysis. Phillips et al. (2008) report that data analysis occurred throughout the study. "After each focus group the researchers met for an initial analysis session to reflect on group interactions" (p. 220). This provided "further revision, grouping and reduction" (p. 220).

The researchers report that data analysis revealed four major themes that were derived using content analysis. These included: targeted education makes a difference, team approach is valued, assessment tools are helpful, and using the right language is essential (Phillips et al., 2008). Although not fully described in this article, the reader is led to believe that through the 3-year project, educational programs, new assessment instruments, and team building are occurring. Assuming that this assumption is correct, then the question that arises is whether stakeholders were actively engaged in the process. The narrative that is included in the report illustrates comments made by the participants who would support this assumption. For the purposes of full understanding of the validity of the findings, inclusion of all steps of the process is critical.

The conclusions provided are true to the data. No theory is developed as a result of the study. The researchers offer that the implications of the study are related to policy making specifically funding. Phillips et al. (2008) do believe that a sustainable change among care providers is in place. They believe that creating a stronger understanding of the needs of palliative patients and building teamwork benefit all those involved.

SUMMARY

*I*n 1999, Jenks reported, "nurse researchers in the United States rarely use action research because they do not regard it as a rigorous form of research" (p. 263). In this chapter, each of the studies offered demonstrates that when action research is implemented appropriately, it is a rigorous methodology that can be useful in creating change. The use of qualitative methods is much more widespread outside of the United States based on the review conducted for this text. The question that looms large is why have action research and other qualitative methodologies gained so much ground abroad, while in the United States use of these methods lags behind. As nursing continues to build its knowledge base, nurse researchers should consider the value of the method in developing more humanistic practice environments. Learning more about the method, understanding its assumptions and characteristics, and applying its framework will not only build the body of nursing knowledge but it will also create practice opportunities for sharing power and knowledge, which will lead to more holistic understanding and care of individuals.

In this chapter, critique has been the focus. Through rigorous review of published studies and careful implementation of the critique process, those unfamiliar with the method will gain an understanding and appreciation of the method as a valuable approach to nursing research.

References

Adams, L., & Canclini, S. (2008). Disaster readiness: A community-university partnership. *Online Journal of Issues in Nursing, 13*. Retrieved August 2, 2009, from http://www.nursingworld.org/MainMenuCategories/ANAMarketplace/ANAPeriodicals/OJIN/TableofContents/vol132008/No3Sept08/ArticlePreviousTopic/Disaster Readiness.aspx)

Coghlan, D., & Casey, M. (2001). Action research from the inside: Issues and challenges in doing action research in your own hospital. *Journal of Advanced Nursing, 35*(5), 674–682.

Davidson, P., DiGiacomo, M., Zecchin, R., Clarke, M., Paul, G., Lamb, K., Hancock, K., Chang, E. & Daly, J. (2008). A cardiac rehabilitation program to improve psychological outcomes of women with heart disease. *Journal of Women's Health, 17*(1), 123–134.

Dickinson, A., Welch, C., & Ager, L. (2007). No longer hungry in hospital: Improving the hospital mealtime experience for older people through action research. *Journal of Clinical Nursing, 17*, 1492–1502.

Gallagher, L., Truglio-Londrigan, M., & Levin, R. (2009). Partnership for healthy living: An action research project. *Nurse Researcher, 16*(2), 7–29.

Glasson, J.B., Chang, E.M.L., & Bidewell, J.W. (2008). The value of participatory action research in clinical nursing practice. *International Journal of Nursing Practice, 14*, 34–39.

Jenks, J. (1999). Action research method. In H. J. Streubert & D. R. Carpenter (Eds.), *Qualitative research in nursing: Advancing the humanistic imperative* (2nd ed., pp. 251–264). Philadelphia, PA: Lippincott Williams & Wilkins.

Jones, S.P., Auton, M.F., Rurton, C.R., & Watkins, C.L. (2008). Engaging service users in the development of stroke services: An action research study. *Journal of Clinical Nursing, 17*, 1270–1279.

Melrose, S. (2006). Facilitating help-seeking through student interactions in a WebCT online graduate study program. *Nursing and Health Sciences, 8*, 175–178.

Minkler, M., & Wallerstein, N. (2008). *Community-based participatory research for health: From process to outcome.* San Francisco, CA: Jossey-Bass.

Phillips, J.L., Davidson, P.M., Jackson, D., & Kristjanson, L.J. (2008). Multi-faceted palliative care intervention: Aged care nurses' and care assistants' perceptions and experiences. *Journal of Advanced Nursing, 62*(2), 216–227.

Taylor, B., Bewley, J., Bulmer, B., Fayers, L., Hickey, A., Hill, L., Luxford, C., McFarland, J., & Stirling, K. (2008). Getting it right under pressure: Action research and reflection in palliative nursing. *International Journal of Palliative Nursing, 14*(7), 326–331.

US Census Bureau (2008). *Older Americans 2000: Key indicators of well-being.* Retrieved August 2, 2009, from http://www.agingstats.gov/agingstatsdotnet/Main_Site/Data/2008_Documents/Population.aspx.

Research Article

Partnership for Healthy Living: An Action Research Project

Louise P. Gallagher, Marie Truglio-Londrigan, and Rona Levin

The purpose of this study was to develop and evaluate an advanced practice nurse case-management intervention programme in a US senior citizen community centre. Researchers Louise Gallagher, Marie Truglio-Londrigan and Rona Levin used a participatory action research method and found that a number of themes emerged to guide nursing interventions

Keywords: action research, case-management, older people, social support

Introduction

Globally, the population is ageing. The world's elderly population is increasing by 795,000 each month (Kinsella and Velkoff 2001). Industrialised nations have demonstrated a tremendous increase in this population. More than 35 million people residing in the US are over 65 years of age and they make up 13 per cent of the population (Federal Interagency Forum on Aging-Related Statistics 2000). The population of people 85 and over increased by 38 per cent from 1990 to 2000 (US Census Bureau 2000). The older American adult population is expected to more than double by the year 2050, with the largest growth spurt taking place between 2010 and 2030 when the baby boom generation enters the 'golden years'.

As people age, chronic illness becomes a major issue. Eighty per cent of older adults suffer from at least one chronic condition and the average 75-year-old has three chronic conditions (Merck Institute of Aging and Health and Centers of Disease Control 2004). Independent functioning in later years can be diminished by chronic illness. Despite the number of older adults with chronic illness, nearly 79 per cent of older adults who need long-term care live at home rather than in institutions (Merck Institutions of Aging and Health and Centers of Disease Control 2004). This would suggest that support for older adults from family, friends and the community is necessary for them to remain in their homes.

There is a lack of research into finding intervention strategies that can assist older adults in identifying and accessing appropriate and affordable community resources for support. The purpose of this pilot action research project was to develop, implement and evaluate the impact of a nurse-run case-management programme in a senior citizen community centre as a form of community support. We used a participatory action research method to accomplish this goal. This method uses collaboration between researchers and participants in all areas of the research design and implementation, from problem identification to evaluation, ultimately

From Gallagher LP, Truglio-Londrigan M, Levin R. *Nurse Researcher*. vol. 16, issue 2, pp. 7–29. Copyright © 2009 by RCN Publishing Company Ltd. Reprinted with permission.

empowering the participants. Participants' reflection is a key aspect of participatory action research, which leads to a greater awareness of their problems or needs.

Background

Many older adults live with chronic illnesses that affect their independence. Despite this, statistics indicate that these same older adults are ageing in place and remaining in their home communities. This leads to the question of what supports are in place.

Social support is the caring interactions that are available and support an individual or that have been received (Pender et al 2002). Barrera (1986) identifies three types of social support: social embedment, or the frequency of contact with others; received support or the amount of tangible support provided by others; and perceived support or subjective satisfaction with support. Social support enhances people's personal strengths and assists them in the achievement of their goals. It also encourages them to engage in healthy behaviour (Pender et al 2002).

The buffering function of social support is also essential. Krause (2005) suggests that emotional support from family and friends helps older adults cope more effectively, especially with financial strain, and that the oldest and old benefit from informal emotional support. Unger et al (1999) notes the importance of social support with coping with the emotional and physical consequences of chronic illness. Cross-national studies have also found a relationship between social support and health, and attribute this to the protective buffering effect of social support (Wu and Rudkin 2000).

Others have shown the positive effects of social support on older adults' cognitive abilities. Whitfield and Wiggins (2003) indicate that there may be a difference in the cognitive abilities of those older adults involved in social activities, resulting in better problem-solving skills. They suggest this may cause these older adults to avoid more formal care.

Social networks are the family members, friends or community agencies with whom an individual interacts (Pender et al 2002). Social supports, therefore, are perceived and received via these networks (Litwin and Landau 2000). Healthy People 2010 (US Department of Health and Human Services 2000) recognised social networks as critical in influencing and promoting health and independence for individuals and contributing to their wellbeing and quality of life. Older adults who are connected to active social networks have been shown to demonstrate better physical and mental health than those who are less connected and involved with others (Antonucci 1990, George 1996). Social support and social networks together are associated with lower risks of morbidity and mortality (Berkman et al 1992), although the reasons for these decreases are not completely understood.

The Convoy Model as a Conceptual Framework

The Convoy Model (Figure 1) is prominent in the literature and attempts to describe and explain support (Antonucci and Akiyama 1987). It depicts support as three concentric circles surrounding an individual. The innermost ring consists of the family as the closest and most important providers of support; the middle ring consists of friends who are important but not the most intimate supporters; and the external ring includes supporters who occupy a role such as co-worker or acquaintance (Antonucci and Akiyama 1987). This outer ring may also include other community

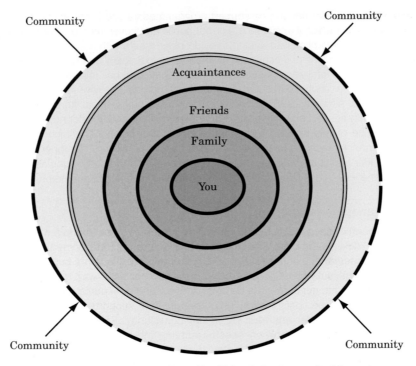

Community   Community

Acquaintances

Friends

Family

You

Community   Community

Note: The black broken line represents the possible addition of a fourth means of social support, which the investigators call community social support.

Figure 1: **Convoy Model of social support with an added dimension of community.**

support services such as recreational activities, spiritual comfort, safety, transportation, education programmes, social services, communication services, programmes to maintain the older adults' physical environment, and a government that is aware of and responsive to older adults' needs (Anderson and McFarlane 2000). Thus, this outer ring represents social supports and the social networking essential for older adults who live in the community.

Overall, it appears that friends provide companionship and short-term crisis intervention while the family's function is to provide more long-term care, such as that necessary when an older adult has a chronic illness (Antonucci and Akiyama 1996). Research into community support that assists older adults to live in their community of choice and the outcomes of this process is limited (Antonucci and Akiyama 1996). Recently, Antonucci et al (2004) supported previous research and spoke of the Convoy Model and the relationships that take place in each of the rings – in particular how these relationships serve to shape and protect individuals.

Anderson and McFarlane (2004) illustrate the multi-dimensional nature of a community in a model to guide nursing practice. This model portrays a community with eight interdependent subsystems surrounding the core or the people of the community. These subsystems include: physical environment; health and social services; education; safety and transportation; politics and government; communication; economics; and recreation. Support programmes can be found in each of these subsystems and include informal support groups such as senior citizen centres, civic clubs and churches. All of these may provide support programmes for social interaction and physical as well as emotional assistance. Formal public and governmental agencies, such as area agencies dealing with ageing, provide older adults with resources and assistance, such as housing and economic or financial help (Lassey and Lassey 2001).

Research into family and friends as providers of support has shown the crucial role they play for older adults, particularly in enhancing their ability to live in the community (Antonucci and Akiyama 1996, Siebert et al 1999). The professional literature concerning community support also highlights its importance in assisting older adults. Despite the existence of this wealth of information, there has been a conspicuous lack of research into community support and how older adults perceive it. If support is necessary for older adults to live independent lives of quality in their communities, would it not be beneficial to ask this population what they find meaningful and helpful?

Case Management

The American Nurses Association (1991) has defined case management as 'a healthcare delivery process whose goals are to provide quality healthcare, decrease fragmentation, enhance the client's quality of life, and contain costs'. Netting and Williams (1999) views case management as a way to advocate for clients who need to negotiate in a complex system and a resource allocation mechanism to contain the cost of care. The literature has supported benefits of case management with older adults living in the community. Schein et al (2005) describes the association between specific nursing interventions performed in the context of case management and noted that coping assistance among frail older adults was associated with a small yet beneficial increase in IADL (independent activities of daily living) function. Marshall et al (1999) also found less impairment in IADL and ADL after two years. Shapiro and Taylor (2002) noted that community-based case management as an intervention for older adults was positively associated with the older adults' subjective wellbeing and negatively associated with permanent nursing home placement and mortality.

Purpose of the Study

The purpose of this pilot action research project was to develop, implement and evaluate the impact of an advanced practice nurse-run case-management programme in a senior citizen community centre.

Method: Design

The researchers used a community-based participatory action research approach coupled with a focus group design as a pilot programme to provide case-management services for elderly residents residing in a county north of New York City. The action research approach is used by practitioners of professional disciplines to achieve a desired social outcome – to solve problems, improve work situations and/or design and implement special projects (Speziale and Carpenter 2003). This approach makes use of traditional research techniques and at the same time involves a community in the development and assessment of a programme. This process creates a situation where knowledge is produced not only for knowledge's sake but for change (Kelly 2005). Ultimately, this method involves stakeholders as active participants in project development and thus 'provides for a sense of ownership amongst those involved in the endeavor' (Nolan and Grant 1993). This ownership is evident as all participants work together as collaborators in equal partnership (Holkup *et al* 2004, Kelly 2005). The action research approach, therefore, was particularly suited to the current project.

There are several classifications of action research. Holter and Schwartz-Barcott (1993) offer three: technical collaboration; mutual collaboration; and enhancement. This project used technical collaboration. In technical collaboration, the researcher often implements a 'predetermined' intervention for testing. In this project, the intervention was a nursing case-management programme, which was delivered at a community senior centre.

There were three categories of primary stakeholders. These stakeholders included the recipients of the service, senior citizen community centre professionals and the primary political leaders of the community. These individuals were partners in the design, implementation and evaluation of the services to be provided. The duration of the project was approximately 2.5 years, from meetings with the stakeholders to the evaluation of the project.

The pilot study consisted of four stages (Figure 2) and included: problem diagnosis; action-plan design; plan implementation; and outcome evaluation (Nolan and Grant 1993).

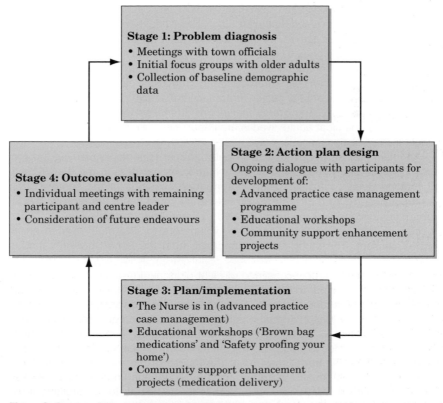

Figure 2: **Stages of the action research process.**

Stage One—Problem Diagnosis

The specific aim of stage one was to diagnose the problem of needed community support through dialogue and interviews with town political officials, community centre professionals, and initial focus groups with elderly community centre participants. The purpose of stage one was to determine whether advanced practice nurse-led case-management was viewed by participants as a viable way to help with their needs, and/or whether they regarded other strategies, such as educational workshops and/community support projects, as desirable additions. The focus groups' reflections provided the researchers with the information they needed to diagnose the community's social problems.

Sampling

Initially, we and two categories of stakeholders tried to determine how to provide case-management services to elderly community residents. These categories were community politicians – the mayor and town supervisor – and senior citizen community centre professionals. We tried to determine with these stakeholders if there was a need in the community, and to gain their support and participation in the project.

The next category of stakeholder to be involved was the older clients of the community centre for whom the case-management services would be provided. The US Census of 2000 revealed that in Mt Kisco, New York, there were 606 males and 905 females over the age of 60. The racial breakdown for older adults was not available but the racial make-up of the population was approximately 78 per cent white, 6 per cent African American, 4 per cent Asian, and 25 per cent Hispanic or Latino of any race. There were approximately 350 older adults between 60 and 90 years of age who used the senior centre facilities and 40 to 60 used the on-site lunch programme daily. The overall majority of attendees were white and female. The majority of the older adults lived in area apartments and belonged to lower and middle income socioeconomic strata.

An initial mailing went to all these potential participants, explaining the proposed project and requesting their participation as partners in the 'Partnership for Healthy Living'. We held several information sessions at the senior citizen community centre for those interested in learning more about the project. Two information sessions were held and between 13 and 15 individuals attended each session. At the end of these sessions, volunteers for the study signed an informed consent. The study received approval from the Pace University institutional review board.

The initial study sample consisted of eight older adults who volunteered to be participants in the action research project. The age range was 60 to 90, and all were Caucasian and female. The sample size experienced vast changes over the course of the study. One individual was lost immediately and did not participate in the first focus group. The remaining seven participated in the first two focus groups. By the third focus group, this decreased to five as a result of one death and one individual moving out of town. Over the course of the year, another member moved to assist her daughter with her ailing husband, and another individual was hospitalised and the centre was never able to locate her. At the completion of the study, only one of the individuals remained.

Data Collection

First, investigators kept a journal of semi-structured interview sessions held with key stakeholders, the community political leaders and senior centre professionals. Each stakeholder group was interviewed once. These semi-structured interview sessions initially assisted us in the early phases of the research with identifying a population and location for the project, and in gaining access to the potential participants. This journal, which became known as *The Journey*, was also used during the case management sessions to document what had transpired each visit.

Second, at the request of participants, we held focus groups throughout the project to determine their needs and work with them using a technical collaboration approach. The focus groups were a descriptive and exploratory process used to assist with the sharing and comparing of ideas among all participants to identify their reflections on problems with community support. We used a rigorous systematic process developed by Krueger (1998) to ensure accurate data collection and interpretation. Participant reflections assisted with the design of programmes and services the older adults identified as necessary to helping them live independently in their community. Initially, these focus groups took place every other week for five months. Towards the end of the project, these focus groups only took place once a month due to the implementation of strategies that the participants identified as well as 'The Nurse is In'. All focus groups with older adult participants were tape-recorded and transcribed.

Several guiding questions were used to help the groups. Examples of guiding questions included: 'What are the most pressing issues you must deal with on a daily basis?'; 'How do these issues affect you and your ability to live independently?'; 'How do you cope or get around these issues?'; 'What do you see as a more permanent answer to these issues?'; and 'Why have you not attempted to resolve these issues in this permanent way?' Observations of these focus groups in terms of participant interactions and responses to dialogue were also documented in *The Journey*.

Data Analysis and Findings Demographics of Elderly Adult Participants

All participants were white females, 60 years of age or older. Out of the eight participants, two lived alone. Three saw their children monthly or not at all. Of the six individuals who indicated that they had a sibling, none saw them monthly. All participants stated that they had been diagnosed with a medical condition. Of the 22 documented medical conditions, 50 per cent or more of the participants indicated a diagnosis of osteoarthritis, hypertension, insomnia, sadness, anaemia or hearing loss. In fact, 50 per cent of the participants indicated ten or more medical conditions and 50 per cent took four or more medications.

Of the eight initial participants, three had been hospitalised during the previous year, and one of these three was readmitted because of an infection at the surgical site. Additionally, three of the eight individuals experienced an unplanned visit to their primary healthcare provider; one of these three individuals had three unplanned visits. Two of the eight participants had visits to the emergency room, with two of the eight participants using the visiting nurse service.

Focus Group Themes

Content analysis of focus group data revealed several themes pertaining to community support: 'Negotiating the health insurance bureaucracy', 'Trials and tribulations of transport' and 'Medication madness'.

Negotiating the Health Insurance Bureaucracy

Participants shared their concerns about health insurance coverage. For example, one participant noted lack of coverage as a problem:

'They are urging us all the time as seniors to have a yearly check-up and over the last five years they are constantly cutting back on just how much they are allowing. You have to give a lot more money in order to get it and I think that is counter-productive.'

Another participant noted a problem with coverage not offered by her private insurance:

'Look at me. I need a battery-powered wheelchair. My insurance sent in someone to evaluate me. They denied me the wheelchair because they said I had strong upper body strength. That may be so but I have a terrible cardiac condition and I cannot use my upper body.

Trials and Tribulations of Transport

Participants overwhelmingly stated that transport as a community support was a major issue. The cost of taxis was one issue:

'It is only supposed to cost you $3.50 but if you do not say anything they will charge you $4.50.'

Another issue was that the taxi service had a policy of picking up other passengers along the way. Participants found this disturbing since they had to get to appointments on time.

'You take a taxi to the doctor so instead of going out to the medical group he takes another road. I said: "I am going to the medical group." He said: "Do you have time to pick up another passenger?" I said: "No, I hired you, I am in a hurry."'

Other means of transport also created difficulties. Buses are limited, particularly at weekends, and the bus and train schedules are not co-ordinated. As an example:

'I transport by buses a lot. It would be great if the bus and the train were co-ordinated. There are people here who are totally dependent on the buses and on Saturday they are every two hours and on Sunday there are none at all.'

Even the simple act of walking is not simple:

'Thank God we are able to walk but what about those who are unable to walk. I mean, dragging up the hill. It's a problem. I mean, I am just thinking going way down the road... like I said me and my husband walk but sometimes walking is not easy.'

Many participants used a volunteer organisation called FISH. This was a group of volunteers who drove older adults to medical appointments. Participants were quick to sing the praises of FISH. They indicated, however, that there were not enough volunteers and that the service was limited – for example, it drove participants to medical appointments, but not to the store for shopping. Participants also noted that this service would pick up a participant and then pick up other passengers. As with the taxi service, this was a particular problem when participants were in a hurry to get to appointments.

Medication Madness

Understanding the purpose and action of medications is a major issue. One participant noted:

> *'My husband was put on medication. We really need someone other than our doctor to come in and dwell on the medications. Should you really be taking certain medications? Maybe the person could talk to the doctors or maybe they could research the medications.'*

Getting to the drug store to purchase one's medications was another issue directly related to the transport problems discussed earlier.

Stage Two—Action Plan Design

After analysing the data collected during initial focus groups and sharing the themes and findings that emerged from these sessions with participants for validation, the project partners (researchers and participants) designed an action plan for providing specific services to address identified needs. In this type of research, the action can only be developed after stage one of the project – problem identification – is completed. For example, Ducharme *et al* (2001) used an action research model to develop an intervention programme to promote the mental health of family caregivers. They based the specific intervention on what they learned from participants in initial focus groups. In our project, the data analysis led us to develop a plan of action specific to the needs participants had identified.

Participants indicated that they wanted their action plan to include two main approaches. The first was to continue the focus groups, which they enjoyed and saw as a way to identify issues that they would be able to work on us. This resulted in educational programmes and community projects. The second approach was to start a programme called 'The Nurse is In'. Participants indicated that they wanted this to be implemented by the two of us who were also nurse practitioners with gerontological expertise. These nurses provided case-management services to the participants one day a week for two hours each day for six months. The setting was an office at the senior citizen community centre. The time of the programme was one hour before and after lunch.

The decision that we would serve as the case managers further illustrates the partnership and collaboration between the action researchers and the participants. Some have questioned whether this kind of close, collaborative relationship creates 'particular consequences' (Williamson and Prosser 2002). To address this issue, the researchers were very clear about their roles and responsibilities. From the onset of the project, we were introduced as nursing faculty members from a local university. In addition, it was explained that we were nurses specialising in gerontology and community nursing. The purpose of community action research was explained, as was the role of participants as partners and collaborators. As the research unfolded, it was the participants' request that 'The Nurse is In' be led by us. It is possible that the participants were comfortable with us and trusted us to perform the role of case manager as a result (Truglio-Londrigan *et al* 2006). Our multiple roles, however, were a constant source of conversation as a potential for role confusion; that is, conflicting roles of researcher and healthcare provider could create challenges regarding confidentiality and anonymity. The researchers were aware of the roles of service provider or the giving of assistance and that of researcher and the need to be focused in one's intention at varying points in time to avoid role confusion.

Stage Three—Plan/Implementation

The specific aim of stage three was to implement the two primary approaches identified above. The first of these was to continue the focus groups, which ultimately resulted in educational workshops and community projects. The second was the 'The Nurse is In' case-management programme.

Educational Workshops

Participants believed that they and their peers who attended the senior citizen centre needed more information about a number of topics to help them remain living in the community independently. To determine what type of educational programmes they wanted, participants worked with us to develop a flyer that listed several key issues that older adults dealt with every day and asked them to identify which of these issues they would like to hear more about. These flyers were distributed to members of the centre, after which we collected and collated them. The programmes that the older adults most wanted information on were 'safety-proofing one's home' and 'brown bag medications'. We developed two, 40-minute programmes, which we then delivered to the entire senior citizen community centre, not just participants of the action research project.

Community Projects

Throughout the focus groups, participants stated that there were three major problem areas for older adults: the need for education and support regarding health insurance, specifically Medicare, the publicly-funded programme for over-65s; the need for medication to be delivered to older adult homes because of transport difficulties; and the need for seating outside public spaces such as shopping centres.

Health Insurance

All focus group participants continually expressed frustration with Medicare. We identified a community programme called Medicare Minute and assisted the centre in gaining access to this by bringing in Medicare Minute representatives each month. These community experts were older adults trained in Medicare issues and facts. Their primary responsibility was to go out into the community and educate others.

Medication Delivery

Participants identified home delivery of medications as a needed community support. We worked with participants to develop a sample letter requesting the home delivery of medication from local pharmacies. All senior citizen community centre clients signed the letters.

We and the participants went to four of the town pharmacies. The participants found that one pharmacy would deliver medications for a two-dollar fee.

Neither the participants nor other older adults attending the centre had known that this service was available. The participants suggested putting the information in the centre's newsletter, which was mailed out to all the centre's users each month.

The other three pharmacies were unable to deliver medications. Two declined the offer without further discussion. A third wanted to assist the participants and tried to develop a delivery system; however, none of the employees had driving licences and many came to work by bike, leaving no way for the pharmacy to deliver medications.

Community Seating

We, the participants and the centre professionals discussed the best way to approach the issue of seating in community places, especially outside food stores where senior citizens needed somewhere to sit while they waited for buses. Store officials indicated that providing seating was a problem because the area would then become 'hang outs' for teenagers and other groups. However, three months later, another pharmacy opened next to the food store and park benches were installed, which older adults used when waiting for the senior citizen bus.

'The Nurse is In'

During the 'The Nurse is In' case-management portion of the project, older adults would arrive to discuss issues with the nurse researchers. The overall themes that unfolded pertained to community support services and were congruent with what was presented in the focus groups.

Negotiating the Health Insurance Bureaucracy

One individual who came to 'The Nurse is In' said that she had to go to a dentist to have a tooth removed. She also said she had to pay the dentist over $500 (£320). This participant was in her nineties and was a retired Bell Telephone worker. She had health insurance but did not know whether she had dental insurance and thus had to pay for dental services herself.

That day, we called the participant's health insurance agency. Navigating the maze of telephone instructions to reach the appropriate department took 20 minutes. We discovered that the participant had dental insurance but needed to download a claim form. The participant did not have a computer and neither did the centre, so we went back to the university office and downloaded the form. We took the form back to the centre at a later date, filled it in and sent it off. Several weeks later, the participant said she had received a cheque from the agency and noted that she would not have been able to obtain this without our assistance.

Medication Madness

During 'The Nurse is In', many older adults expressed concern about medications – they did not fully comprehend the medications, their side effects and costs. Two people who came to 'The Nurse is In' were not participants in the project yet came several times with concerns about medication use. When questioned about whether they wanted to become a part of the group, both refused.

Stage Four—Outcome/Evaluation

The aim of stage four was to review outcomes and evaluate the effectiveness of the intervention, assess participants' satisfaction, and determine the feasibility of implementing the project in the larger community.

During the final stage of the project, interviews were held with participants to assess qualitatively the success of the intervention strategy and whether participants thought it was helpful. An external interviewer was used for this aspect of the study to control for social desirability. Questions posed in this interview covered participants' overall impression of the programme, ways in which it had been of benefit, observations on the most and least successful aspects of the programme, and any actions we could take to strengthen the programme.

At the end of the study, only two people were available for interview. The first was the head of the centre. Her overall evaluation was that the programme had the potential to be very successful. She said 'The Nurse is In' was particularly effective. The fact that fewer people had participated than she had anticipated concerned her. She did not understand why more had not availed themselves of the service, but said this had been a constant enigma for the centre. She said: 'Many times these individuals complain, yet when something is being offered they do not partake. I just do not understand.'

The head of centre had not revealed these concerns earlier in the project, although we had not raised questions about the older adults' potential participation. We would certainty include such questions in future projects.

The second person to evaluate the programme was the only remaining participant of the original eight. She also indicated that she thought the programme was very valuable and did not understand why people failed to participate.

Both individuals identified several reasons for this limited participation. First, the community in which the centre is located is primarily a middle-income area, and all individuals had health insurance and primary healthcare providers. So while there may have been needs, participants were not in crisis. Second, both individuals indicated that one potential problem was the purpose of the centre. Since the centre was seen as a place to socialise, unwind and have fun, it may not have been viewed as a place where health issues could be addressed. Finally, both individuals who evaluated the programme shared the view that older adults who use the centre may not participate in programmes because they interpret participation as a form of weakness, which they do not want to portray to anyone.

Discussion

The major limitations of this action research project were the small number of participants, the attrition and its restricted generalisability. Also, the limited human resources of this project meant the advanced practice nurse case managers were on site for only two hours each week. Thus, fewer older adults might have accessed services than would have been the case if there had been a more visible cadre of providers. While we, the town political officials and the centre professionals thought the nutrition site was an appropriate venue for this inquiry and programme, the participation rate indicated otherwise. Throughout the project, participants were involved and information was shared continuously. We made attempts to identify from the participants methods to encourage centre participation.

Despite the limitations of the study, it seems clear that older adults' needs for community support are not being met. Kelly (2005) notes that an overall goal of an action research project is to work 'with' the community to implement an action so that social change can take place to resolve an issue. In this particular project, there were two major actions to be implemented 'with' the community to try to resolve issues. The first was the focus groups that resulted in the educational programmes and the community projects. The second was the 'The Nurse is In' case-management project. While the educational programmes took place and were well received and attended, the community projects and 'The Nurse is In' had limited success.

Holkup et al (2004) elaborate on a process they note as a spiral. This process involved planning for change, incorporating the change, reflecting on the processes and then re-planning. On reflection, we identified an overall lack of understanding by the general community as to what is meant by community support as well as the specific needs of this particular population. For example, the community lacked an understanding of ageing changes, chronic illness and endurance, as well as how the community can support older adults regarding these issues. The community also failed to recognise that park benches were not just a nicety but a necessity for some. If there was a problem with the park benches – for example, they were a hang-out for others – the act of removing the benches only created another problem for an entirely different group of citizens in the community – the older adults. In addition, the importance of social networks became very evident as the project unfolded.

Implications

Community social networks should be in place and seamless to meet the types of needs that participants identified in this study. For example, when we first made contact with the community political leaders, one of their immediate responses was that there was a need for case-management services for older adults in the community. But they were also quick to tell us that the community had multiple supports in place. They seemed to think that the advanced practice nurse case manager only had to point older adults in the right direction for them receive and use community support. As this project unfolded, it was clear that although community supports were in place, the needs of only a few were being met and only some of the time.

The community in which this research project took place is similar to many other middle- to upper-class communities and prides itself on the number and type of services offered. In essence, the number of community supports was not the issue. Rather, the community's development of a solid continuous network that meets the needs of each citizen was present but spotty at best, thus not affording seamless care delivery. These results present multiple issues despite the resources available to older citizens.

A primary concern is the community's inability to address community support issues where they count the most: issues that have a direct bearing on quality of life. For example, a pharmacy trying to help older adults by delivering medications to their homes is unable to do so because their employees, like older adults in the community, do not have access to transport because there is no network that would permit this to happen.

Another example of the importance of networks involves buses as a community support. It is not enough for a community to buy a bus for older adults and feel that their needs will be met. Rather, specific questions must be asked that will help define what is needed for this specific population. How often does this bus make trips? Where does the bus pick people up? Is there a place for people to sit who are waiting for the bus? How much is the bus? Where does the bus go? How long do the individuals have once the bus arrives at the end destination before they must return to the bus to be taken home? Does the bus run at weekends? These questions would give rise to community support involving a transport system that would be tightly networked and thus usable by the population in question. Essentially, the supports that are in place are not networked.

Nurse case managers may take note of what Holkup *et al* (2004) say regarding the process of change, incorporating the change, reflecting on the processes and then re-planning. They can be leaders in community endeavours to provide much needed community social networks to older citizens. One way to accomplish this may be to become members of the community advisory board, thus providing a way to educate the community about the needs of specific groups and what this means in terms of establishing programmes with networks that are seamless.

Conclusion

If it takes a village to raise a child, then it also takes a village to support older adults in living in their home communities. Healthcare professionals, leaders in the community and the people themselves – in this case community-dwelling older adults – must peck away at the apparent lack of knowledge and misunderstanding about what community support means. All stakeholders must take an active part in creating networks and participating in community development issues. Healthcare professionals, especially nurses who make up a very large segment of this professional group, must continually help others understand what a community is and how communities can be designed to support the independent dwelling of older adults.

We are organising a presentation to the town board with the professionals from the senior site. The purpose of this presentation is to educate. The individuals who make decisions must understand the when, where and how of supports that are in place in the community. In addition, healthcare professionals have a responsibility to teach older adults how to verbalise and express their needs and make their voices heard, particularly in a political sense. Although only one of the original eight participants remained, that person's voice will be prominent at the presentation.

One point that bears discussion is that the political leaders who were initially in office and stakeholders in the project have been voted out of office. This does not mean that the presentation is lost, only that we, participants and town officials must re-acquaint ourselves as well.

Finally, what became clear for us was that you cannot work alone in the community. Issues are much too complex and require a way to develop coalitions and partnerships with multiple organisations. This is an area you may be uncomfortable with and you may not have the necessary skills. This does not mean you should shy away from such endeavours and you can develop the appropriate skills, potentially as an initial step in nursing education. There is an understanding among us and the participants in this project that community support is important, and that the effects of this type of support for older adults are only forthcoming, and there is an urgent need for further work.

Louise P Gallagher EdD, FNP, RN, is professor at Pace University, Lienhard School of Nursing, New York, US

Marie Truglio-Londrigan PhD, GNP, RN, is associate professor at Pace University, Lienhard School of Nursing, New York, US

Rona Levin PhD, RN, is professor and project director for the Joan M Stout RN Evidence-Based Practice Initiative at Pace University, Lienhard School of Nursing, Visiting Faculty, Visiting Nurse Service of New York, US

This article has been subject to double-blind review.

References

American Nurses Association (1991) *CHN Communiqué*. Council of Community Health Nursing.

f Aging and the Social Sciences. Fourth edition. Academic Press, New York.

Holkup RA, Tripp-Reimer T, Salois EM *et al* (2004) Community-based participatory research: an approach to intervention research with a Native American community. *Advances in Nursing Science*. 27, 3, 162–175.

Holter IM, Schwartz-Barcott D (1993) Action research: what is it? How has it been used and how can it be used in nursing? *Journal of Advanced Nursing*. 18, 2, 298–304.

Kelly PJ (2005) Practical suggestions for community interventions using participatory action research. *Public Health Nursing*. 22, 1, 65–73.

Kinsella K, Velkoff V (2001) *An Aging World: 2001* (US Census Bureau Series p95/01-1). US Government Printing Office, Washington DC.

Krause N (2005) Exploring age differences in the stress-buffering function of social support. *Psychology and Aging*. 20, 4, 714–717.

Krueger RA (1998) *Analyzing and Reporting Focus Group Results*. Sage, Thousand Oaks CA.

Lassey WR, Lassey ML (2001) *Quality of Life for Older People: An International Perspective*. Prentice Hall, Upper Saddle River NJ.

Litwin H, Landau R (2000) Social network type and social support among the old-old. *Journal of Aging Studies*. 14, 2, 213–229.

Marshall BS, Long MJ, Voss J *et al* (1999) Case management of the elderly in a health maintenance organization: the implications for program administration under managed care. *Journal of Healthcare Management*. 44, 6, 477–493.

Merck Institute of Aging and Health and Centres for Disease Control (2004) *The State of Health and Aging in America 2004*. Merck Institute of Aging and Health and Centres for Disease Control, Washington DC.

Netting FE, Williams FG (1999). Implementing a case management program designed to enhance primary care physician practice with older persons. *Journal of Applied Gerontology*. 18, 1, 25–45.

Nolan M, Grant G (1993) Action research and quality of care: a mechanism for agreeing on basic values as a precursor to change. *Journal of Advanced Nursing*. 18, 2, 305–311.

Pender N, Murdaugh C, Parsons MA (2002) *Health Promotion in Nursing Practice*. Prentice Hall, Upper Saddle River NJ.

Schein C, Gagnon AJ, Chan L *et al* (2005) The association between specific nurse case management interventions and elder health. *Journal of the American Geriatrics Society*. 53, 4, 597–602.

Shapiro A, Taylor M (2002) Effects of a community-based early intervention program on the subjective well-being, institutionalization, and mortality of low-income elders. *The Gerontologist*. 42, 3, 334–341.

location of a boat by adding different compass readings, the researcher applying principles of triangulation to a study design adds new confidence to the reliability and validity of data.

Campbell and Fiske (1959) were the first to apply the navigational term *triangulation* to research. The metaphor is a good one because a phenomenon under study in a qualitative research project is much like a ship at sea. The exact description of the phenomenon is unclear. To gain clarity about the phenomenon, researchers study the phenomenon from a particular vantage point, from which they learn additional information about the phenomenon. However, the information at this point is not precise. Like navigators, researchers then move to a different vantage point to study the phenomenon. Information from the second vantage point provides additional data about the phenomenon, hence making the description clearer. A third vantage point makes the description of the phenomenon far clearer than either of the first two vantage points. As in compass readings, techniques of qualitative research have their margins of error. The goal in choosing different strategies in the same study is to balance them so that each counterbalances the margin of error in the other (Fielding & Fielding, 1989).

Proponents of triangulation recognize that application of multiple approaches to an investigation can improve reliability and validity of data because the strengths of one method may help to compensate for the weaknesses of another. The ultimate goal of triangulation is to "overcome the intrinsic bias that comes from single-method, single-observer, and single-theory studies" (Denzin, 1989, p. 313). Four types of triangulation for qualitative research have been described: (1) data triangulation; (2) investigator triangulation; (3) theoretical triangulation; and (4) method triangulation (Denzin, 1989). This chapter examines the four types of triangulation described by Denzin (1989). Mitchell (1986) and Denzin (1989) have also suggested a fifth type, multiple triangulation, whereby combinations of triangulation strategies are used. This is a complex approach, using a combination of two or more triangulation techniques in one study. For example, using multiple triangulation, the study design may include more than one data source as well as more than one researcher (Denzin, 1989; Polit, Beck, & Hungler, 2004).

CHOOSING TRIANGULATION AS A RESEARCH STRATEGY

Qualitative investigators may choose triangulation as a research strategy to ensure completeness of findings or to confirm findings (Campbell & Fiske, 1959; Miles & Huberman, 1989; Patton, 1983; Polit et al., 2004; Risjord, Dunbar, & Moloney, 2002). Ensuring complete and thorough findings provides breadth and depth to an investigation, offering researchers a more accurate picture of the phenomenon (Denzin & Lincoln, 1994). Further, triangulation approaches reveal the varied dimensions of a phenomenon and help to create a more accurate description (Fielding &

Fielding, 1989). The metaphor of a group of visually impaired people describing an elephant based on the area they touch provides a good description of completeness. The person touching the trunk describes the elephant based on what that person feels. The person touching the foot provides a different description because of what he or she feels. The person touching the tail provides a third description. The most accurate description of the elephant comes from a combination of all three individuals' descriptions. None of the three alone is complete or accurate. Combining data from the vantage point of all three people results in a more complete and holistic description of the elephant.

Researchers might also choose triangulation to confirm findings and conclusions. Any single qualitative research strategy has its limitations. By combining different strategies, researchers confirm findings by overcoming the limitations of a single strategy (Breitmayer, Ayres, & Knafl, 1993). Confirmation occurs when investigators compare and contrast the information from different vantage points. Uncovering the same information from more than one vantage point helps researchers describe how the findings occurred under different circumstances and assists them to confirm the validity of the findings.

TYPES OF TRIANGULATION

*I*nvestigators have the option of using several different types of triangulation to confirm or ensure completeness of findings. The triangulation approach selected depends on the research question asked and the complexity of the phenomenon under study. When planning a study, researchers carefully consider the research methodology necessary to adequately answer a research question. Qualitative researchers may choose to use triangulation as a strategy in any investigation in which their goal is to provide understanding or to obtain completeness and confirmation. In designing their study, researchers may use data triangulation, methodological triangulation, investigator triangulation, and theoretical triangulation, or a combination. Each type of triangulation possesses both strengths and weaknesses. Table 15-1 illustrates the strengths and weaknesses of each approach. A discussion of each triangulation type follows.

Data Triangulation

Using data triangulation, researchers include more than one source of data in a single investigation. Denzin (1989) described three types of data triangulation: (1) time; (2) space; and (3) person. Researchers choose the type of data triangulation that is relevant to the phenomenon under study. Using *time triangulation*, researchers collect data about a phenomenon at different points in time. Time of day, day of week, and month of year are examples of times researchers would collect data for triangulation. Studies based on

Table 15-1 • Strengths and Weaknesses of Four Types of Triangulation		
Type of Triangulation	*Strengths*	*Weaknesses*
Data Triangulation	Extensive data	False interpretation due to overwhelming amount of data
	Data convergence and divergence	
	Increased confidence in the research data	Difficulty dealing with vast amounts of data
	Creative, innovative ways of phenomena	Fitting qualitative data into a quantitative mold
Investigator Triangulation	Expertise of more than one researcher in more than one methodology	Investigator bias
		Disruptive during interview
		Potential disharmony based on investigator biases
Method Triangulation	Exposing different types of information that contribute to overall understanding of the research problem	Multimethod research is expensive
		Difficulty meshing narrative and numerical data
Theoretical Triangulation	Broader analysis of findings	Adds to confusion if there are conflicts due to theoretical frameworks
		Lack of understanding as to why triangulation strategies were used

Adapted from Thurmond, V. A. (2001). The point of triangulation. *Journal of Nursing Scholarship*, 33(3), 253–258.

longitudinal designs are not considered examples of data triangulation for time because they are intended to document changes that occur over time, rather than specific time intervals for data collection (Kimchi, Polivka, & Stevenson, 1991).

Space triangulation consists of collecting data at more than one site. For example, a researcher might collect data at multiple units within one hospital or in multiple hospitals. At the outset, the researcher must identify how time or space relates to the study and make an argument supporting the use of different time or space collection points in the study. For example, a researcher studying decision making on a nursing unit might collect data on six different nursing units to triangulate for space. The researcher might also collect data on each shift and on weekdays and weekends to triangulate for time. The rationale for using the various collection spaces and times is to compare and contrast decision making at each time and in each location. By collecting data at different points in time and in different spaces, the researcher gains a clearer and more complete description of decision making and is able to differentiate characteristics that span time periods and spaces from characteristics specific to certain times and spaces.

Using *person triangulation*, researchers collect data from more than one *level of person*, that is, a set of individuals, groups, or collectives (Denzin, 1989). *Groups* can be dyads, families, or circumscribed groups. *Collectives* are communities, organizations, or societies. Investigators choose the various levels of person relevant to the study. In the previous example of studying decision making on a nursing unit, the level of person might be individual nurses, the staff working on a given shift, or the staff assigned to a given unit. Researchers use data from one level of person to validate data from the second or third level of person. Researchers might also discover data that are incongruent among levels. In such a case, researchers would collect additional data to reconcile the incongruence.

Reising (2002) conducted a grounded theory study to explore the early socialization of new critical care nurses. She used data triangulation in her research by interviewing both critical care nurses and their preceptors regarding the experience of socialization to the critical care area. The interviews with the preceptors were conducted following the conclusions of data collection with the critical care nurses. This was done "to help clarify the orientation process from the preceptors' points of view" (p. 21). Person triangulation added to the trustworthiness of Reising's findings by confirming and clarifying data. Kan and Parry (2004) used data triangulation to investigate the types of nursing leadership that are used to overcome resistance to change in the hospital setting. Data sources for this study included nonparticipant observation, informal/unstructured and formal/semistructured interviews, document analysis, and the Multifactor Leadership Questionnaire. Data triangulation added to the breadth and depth of the findings in this grounded theory investigation.

When carried out responsibly, data triangulation contributes to the rigor of a qualitative study. When planning a study, investigators should consider their data carefully. They should decide if time, space, or level of person is relevant to the data. They should plan to collect data from all appropriate sources, at all appropriate points in time, and from all appropriate levels of person. The result will be a broader and more holistic description of the phenomenon under study.

Methodological Triangulation

Qualitative researchers use methodological triangulation when they incorporate two or more research methods into one investigation. Method triangulation can occur at the level of design or data collection (Kimchi et al.,

1991). Method triangulation at the design level has also been called *between-method triangulation,* and method triangulation at the data collection level has been called *within-method triangulation* (Denzin, 1989). Triangulation design method most often uses quantitative methods combined with qualitative methods in the study design. Sometimes triangulation design method might use two different qualitative research methods. For example, Wilson and Hutchinson (1991) described how researchers might use two qualitative research methodologies, Heideggerian hermeneutics and grounded theory, in qualitative nursing studies. They explained that using two unique methods in one study can explicate realities of the complex phenomena of concern to nursing that might remain illusive if researchers used either method alone. "Hermeneutics reveals the uniqueness of shared meanings and common practices that can inform the way we [nurses] think about our practice; grounded theory provides a conceptual framework useful for planning interventions and further quantitative research" (p. 263).

When researchers combine methods at the design level, they should consider the purpose of the research and make a cogent argument for using each method. Also, they should decide whether the question calls for simultaneous or sequential implementation of the two methods (Morse, 1991). If they choose *simultaneous implementation,* they will use the qualitative and quantitative methods simultaneously. In *sequential implementation,* they will complete one method first, then, based on the findings of the first technique, plan and implement the second technique. Using simultaneous implementation, researchers must remember that they must limit interaction between the two data sets during data generation and analysis because the rules and assumptions of qualitative methods differ (Morse, 1991, 1994). For example, it is usually impossible to implement qualitative and quantitative methods on the same sample. Qualitative methods require a small, purposive sample for completeness, whereas quantitative methods require large, randomly selected samples. In simultaneous triangulation, the qualitative sample can be a subset of the larger quantitative sample, or researchers might choose to use different participants for each sample. An exception occurs if the quantitative measure is standardized. In this case, researchers would have the participants in the qualitative sample complete the quantitative measure and then would compare the findings with the standardized norms (Morse, 1994). If the measure is not standardized, then researchers must use a sequential triangulation technique as well as a much larger sample for the quantitative measure.

Combining quantitative and qualitative data can be particularly valuable in providing detailed descriptions of phenomena. Combining methods once again provided a more complete understanding and description of the problem. Cavendish, Konecny, Luise, and Lanza (2004) used method triangulation in their study dealing with prayer, empowerment, and performance enhancement. In contrast, researchers using a sequential triangulation technique begin by collecting either quantitative or qualitative data.

If substantial theory has already been generated about the phenomenon, if the researchers can identify testable hypotheses, or if the nature of the phenomenon is amenable to objective study, the investigation would begin with a quantitative technique. If there is no theory, the theory is not well developed, or the phenomenon is not amenable to objective study, researchers would begin with a qualitative technique (Morse, 1991). Researchers who begin a study with a qualitative approach do so to further explore unexpected findings following the completion of a quantitative analysis. A study might begin with a qualitative technique to generate testable hypotheses that a researcher will then study quantitatively.

Im, Lee, Park, and Salazar (2004) used sequential method triangulation at the design level in an investigation exploring the cultural meanings of breast cancer among Korean women. This descriptive, longitudinal study used methodological triangulation to gather both quantitative and qualitative data regarding Korean women's breast cancer experience.

When combining research methods, it is essential that investigators meet standards of rigor for each method. Using qualitative methods, researchers should ensure sampling is purposive and should generate data until saturation occurs. Using quantitative methods, researchers should ensure sample sizes are adequate and randomly chosen. Theory should emerge from the qualitative findings and should not be forced by researchers into the theory they are using for the quantitative portion of the study (Morse, 1991). Likewise, investigators should appropriately use validity and reliability measures to ensure rigor of quantitatively derived data. Analysis techniques should be separate and appropriate to each data set. The blending of qualitative and quantitative approaches does not occur during either data generation or analysis. Rather, researchers blend these approaches at the level of interpretation, merging findings from each technique to derive a cohesive outcome. The process of merging findings "is an informed thought process, involving judgment, wisdom, creativity, and insight and includes the privilege of creating or modifying theory" (Morse, 1991, p. 122). If contradictory findings emerge or researchers find negative cases, the investigators most likely will need to study the phenomenon further. If knowledge gained is incomplete and saturation has not occurred, additional data collection and analysis should reconcile the differences and result in a more complete understanding.

In another study, Dreher and Hayes (1993) used method triangulation at the design level to study the effects of marijuana use during pregnancy and lactation on children from birth to school age. The researchers planned to study two groups of Jamaican women: marijuana users and nonmarijuana users. However, the tool they had expected to use had been developed in the United States and, thus, was culturally inappropriate to Jamaican society. Instead, the researchers used ethnographic interview and observation of Jamaican women to revise the tool for culture appropriateness. The ethnographic data helped the researchers refine the language and relevancy

potentially have on a professional career, selecting an area of research must be guided by several factors. More important, one's career will be affected negatively if qualitative research is "poorly valued in university communities, where researcher prestige is given according to the number of research dollars obtained, not by the worthiness of the completed research and the impact it has on the discipline" (Morse, 2003a, p. 834). First and foremost, the researcher must be immersed enough in the nursing research literature to know what areas of research are more fully developed and where research is still needed. Because research in nursing is still evolving, many opportunities exist to select an area of interest and develop a research agenda that is relevant and that will make a meaningful contribution to nursing's substantive body of knowledge. Second, it is critical to select an area of research that is meaningful not only to the discipline but also to the researcher. One's research agenda should complement one's professional career in nursing practice, education, or administration. The effort needed and the significant amount of time required to develop a research agenda demand that the researchers become immersed in and feel connected to what they are doing. Boyd and Munhall (2001) articulate this position skillfully:

> On some level, most researchers settle on a research topic because of some personal reason. Even for the opportunistic researcher with an eye on funding priorities, personal interest is usually aroused with ties to the researcher as person. For the qualitative researcher, personal interest is a strategic tool in the research project; it provides the energy and the motivation to persevere with the challenges and tedium inherent in any scholarly work. More importantly, however, personal interest can position the researcher to attend to the phenomenon under study in a certain way; it establishes figure and ground for the research endeavor in what can be highly personalized ways that make the research a passion, a preoccupation, an intimate companion. (p. 615)

Additionally, establishing an area of research requires that the investigator confirm the significance of the problem and articulate not only why the study needs to be done but also why the study requires a qualitative format. This stage is complex and requires diligence and clarity of thought. The process is one that takes time and requires an ongoing process of evaluation. Reading, sharing ideas with colleagues, writing, and rewriting are all necessary aspects of the refinement of one's research agenda. When conducting a qualitative study for the first time, investigators inexperienced in this methodology should consider enlisting the help of a seasoned qualitative researcher to serve as a mentor during the development of a new project.

GENERAL CONSIDERATIONS

*I*dentifying a research agenda requires that the researcher clarify the problem or phenomenon of interest to be studied. Articulating the need for a particular study and articulating one's purpose will provide the appropriate direction needed to proceed with proposal development. Ideas must be logically developed and conceptually linked.

Determining scientific merit and quality of the proposal is guided by the researcher's ability to communicate the research paradigm and method. The conduct of any research study requires precision and rigor. The proposal must be clear, concise, and complete (Dexter, 2000). Knowledge of qualitative methodology, prior experience with the methodology, and availability of appropriate resources to successfully complete the study are important considerations. The extensiveness of a research proposal is essentially determined by its ultimate purpose. Variation exists depending on whether you are preparing a proposal for a dissertation, a grant, or an individual research project. For academics, guidelines can generally be obtained from the office of research services. If you are writing a grant proposal, then the granting agency's requirements determine how you prepare your materials. The content of the proposal must address all the stipulations set forth in enough depth to be meaningful, clear, and educational. To begin, it is helpful to prepare a basic outline or plan for the research idea. The detailed plan will then develop into a research proposal as each step in the outline is narrated and gaps are filled to illustrate logical and consistent expansion of an idea from question to answer (Brink & Woods, 2001).

Very often, members of Institutional Review Boards are grounded in quantitative research approaches. Therefore, the composition of the board may result in qualitative research proposals that face unnecessary obstacles. Qualitative research cannot be evaluated from a quantitative paradigm. This should be clear at this point in the textbook. The abstract nature of many qualitative approaches is so different from a qualitative worldview that the proposal will require excellent rationale and explanation of qualitative method applications. The proposal should be written in such a way that it provides enough theoretical support for the research paradigm so as to answer the questions of individuals reviewing the project who may not be familiar with qualitative approaches. The content of any proposal must always be written with the interest and expertise of the reviewers in mind. Morse (2003a) delineates criteria that could be used to evaluate qualitative proposals in terms of relevance, rigor, and feasibility. According to Boyd and Munhall (2001), when the *"guardians of the dominant paradigm"* (p. 614) are reviewing your qualitative research proposal, the readers should be provided with the following:

- Education about and description of the method from its aim to its outcome. Such detail also enhances confirmability by leaving a decision trail.

- Justification for using the method through a logically developed explanation of why the researcher has chosen to use it.
- Translation of language unique to the method in terms that are likely to be understood by readers (p. 614).

The overall appearance of the proposal is an additional consideration. It is expected that the work is completed professionally. Therefore, in addition to clear and accurate content, the writer must also ensure that there are no spelling, punctuation, or grammatical errors. The document must be aesthetically appealing in addition to being described clearly (Dexter, 2000).

The reader will now be provided with an overview of the essential components of the research proposal. The detail needed to complete a written account of each aspect of the proposal can be found in method-specific chapters.

ELEMENTS OF THE RESEARCH PROPOSAL

*T*he purpose of the research proposal is similar for both quantitative and qualitative research paradigms; however, evaluation criteria used by review boards must be significantly different. The document must communicate to the reviewers the essential elements of the study in such a way that the study's purpose, method, data generation, and treatment strategies are clear and methodologically precise. Further, the document must communicate to the reader that the participants in the project will be protected from harm. An overview of each component of the proposal follows. Box 16-1 lists the elements that should be included in a complete proposal. As with any document, the writer should begin with an introduction and overview of the project.

Introduction and Overview of the Project

All research must begin with a judgment regarding the importance of the project to the development of knowledge in the discipline. Introducing the study requires identification of the *phenomenon of interest, the problem statement,* and purpose. The researcher must clearly describe the background and significance of the project. Linking the proposed investigation to the current body of nursing knowledge adds to the development of the significance of the research for the discipline of nursing and verifies that what is currently known about the topic is insufficient, requiring additional investigation. The researcher must identify where gaps in the literature exist, how the study will potentially contribute to scientific understanding, and ultimately how our substantive body of knowledge regarding the topic will be advanced. "The onus is on the investigator to convince the reviewers that the project is vital for the advancement of their disciplinary goals" (Morse, 2003a, p. 837).

The *literature review* refines the questions and builds the case for the conduct of the study. It is important to prepare the literature review in a way

Box 16-1

Elements of the Research Proposal

The Introduction
1. Identification of the phenomenon or problem of interest
2. Statement of purpose
3. Rationale for research approach
4. Significance of the phenomenon to nursing

The Literature Review
1. Review of relevant theoretical and research literature
2. Discussion of literature review and how it will be used in the qualitative investigation

The Research Design
1. Introduce the research design (phenomenology, grounded theory, ethnography, action research, historical research)
2. Describe the philosophical underpinnings
3. List the procedural steps
4. Describe strengths and potential limitations of the design

Methodology
1. Researcher's role and credentials
2. Participant selection/sample
3. Gaining access, entering the setting for data generation
4. Protection of participants and ethical considerations relevant to qualitative inquiry
5. Data generation and treatment (process, data collector's training, data management, data analysis)

Discussion of Communication of the Findings
1. Within the proposal, briefly address how the findings will be addressed within the context of the literature review
2. Address rigor in relationship to the method
3. Discuss implications for nursing practice, education, and administration
4. What are the implications for future research?

References

Appendices
1. Consent forms
2. Any other relevant supporting documents

that will familiarize the reader with the selected area of study. Additionally, this section of the proposal should clarify what is known about the phenomenon under investigation and the rationale for selecting a qualitative approach. Chapter 2 addresses issues related to the conduct of the literature review in a qualitative investigation. The discussion addresses the fact that often qualitative researchers do not begin with an extensive literature review to reduce the likelihood that researchers might bias their data collection or analysis through development of preconceived notions about the topic under investigation. Should the qualitative researcher choose to maintain this standard, then rationale should be provided for the reviewers. In any case, the researcher should include a cursory review of the literature. The goal of the literature review is the development of an argument backed by adequate evidence to create and support a clear purpose statement. The writing style must be compelling and convince reviewers that the study is critically needed (Penrod, 2003).

Research Approach

Following the study's introduction, it is important to discuss the rationale for selecting a qualitative format and the philosophical underpinnings that support the approach. Qualitative research approaches vary, and consequently the conceptual foundations that support the approaches vary as well. The underlying assumptions relevant to the qualitative approach selected must be described in detail. See Chapter 2 for a detailed discussion of how different qualitative approaches may be used to study particular phenomena.

Method

Once the phenomenon of interest has been fully described and the research approach selected, the investigator should then proceed with a detailed discussion of the actual application of the design. This is an essential component of the proposal, and it is critically important that this section should "flow from the developed background and significance and that the methods be congruent with the desired product of the project" (Penrod, 2003, p. 825). Often, research methods are grounded in specific philosophical perspectives such as feminist inquiry or critical theory. When developing the method section, the researcher must make clear to the reader the philosophical underpinnings of the work. Discussion of the research protocol will ensure consistent application of the method. Decisions made related to method application are essential to the overall cohesiveness of the project. They culminate in a road map of how the study will be conducted. The method section should also address resources needed to conduct the study, such as time, money, and personnel.

Within the section addressing method, the strengths and weaknesses of the research design must also be addressed. A level of expertise in the application of qualitative methods is expected from the researcher and should be evident in a description of the researcher's credentials. If the individual is not a skilled qualitative researcher, then the mentor's credentials should be included. The emerging nature of a qualitative investigation should also be addressed. Explicit description of the philosophical stance guiding method application will enhance the credibility of the proposal. The researcher should also address the possibility that the study may need to be modified for implementation. The rationale for potential modifications must be provided (Sandelowski, Davis, & Harris, 1989).

In addition to the researcher's credentials, the proposal must include how participants will be selected, how the researcher will gain entry into the setting where data will be collected, and once there, how the rights of participants will be protected. "Threats to validity are addressed as potential limitations of the study to demonstrate the researcher's attention to methodological rigor" (Penrod, 2003, p. 825). For a detailed discussion of protection of human subjects and the ethical issues facing qualitative researchers, the reader is referred to Chapter 4.

Data generation and treatment in a qualitative investigation generally consist of in-depth interviewing. Often the interviews are tape-recorded and can range from very open-ended to very structured interviews. Data analysis techniques should be discussed along with issues related to how the researcher will ensure authenticity and trustworthiness of the data (see Chapter 4).

Protection of Human Subjects

Protection of human subjects is without question a critical component of any research study and must be addressed completely in the proposal. "The government's system for regulating research involving human subjects was born out of fear that researchers might, whether wittingly or not, physically or mentally injure the human beings that they study" (American Association of University Professors, 2001, p. 55). This report further notes that "IRBs, in carrying out their responsibilities, too often mistakenly apply standards of clinical and biomedical research to social science research, to the detriment of the latter" (p. 56). Protection of human subjects essentially ensures that participants are informed, that they consent to participation in the study, and that they are aware that they may withdraw from the study at any time. Although generally low risk, qualitative studies pose unique concerns for participants. These concerns are discussed in detail in Chapter 4. Because of the open-ended process of data collection used in qualitative research, interviews and observations may move in unanticipated directions. Therefore, informed consent takes on a new and different meaning when applied to qualitative studies as opposed to clinical or biomedical research. For this reason, Boyd and Munhall (2001) have suggested that qualitative researchers address the idea of *process consent* as opposed to *informed consent*. This essentially involves renegotiating informed consent throughout the study as data emerge and the research evolves. If the proposal author plans to use process consent, then this type of consent should be explained fully to proposal reviewers in terms of its definition and application.

Qualitative Research Findings

The proposal is prepared to gain permission to conduct a formal study and in some cases obtain funding for the research. Although the results cannot be addressed in the proposal, a brief discussion of why the findings will be important and how they will be used may be helpful in adding a sense of completeness to the proposal. Addressing how the results will ultimately be disseminated will strengthen the value of the research and its potential ability to contribute to nursing's substantive body of knowledge. Again, the writer must be sure to address the specific guidelines provided as they relate to the type of proposal being written.

Appendices and References

Appendices and references of the proposal should include an example of the consent form to be used as well as any other supplemental material to be included in the research. For example, if participants will be asked to write detailed responses to open-ended questions, the format and items to be included should be placed in the appendix. The reference list provided will verify the need for the study and will substantiate the researcher's expertise in the research area as well as the methodology planned.

SUMMARY

*T*he researcher completing a funding proposal for a qualitative study for the first time should be aware that despite precise attention to all the elements of the proposal, qualitative research is often reviewed by unqualified individuals (Morse, 2003b). Seasoned qualitative researchers continue to raise their voices about the injustices in a system that values measurement over understanding. To improve one's chances for funding, it is essential to search for organizations and agencies that have demonstrated a commitment to fund qualitative proposals so as not to spend protracted periods of time developing proposals that will not be supported.

This chapter has addressed issues related to the development of a qualitative research proposal. The fundamental elements necessary for proposal development are highlighted, along with some suggestions for avoiding roadblocks with Institutional Review Boards. Detailed discussions of all elements of the proposal are included within individual chapters of this book. Further, application is addressed in the sample grant found at the end of this chapter.

References

American Association of University Professors. (2001). Protecting human beings: Institutional review boards and social science research. *ACADEME* (May–June), 55–67.

Beck, C. T. (1997). Developing a research program using qualitative and quantitative approaches. *Nursing Outlook, 45*, 265–269.

Boyd, C. O., & Munhall, P. L. (2001). Qualitative research proposals and reports. In P. L. Munhall (Ed.), *Nursing research: A qualitative perspective* (3rd ed., pp. 613–638). Boston, MA: Jones and Bartlett.

Brink, P. J., & Woods, M. J. (2001). *Basic Steps in Planning Nursing Research: From Question to Proposal.* Boston, MA: Jones and Bartlett.

Dexter, P. (2000). Tips for scholarly writing in nursing. *Journal of Professional Nursing, 16*(1), 6–12.

Morse, J. M. (2003a). A review committee's guide for evaluating qualitative proposals. *Qualitative Health Research, 13*(6), 833–851.

Morse, J. M. (2003b). The adjudication of qualitative proposals. *Qualitative Health Research, 13*(6), 739–742.

Penrod, J. (2003). Getting funded: Writing a successful qualitative small-project proposal. *Qualitative Health Research, 13*(6), 821–832.

Sandelowski, M., & Barroso, J. (2003). Writing the proposal for a qualitative research methodology project. *Qualitative Health Research, 13*(6), 781.

Sandelowski, M., Davis, D. H., & Harris, B. G. (1989). Artful design: Writing the proposal for research in the naturalist paradigm. *Research in Nursing and Health, 12*(2), 77–84.

Agazio Project

OMB No. 0925-000'

Department of Health and Human Services Public Health Services **Grant Application** *Do not exceed character length restrictions indicated.*	LEAVE BLANK—FOR PHS USE ONLY.		
	Type	Activity	Number
	Review Group		Formerly
	Council/Board (Month, Year)		Date Received

1. TITLE OF PROJECT *(Do not exceed 81 characters, including spaces and punctuation.)*
Deployment of military mothers during wartime

2. RESPONSE TO SPECIFIC REQUEST FOR APPLICATIONS OR PROGRAM ANNOUNCEMENT OR SOLICITATION ☐ NO ☐ YES
(If "Yes," state number and title)
Number: Title:

3. PROGRAM DIRECTOR/PRINCIPAL INVESTIGATOR | New Investigator ☒ No ☐ Yes

3a. NAME (Last, first, middle) Agazio, Janice Blair	3b. DEGREE(S) PhD MSN CRNP	3h. eRA Commons User Name AGAZIOJ

3c. POSITION TITLE
Assistant Professor

3d. MAILING ADDRESS *(Street, city, state, zip code)*
The Catholic University of America
School of Nursing Gowan Hall Room 409
620 Michigan Avenue, N.E.
Washington, DC 200654

3e. DEPARTMENT, SERVICE, LABORATORY, OR EQUIVALENT
School of Nursing, The Catholic University of America

3f. MAJOR SUBDIVISION

3g. TELEPHONE AND FAX *(Area code, number and extension)*
TEL: 202-319-5719   FAX: 202-319-6485

E-MAIL ADDRESS:
agazio@cua.edu

4. HUMAN SUBJECTS RESEARCH
☐ No ☒ Yes

4a. Research Exempt
☒ No ☐ Yes

If "Yes," Exemption No.

4b. Federal-Wide Assurance No. 00004459	4c. Clinical Trial ☒ No ☐ Yes	4d. NIH-defined Phase III Clinical Trial ☒ No ☐ Yes

5. VERTEBRATE ANIMALS ☐ No ☐ Yes | 5a. Animal Welfare Assurance No.

6. DATES OF PROPOSED PERIOD OF SUPPORT *(month, day, year—MM/DD/YY)*		7. COSTS REQUESTED FOR INITIAL BUDGET PERIOD		8. COSTS REQUESTED FOR PROPOSED PERIOD OF SUPPORT	
From	Through	7a. Direct Costs ($)	7b. Total Costs ($)	8a. Direct Costs ($)	8b. Total Costs ($)
9/01/2009	8/31/2011	58,257	83,419	71,674	102,815

9. APPLICANT ORGANIZATION
Name   The Catholic University of America
Address   620 Michigan Avenue, N.E.
Washington, DC 200654

10. TYPE OF ORGANIZATION
Public: → ☐ Federal   ☐ State   ☐ Local
Private: → ☒ Private Nonprofit
For-profit: → ☐ General   ☐ Small Business
☐ Woman-owned ☐ Socially and Economically Disadvantaged

11. ENTITY IDENTIFICATION NUMBER
53-0196583
DUNS NO. 04-196-2788   Cong. District DC 001

12. ADMINISTRATIVE OFFICIAL TO BE NOTIFIED IF AWARD IS MADE
Name   Mr. Ralph Albano
Title   Associate Provost for Research
Address   Office of Sponsored Programs & Research Services
620 Michigan Avenue, N.E.
Washington, D.C. 20064
Tel: 202-319-5218   FAX: 202-319-4495
E-Mail: albano@cua.edu

13. OFFICIAL SIGNING FOR APPLICANT ORGANIZATION
Name   Mr. Ralph Albano
Title   Associate Provost for Research
Address   Office of Sponsored Programs & Research Services   620 Michigan Avenue, N.E.
Washington, D.C. 20064
Tel: 202-319-5218   FAX: 202-319-4495
E-Mail: albano@cua.edu

14. APPLICANT ORGANIZATION CERTIFICATION AND ACCEPTANCE: I certify that the statements herein are true, complete and accurate to the best of my knowledge, and accept the obligation to comply with Public Health Services terms and conditions if a grant is awarded as a result of this application. I am aware that any false, fictitious, or fraudulent statements or claims may subject me to criminal, civil, or administrative penalties.

SIGNATURE OF OFFICIAL NAMED IN 13.
(In ink. "Per" signature not acceptable.)

DATE

Reprinted with permission of the author.

Program Director/Principal Investigator (Last, First, Middle): Agazio, Janice Blair LTC (Ret), AN

PROJECT SUMMARY (See instructions):

      The purpose of this study is to describe the perceptions of military mothers regarding separation from their children over the trajectory of the deployment experience during wartime. this study will answer the following research questions: a) What is the process of managing a deployment for military mothers and their children? b) How do military mothers describe the effects of a deployment upon themselves and their children? c) How do military mothers prepare themselves and their children for deployment? d) How do military mothers manage the separation from their children during deployment? e) How do military mothers manage their relationship with their children during and following deployment? and f) What strategies were effective in maintaining relationship with children during deployment? Using a grounded theory design, approximately 35-40 active duty and reserve component women with children who have been deployed to Iraq or Afghanistan will participate in an interview structured around the stages of deployment to explore the process of maintaining relationships. Interviews will be transcribed verbatim and the constant comparative method will be used to analyze the data in order to identify core processes through a combination of open, axial, and selective coding in order to construct a theoretical model of their deployment separation. Participants will be recruited from clinics at two military medical centers and through media such as military publications, websites, and post newspapers. Theoretical sampling will allow saturation of the data to build substantive theory along with identifying concrete, helpful strategies proven to be useful in helping mothers maintain relationship with their children during the separation, and hopefully reducing the stress of the experience for both military mother and their children.

RELEVANCE (See instructions):

Research has mainly focused upon father separations during wartime. This study will fill a gap in increasing understanding of mother separation in wartime deployments. The findings will identify strategies military women to use before and during wartime deployments; provide evidence based indications for policy development; and guide support networks working with families and children.

PROJECT/PERFORMANCE SITE(S) (if additional space is needed, use Project/Performance Site Format Page)

Project/Performance Site Primary Location

Organizational Name: The Catholic University of America

DUNS:

Street 1: 620 Michigan Ave NE		Street 2:		
City: Washington	County:		State: DC	
Province:	Country: USA		Zip/Postal Code: 20064	

Project/Performance Site Congressional Districts: DC 001

Additional Project/Performance Site Location

Organizational Name: Walter Reed Army Medical Center

DUNS:

Street 1: 6900 Georgia Ave NE		Street 2:		
City: Washington	County:		State: DC	
Province:	Country: USA		Zip/Postal Code: 20307	

Project/Performance Site Congressional Districts:

PHS 398 (Rev. 11/07) Page 2 Form Page 2

Program Director/Principal Investigator (Last, First, Middle): Agazio, Janice Blair LTC (Ret), AN

Use only if additional space is needed to list additional project/performance sites.

Additional Project/Performance Site Location

Organizational Name: Womack Army Medical Center

DUNS:

Street 1:	Street 2:	
City: Ft Bragg	County:	State: NC
Province:	Country: USA	Zip/Postal Code: 28310

Project/Performance Site Congressional Districts:

Additional Project/Performance Site Location

Organizational Name: DiLorenzo Tri-Care Health Clinic

DUNS:

Street 1: 5811 Army Pentagon Room MG914A.5	Street 2:	
City: Washington	County:	State: DC
Province:	Country:	Zip/Postal Code: 20310-5801

Project/Performance Site Congressional Districts:

Additional Project/Performance Site Location

Organizational Name:

DUNS:

Street 1:	Street 2:	
City:	County:	State:
Province:	Country:	Zip/Postal Code:

Project/Performance Site Congressional Districts:

Additional Project/Performance Site Location

Organizational Name:

DUNS:

Street 1:	Street 2:	
City:	County:	State:
Province:	Country:	Zip/Postal Code:

Project/Performance Site Congressional Districts:

Additional Project/Performance Site Location

Organizational Name:

DUNS:

Street 1:	Street 2:	
City:	County:	State:
Province:	Country:	Zip/Postal Code:

Project/Performance Site Congressional Districts:

Program Director/Principal Investigator (Last, First, Middle): Agazio, Janice Blair LTC (Ret), AN

SENIOR/KEY PERSONNEL. See instructions. *Use continuation pages as needed* to provide the required information in the format shown below.
Start with Program Director(s)/Principal Investigator(s). List all other senior/key personnel in alphabetical order, last name first.

Name	eRA Commons User Name	Organization	Role on Project
Agazio, Janice	AGAZIOJ	The Catholic University of America	Principal Investigator
O'Brien, Mary Elizabeth		The Catholic Univerisity of America	Associate Investigator
Padden, Diane		Uniformed Services University	Associate Investigator
Ricciardi, Richard		Walter Reed Army Medical Center	Associate Investigator

OTHER SIGNIFICANT CONTRIBUTORS
Name	Organization	Role on Project

Human Embryonic Stem Cells ☐ No ☐ Yes

If the proposed project involves human embryonic stem cells, list below the registration number of the specific cell line(s) from the following list:
http://stemcells.nih.gov/research/registry/. *Use continuation pages as needed.*

If a specific line cannot be referenced at this time, include a statement that one from the Registry will be used.

Cell Line

Form Page 2-continued
Number the *following* pages consecutively throughout
the application. Do not use suffixes such as 4a, 4b.

The name of the program director/principal investigator must be provided at the top of each printed page and each continuation page.

RESEARCH GRANT
TABLE OF CONTENTS

Appendix *(Five identical CDs.)*

☒ Check if
Appendix is
Included

A. Timeline; p.68
B. Invitational letter: p.69
C. Draft of consent form: p. 70
D. Focused interview guide: p.74
E. Demographic data form: p.75
F. Instructional letter for mailed packets: p.77
G. Draft advertisement: p. 78
H. Letters of support: p.79

Program Director/Principal Investigator (Last, First, Middle): Agazio, Janice Blair LTC (Ret), AN

DETAILED BUDGET FOR INITIAL BUDGET PERIOD DIRECT COSTS ONLY				FROM 9/1/09		THROUGH 8/31/10		

PERSONNEL (Applicant organization only)		Months Devoted to Project				DOLLAR AMOUNT REQUESTED (omit cents)		
NAME	ROLE ON PROJECT	Cal. Mnths	Acad. Mnths	Summer Mnths	INST.BASE SALARY	SALARY REQUESTED	FRINGE BENEFITS	TOTAL
Agazio, Janice	PD/PI		8.5	3	63,646	20,950	4714	25,664
O'Brien, Mary Elizabeth	Associate Investigator		8.5	3	0	0	0	0
Padden, Diane	Associate Investigator	11.5			WOC	WOC	WOC	WOC
Ricciardi, Richard	Associate Investigator	11.5			WOC	WOC	WOC	WOC
TBD	RA	8.5			18,000	18,000	1377	19,377
SUBTOTALS ⟶						38950	6091	45041

CONSULTANT COSTS	
	0

EQUIPMENT (Itemize)	
	0

SUPPLIES (Itemize by category)
General office supplies $500; paper $80; tapes & batteries $75;print toner $130; promotional materials for recruitment $200; envelopes for mailing recruitment materials $50 ;upgrade to NVIVO 8 software $300; storage hard disk $100; Flash drives $64,digital tape recorder $130; locking file cabinet $100

	1729

TRAVEL
Travel to Ft Bragg for recruitment and data collection $1600

	1600

PATIENT CARE COSTS	INPATIENT	
	OUTPATIENT	

ALTERATIONS AND RENOVATIONS (Itemize by category)

OTHER EXPENSES (Itemize by category)
Phone cards for interviews $120: Transcription cost for interviews $7600; Courier for tape transcription $400; Recruitment materials mailing $50; advertisements $1417; pens with logo $300.

	9887

CONSORTIUM/CONTRACTUAL COSTS	DIRECT COSTS	

SUBTOTAL DIRECT COSTS FOR INITIAL BUDGET PERIOD (Item 7a, Face Page)	$	58257

CONSORTIUM/CONTRACTUAL COSTS	FACILITIES AND ADMINISTRATIVE COSTS

TOTAL DIRECT COSTS FOR INITIAL BUDGET PERIOD	$	58257

BUDGET FOR ENTIRE PROPOSED PROJECT PERIOD
DIRECT COSTS ONLY

BUDGET CATEGORY TOTALS		INITIAL BUDGET PERIOD *(from Form Page 4)*	ADDITIONAL YEARS OF SUPPORT REQUESTED			
			2nd	3rd	4th	5th
PERSONNEL: *Salary and fringe benefits. Applicant organization only.*		45241	11337			
CONSULTANT COSTS						
EQUIPMENT						
SUPPLIES		1729	580			
TRAVEL		1600	1500			
PATIENT CARE COSTS	INPATIENT					
	OUTPATIENT					
ALTERATIONS AND RENOVATIONS						
OTHER EXPENSES		9887				
CONSORTIUM/ CONTRACTUAL COSTS	DIRECT					
SUBTOTAL DIRECT COSTS *(Sum = Item 8a, Face Page)*		58257	13417			
CONSORTIUM/ CONTRACTUAL COSTS	F&A					
TOTAL DIRECT COSTS		58257	13417			

TOTAL DIRECT COSTS FOR ENTIRE PROPOSED PROJECT PERIOD	$ 71,674

JUSTIFICATION. Follow the budget justification instructions exactly. Use continuation pages as needed.

See separate document

Section 1. Budget Justification

Principal Investigator: LTC (Ret) Janice Agazio is currently an Assistant Professor in the School of Nursing at the Catholic University of America since 2004 having previously taught in the Department of Nursing Research at the Uniformed Services University of the Health Sciences for four years. She retired from active duty in 2000 after 22 years of active duty service in the Army Nurse Corps. Her program of research includes content and methods reflective of the current proposal. She builds upon previous research completed as regarding Nursing during Wartime and OOTW and health promotion in Military women. Beginning with her thesis focus on Korean American families and dissertation on the effect of termination of home care on families, her research reflects an ongoing interest in military families, military women, and military mothers. Her interest in military readiness and deployment is evidenced in her project on the use of virtual reality in readiness training; COL Jan Harris' study of ethical issues in Army nursing; COL Gurney's study of adaptation to combat; MAJ Lasome's project on computer mediated communication in military nursing management; and the most recent project on nursing in wartime and OOTW. She has experience in grounded theory methods and is comfortable in using NVIVO for qualitative data management and has used the program for multiple studies. LTC (Ret) Agazio's responsibilities on this grant will include hands-on project management, recruitment, data collection, data management and analysis, writing the grant, mentorship, supervising personnel, budgetary management, and writing reports and manuscripts. The PI will be responsible for the budgetary oversight, all delieverables, and for maintaining security for data and consent forms. During the academic year, Dr. Agazio will be costed at 20% effort over 8.5 months and during the summer her effort will increase to 75% effort for 3 months. The second year of the study, 6 months are planned at 20% effort. Salary is calculated based upon her CUA salary (8.5 month contract) plus 22.5% fringe rate. The second year reflects a 3% increase in salary per CUA merit increase guidelines.

    Associate Investigator: Dr. Mary Elizabeth O'Brien, Ordinary Professor, School of Nursing, at the Catholic University of America brings a wealth of qualitative methods and grounded theory experience to the project to provide oversight and guidance with grounded theory methods and analysis. She has completed numerous projects using the grounded theory method to include studies with migrant workers, HIV patients and their families, and most recently in development of her theory of spirituality in illness. She is an expert in grounded theory methods and in use of qualitative data management software. As senior scientist on the team, In addition, she is a retired Naval Reserve officer so has an understanding of military issues. Dr. O'Brien will provide expert review and oversight to insure grounded theory methods are followed meticulously and provide guidance through analysis. Dr. O'Brien will provide consultation time without cost (in kind) at 5% effort over 11 months of the project during the intensive portion of data collection and analysis.

    Associate Investigator: Dr. Diane Padden is an Assistant Professor, Chair of the Department of Health, Injury, and Disease Management, and master and doctoral education faculty at the Uniformed Services University of the Health Sciences, Graduate School of Nursing (GSN). As a Certified Registered Nurse Practitioner credentialed at Kimbrough Ambulatory Care Center at Ft. Meade, MD she is acutely aware of the health issues facing both active duty service members as well as military families. She completed her doctoral work in May of 2006 where she studied the effects of perceived stress, coping and health promoting behaviors on general well being in military spouses during deployment separation. Her research interests include stress and coping as well as health promotion and health prevention in primary care. She is a Co-Investigator of a grant entitled "Access to Care and Utilization of Clinical Preventive Services in Older Adults" and previously on a grant entitled "Identification and Description of Clinical Databases". Bringing a background in descriptive qualitative methods, she will be mentored in grounded theory methods and the use of the NVIVO program on the project and will participate in recruitment, data collection, data analysis, and theory construction. Dr. Padden will devote 10% effort over the 18 months of the project and is without cost as a federal employee.

Associate Investigator: Richard Ricciardi, COL, AN serves as Chief, Nursing Research Service at Walter Reed Army Medical Center after completing his PhD at Uniformed Services University in 2006. His dissertation research project "The Impact of Body Armor on Physical Work Performance" was funded through the Triservice Nursing Research program. COL Ricciardi brings a myriad of readiness and deployment experience to contribute to the project and will be heavily relied upon for data interpretation. He was deployed to Bosnia as head nurse/advance practice nurse of emergency treatment section in the 21st Combat Support Hospital from Oct 1996-May 1997 and served as Head Nurse of Emergency Medical Treatment Section of 21st CSH for 2 years. Also, he participated in multiple field assignments while in Germany June 1991-June 1994. With his previous research focus upon physiological measurement, the mentorship provided in this project will expand his research "toolkit" to include qualitative analysis. In addition, Colonel Ricciardi is an Adjunct Associate Professor at the Uniformed Services University and serves as an associate investigator on a TSNRP funded qualitative study (PI CAPT Patricia Kelley) entitled "Clinical Knowledge Development: Continuity of Care for War Injured Service Members." He will serve as site PI at Walter Reed Army Medical Center and act as liasion to the Pentagon Health Clinic. He will be mentored in grounded theory methods and the use of the NVIVO program on the project. He will also be actively involved in recruitment, data collection, data analysis, and theory development. COL Ricciardi will devote 10% of his time over the 18 months dedicated to the project and is without cost as a federal employee. COL Ricciardi is stabilized until his retirement in 2010. MAJ Meryia Throop will be reporting to Walter Reed in the Nursing Research Service upon completion of her doctoral program at CUA in fall 2010 and, with TSNRP and IRB approval through an addendum, assume the co-investigator and site PI position on the project.

Research Assistant

One research assistant is requested in support of this project. Priority will be given to military nurses and graduate students who are currently attending CUA. Reserve nurses could accept a stipend and any student hired into the position would also be given tuition remission in exchange for 20 hours per week on the project during the academic year. The RA would assist with dissemination of recruitment and survey materials; data checking; formatting of qualitative data for entry into NVIVO; participate in analysis of data; updating of study records; preparation of reports and manuscripts; transcription rechecking; and code entry into NVIVO. Base salary will be costed at $18,000 at 20 hours per week for the 8.5 month academic year; fringe benefits are costed at 7.65% of salary. They will only work the first year of the study.

Equipment: None requested

Supplies

Pricing is based on www.staples.com accessed February 2009. The team requests a backup mini 250GB Maxor hard drive ($100) and a 2GB flash drive for each team member to store the data sets and qualitative data ($64 each × 4).

Audiotapes for interviews will be needed ($10 for 9 pk × 50 tapes). Extra batteries will also be needed for the tape recorders ($25). One digital tape recorder ($129.99) in the first year (one micocassette recorder was purchased the PI's previous project and is available to support this project). Would request an upgrade to NVIVO 8 from existing NVIVO 2 software ($300). NVIVO 8 allows better visualization of coding stripes; compound queries of the data; and advanced find features that will facilitate qualitative analysis. SPSS is already available on the existing laptop computer and available through the university for descriptive data analysis.

General office supplies required annually include paper ($80) and file folders, highlighters, and other general supplies will also be required ($500 in the first year; $500 in the second year). Promotional materials (flyers, brochures, plastic holders) will be needed in the first year to advertise the study in units and medical facilities ($200). Envelopes will be needed for distribution and receipt of the promotional materials ($50). Extra print toner will be needed to support the study ($130 each year). A locking file cabinet is requested to secure data and project files ($100).

Travel: Two trips to Ft Bragg are planned for the PI over the course of the study. Once to advertise and recruit participants; and once for in-person interviews during data collection. Mileage is costed at $.55 (GSA FY09) per mile for a round trip distance of 726 miles ($399 each trip): per diem for lodging and meals is costed at $134 per the 2009 GSA rates for a 3 day stay each visit ($402 × 2 = $804). The total cost for each trip will be $ 800.

Travel is also budgeted at $1500 to cover air, per diem, and registration for PI to present the study results at professional conference to be determined during the second year.

Other: Promotional materials will be mailed out to medical facilities ($50) in advance of the recruitment visits. Interviews will be conducted by phone for those not currently stationed in the local area. Two 600 minute phone cards should be sufficient to conduct the interviews and cover phone contacts to research sites during the study ($60 each × 2 = $120 first year only). As a token of thanks, a pen embossed with the study logo and used for completing the consent and demographic sheet, will be presented as a token gift of thanks for participating in the study (Office Depot, $300)

Transcription of audiotapes and team meetings will be sent out to the Carol J Thomas Stenotype Services in Fairfax, Virginia (or comparable agency). The PI has used this service for five previous studies and they have always provided accurate written transcripts of the tapes within a two week time period. Along with the returned interview tapes, the service also provides a printed copy of the transcript and file copy on disk that facilitates entry into QSR NVIVO software. Transcription is priced at $3.50 per page with an estimation of 40 pages of transcript per hour. A 60–90 min interview would be approximately 40–60 pages of transcription for a cost of $ 140-210 per interview. Estimating 40 interviews at an average cost of $190 would total a maximum of $7600 for interview transcriptions. Tapes would be delivered by courier ($40 for pickup) and the transcripts would be returned by encrypted email for fast turn around to be available to analysis (constant comparison). To ensure timely transcription we would estimate 10 courier trips ($100) with the remainder of tapes delivered and/or picked up by a member of the research team.

Recruitment ads will be placed in post newspapers at Womack (The Parachute) and Walter Reed (The Stripe). Additionally, an ad will be placed on a periodic basis in more widely read publications, The Army Times, The Navy Times, Marine Corps Times, and The Air Force Times. A classified advertisement is $26.10 per line. A line is approx. 20 characters including spaces. The proposed ad will be approximately 18 lines at $472 per ad. The ad would run in all Military Times publications for the week of issue. (Personal communication, Jeanette Chandler, Senior Advertising Sales Executive, Army Times Publishing Co). Would request placement of ads 3 times across the length of the recruitment period ($1417). Other ads may be placed in military family or other military organization websites with permission and only if at no cost.

Program Director/Principal Investigator (Last, First, Middle):   Agazio, Janice Blair LTC (Ret), AN

RESOURCES

FACILITIES: Specify the facilities to be used for the conduct of the proposed research. Indicate the project/performance sites and describe capacities, pertinent capabilities, relative proximity, and extent of availability to the project. If research involving Select Agent(s) will occur at any performance site(s), the biocontainment resources available at each site should be described. Under "Other," identify support services such as machine shop, electronics shop, and specify the extent to which they will be available to the project. Use continuation pages if necessary.

Laboratory:

Clinical:

Animal:

Computer:
Toshiba laptop purchased on previous TSNRP grant is available to support this project. It has Microsoft Office, NVIVO, and SPSS installed and is equipped with wireless Internet access for communication with research team. HP laser printer (TSNRP grant) will support the printing needs of the project.

Office:
Office, desk, chair, telephones, electronic mail, conference table, fax machine, and copier are available in the College of Nursing and are sufficient to support the project.

Other:

MAJOR EQUIPMENT: List the most important equipment items already available for this project, noting the location and pertinent capabilities of each.
Toshiba laptop and Hewlitt Packard printer located in College of Nursing. Both items previously purchased in support of TSNRP project. File cabinet also available to secure data.

The Catholic University of America

The Catholic University of America, situated on 144 landscaped acres in Washington, D.C., offers a traditional, medium-size college campus, the resources of a major research university and the excitement of the nation's capital. Founded by the U.S. Catholic Bishops in 1887, CUA is the national university of the Catholic Church. It is accredited by the Middle States Association of Colleges and Schools and is a founding member of the Association of American Universities. The university emphasizes Catholic values and intellectual development and welcomes students from all religious traditions. Students from every state and more than 100 countries come to CUA to pursue higher education and to take advantage of the resources of the Washington, D.C., area. CUA has its own university press. Among the journals it publishes are *Anthropological Quarterly* and *The Catholic Historical Review*. Among other works published or edited on campus are *Review of Religious Research, Law and Policy, The New Catholic Encyclopedia* and *The Journal of Chinese Philosophy*. CUA hosts a number of research centers and facilities. Among them are the Center for Advanced Training in Cell and Molecular Biology, the Center for Irish Studies, the Institute for Communications Law Studies and the Institute for Social Justice.

The School of Nursing, established in 1932, has long provided outstanding nursing education that clearly emphasizes the role of ethics, values and spirituality in health care. The School of Nursing offers undergraduate, graduate master's and doctoral programs. Students in CUA's nursing programs gain clinical experience in 100 of the Washington Metropolitan area's premier health care facilities often with alumni preceptors. Our research-intensive doctoral program is located within easy access of premier research and health facilities, including the National Institutes of Health and the Institute of Medicine. The SON is housed in Gowan Hall and in part of the adjacent Nursing-Biology wing. The Office of the Dean, the offices of the two Associate Deans, and the offices of their support staffs are located on the first floor of Gowan Hall. This floor also provides space for the following services: Gowan Auditorium (capacity 279), a faculty conference room, copying room, a file and records room, and the newly renovated Donley Technology Center. The second floor of Gowan contains the first level of the Nursing-Biology Library and faculty offices. Portable AV equipment is available for checkout from the Donley center. This includes 5 laptops and LCD projectors; plus video and DVD players. Classrooms are equipped with desks, blackboards, and projection screens. Conference/seminar rooms have tables, chairs, blackboards, and projection screens. Currently all faculty have private offices equipped with computers, telephones, internet connections and private printers. The Copier room contains a FAX machine, and a copier. A scanner and Scantron are available to faculty for transferring documents and for scoring tests. Offices are available for teaching and research assistants.

Information Technology

The Center for Planning and Information Technology (CPIT) provides computing and network facilities to students and faculty for their educational and research activities, supports the university's management information systems, manages the campus network and provides telecommunication services and leadership on the ethical use of computing. Numerous public lab areas and classrooms are equipped with networked desktop computers. All residence hall rooms have network connections via a gigabit Ethernet campus backbone. The center supports Internet tools such as World Wide Web browsers and electronic mail. Numerous Web tools are also available for instructional and research purposes. Popular software programs for Windows and Macintosh are supported in the public users' areas.The campus network consists of Sun and Intel servers running Solaris, Windows and Linux operating systems, numerous workstations and more than 2,000 networked Windows-based PCs and Macintosh desktop computers with direct access to the Internet, Internet2 and the Washington Research Library Consortium. The central systems are accessible via direct connections on campus and via the Web. CPIT has a wide range of technology resources available for faculty and students to enhance the pedagogical environment.

In the School of Nursing, the Donley Technology Center houses twelve computers for student use and connected to the university's fiber optic network. The center is located on the first floor of Gowan Hall across the hall from the PI"s office. The school employs a full time lab director with a master's degree in Computer Systems Management, Alice Myers, who is responsible for maintaining the computers in the lab, other computers throughout the SON, and the audiovisual equipment in the school. The director is also the SON liaison with CPIT and is responsible for maintaining the schools website and providing instruction in computers and computer-related matters to faculty and students. In the SON and Donley Center, all the network-connected computers run Windows XP. General purpose software available to students and faculty include the Microsoft Office 2003 suite (Access, Word, Powerpoint, Excel, and Publisher), SPSS, Internet Explorer, email, Mozilla Firefox and Netscape Navigator.

Library Services

The library system of CUA offers academic resources and services to support student, faculty and staff research. The John K. Mullen of Denver Memorial Library is the main campus library and maintains collections in the humanities, social sciences, library science, chemistry, religious studies, philosophy, and canon law. Altogether, the CUA library systems own about 2,3 million items. The special libraries include: Engineering/Architecture/Mathematics, Music, Nursing/Biology, and Physics. There are also two separately administered libraries: the Oliveira Lima Library and the Judge Kathryn J. DuFour Law Library. Students and faculty have on-campus and remote access to ALADIN as a benefit of CUA's membership in the Washington Research Library Consortium. ALADIN includes the online library catalog for CUA and seven local universities, full-text electronic journals, article databases and digitized special collections of photographs and other research materials. CUA students and faculty may borrow books and photocopy articles when visiting the consortium libraries, all located in the D.C. metropolitan area, or may request through ALADIN that items be delivered. Assistance with research is available by e-mail and phone, in person at the information/reference desks in Mullen Library and the campus libraries, through the "IM@theLibrary" instant messaging service and as part of the library instruction program. In addition, there is convenient access to the library resources of the Washington metropolitan area. These include the Library of Congress, the National Library of Medicine, and the National Institutes of Health.

The Nursing-Biology Library occupies one full wing (2 floors) on the second and third floor of the SON building, Gowan Hall. The library is a satellite of the main library located in the Mullen building and is a member of the Washington research consortium. It is generally open 73 hours per week during the regular semesters. The Nursing-Biology Library currently has on site about 34,000 items, approximately two-thirds of the space and collection is designated for the nursing portion of the library. The library subscribes to about 320 print journals and has access to about 450 electronic journals, which include most of those nursing journals published in the English language, as well as selected medical and biological journals. Online access is available via Aladin to CINAHL, Medline, Health and Psychosocial Instruments (HAPI), Eric, PsychInfo, Journals@Ovid, the Cochrane Library for Evidence Based Practice, and other databases. Internet access is available on four public terminals in the library.

Walter Reed Army Medical Center

Walter Reed Army Medical Center (WRAMC) is a 350 bed tertiary care medical facility located in Washington, DC serving active and retired military beneficiaries as well as Congressionally-designated beneficiaries. It is the US Army's leading center of support to meet three critical goals-to provide the best in patient care, to encourage the education and training of tomorrow's health professionals, and to expand the field of healthcare knowledge through research. WRAMC features acute and intensive care beds and 16 operating rooms. It admits 25,000 patients annually and sees 540,000 as outpatients. Approximately 430 physicians in 50 specialties and subspecialties (including obstetrics and neonatology) train there as well as 12 dental residents in selected specialties.

The **Nursing Research Service (NRS)** provides a superb environment for research and scholarly interchange. Staffed usually by 2-3 doctorally-prepared nurse researchers, it serves as a bustling nerve center for a variety of active and ongoing studies as well as other research. Because WRAMC is a state-of-the-art facility in education and research it's expansive medical library maintains most leading journals both clinical and research as well as remote access to Medline, Grateful Med and multiple other medical literature databases. The Department of Clinical Investigation (DCI) assures research meets scientific and human subjects requirements and oversees 20 research laboratories. It provides multiple PC terminals in a computer center able to handle small to moderate-sized data sets. DCI's staff biostatistician is available for statistical consultation on approved protocols. The NRS fosters an open atmosphere of formal and informal consultation based upon their methodological, theoretical, and clinical strengths. The office is equipped with a personal desktop computer for each researcher and the department's editorial assistant.

Womack Army Medical Center

According to the Womack Army Medical Center website (http://www.wamc.amedd. army.mil/), "The Mission of Womack Army Medical Center is to provide the highest quality healthcare, maximize the medical deployability of the force, ensure the readiness of Womack Personnel, and sustain exceptional education and training programs. The site is a 163-acre wooded site north of Albritton Junior High School bordered by Normandy Drive to the south, Longstreet Road to the north, Reilly Road to the east and the All American Expressway to the west. The new health care complex has increased quality care and access to beneficiaries by bringing more medical and specialized resources to Fort Bragg. Some of the specialties added since the current facility became a medical center include cardiology, hematology-oncology and pulmonology. The Army Medical Department is committed to providing quality, cost-efficient care for "The Total Army Family." Womack Army Medical Center is proud to serve the more than 160,000 eligible beneficiaries in the region, the largest beneficiary population in the Army. This facility has three connecting buildings. Building "A" is the clinic mall area at the All American Expressway entrance and it houses the outpatient clinics. Building "B", which is the building in the middle, houses most of our ancillary clinics and departments. Building "C", the inpatient tower, is located at the Reilly Road entrance. The inpatient tower is seven floors with an interstitial space between each floor that allows computer, equipment, plumbing etc... to be repaired without interrupting patient care. The new Womack is 1,020,359 square feet."

DiLorenzo Tricare Health Clinic

The DiLorenzo Tricare Health Clinic is located in side the north face of the Pentagon offering on-site care to eligible beneficiaries and their dependents stationed at the Pentagon. The population served is multi-service. Their mission, according to their website (http://www.tricare.mil/MTF/facility.aspx?fid=3) is to "provide compassionate, quality outpatient and preventive medical care to our beneficiaries and first echelon emergency medical support at this national landmark while promoting the personal and professional readiness of the DiLorenzo Tricare Health Team."

Program Director/Principal Investigator (Last, First, Middle): **Agazio, Janice Blair**

CHECKLIST

TYPE OF APPLICATION *(Check all that apply.)*

☒ NEW application. *(This application is being submitted to the PHS for the first time.)*

☐ RESUBMISSION of application number: _____
(This application replaces a prior unfunded version of a new, renewal, or revision application.)

☐ RENEWAL of grant number: _____
(This application is to extend a funded grant beyond its current project period.)

☐ REVISION to grant number: _____
(This application is for additional funds to supplement a currently funded grant.)

☐ CHANGE of program director/principal investigator.

Name of former program director/principal investigator: _____

☐ CHANGE of Grantee Institution.   Name of former institution: _____

☐ FOREIGN application   ☐ Domestic Grant with foreign involvement   List Country(ies) Involved: _____

INVENTIONS AND PATENTS *(Renewal appl. only)*   ☐ No   ☐ Yes

If "Yes,"   ☐ Previously reported   ☐ Not previously reported

1. PROGRAM INCOME (See instructions.)
All applications must indicate whether program income is anticipated during the period(s) for which grant support is request. If program income is anticipated, use the format below to reflect the amount and source(s).

Budget Period	Anticipated Amount	Source(s)
none		

2. ASSURANCES/CERTIFICATIONS (See instructions.)
In signing the application Face Page, the authorized organizational representative agrees to comply with the policies, assurances and/or certifications listed in the application instructions when applicable. Descriptions of individual assurances/certifications are provided in Part III and listed in Part I, 4.1 under Item 14. If unable to certify compliance, where applicable, provide an explanation and place it after this page.

3. FACILITIES AND ADMINSTRATIVE COSTS (F&A)/ INDIRECT COSTS. See specific instructions.

☒ DHHS Agreement dated: **6-5-2005**   ☐ No Facilities And Administrative Costs Requested.

☐ DHHS Agreement being negotiated with _____ Regional Office.

☐ No DHHS Agreement, but rate established with _____ Date _____

CALCULATION* *(The entire grant application, including the Checklist, will be reproduced and provided to peer reviewers as confidential information.)*

a. Initial budget period:	Amount of base $	38,950	x Rate applied	64.6	% = F&A costs	$	25,162
b. 02 year	Amount of base $	9255	x Rate applied	64.6	% = F&A costs	$	5978
c. 03 year	Amount of base $		x Rate applied		% = F&A costs	$	
d. 04 year	Amount of base $		x Rate applied		% = F&A costs	$	
e. 05 year	Amount of base $		x Rate applied		% = F&A costs	$	

TOTAL F&A Costs $ **31,141**

*Check appropriate box(es):

☒ Salary and wages base   ☐ Modified total direct cost base   ☐ Other base *(Explain)*

☐ Off-site, other special rate, or more than one rate involved *(Explain)*

Explanation *(Attach separate sheet, if necessary.)*:

4. DISCLOSURE PERMISSION STATEMENT: If this application does not result in an award, is the Government permitted to disclose the title of your proposed project, and the name, address, telephone number and e-mail address of the official signing for the applicant organization, to organizations that may be interested in contacting you for further information (e.g., possible collaborations, investment)?   ☐ Yes   ☐ No

Program Director/Principal Investigator (Last, First, Middle):   Agazio, Janice Blair

Place this form at the end of the signed original copy of the application.
Do <u>not</u> duplicate.

PERSONAL DATA ON
PROGRAM DIRECTOR(S)/PRINCIPAL INVESTIGATOR(S)

The Public Health Service has a continuing commitment to monitor the operation of its review and award processes to detect—and deal appropriately with—any instances of real or apparent inequities with respect to age, sex, race, or ethnicity of the proposed program director(s)/principal investigator(s).

To provide the PHS with the information it needs for this important task, complete the form below and attach it to the signed original of the application after the Checklist. When multiple PDs/PIs are proposed, complete a form for each. **Do not attach copies of this form to the duplicated copies of the application.**

Upon receipt of the application by the PHS, this form will be separated from the application. This form will **not** be duplicated, and it will **not** be a part of the review process. Data will be confidential, and will be maintained in Privacy Act record system 09-25-0036, "Grants: IMPAC (Grant/Contract Information)." The PHS requests the last four digits of the Social Security Number for accurate identification, referral, and review of applications and for management of PHS grant programs. Although the provision of this portion of the Social Security Number is voluntary, providing this information may improve both the accuracy and speed of processing the application. Please be aware that no individual will be denied any right, benefit, or privilege provided by law because of refusal to disclose this section of the Social Security Number. The PHS requests the last four digits of the Social Security Number under Sections 301(a) and 487 of the PHS Acts as amended (42 U.S.C 241a and U.S.C. 288). All analyses conducted on the date of birth, gender, race and/or ethnic origin data will report aggregate statistical findings only and will not identify individuals. If you decline to provide this information, it will in no way affect consideration of your application. Your cooperation will be appreciated.

DATE OF BIRTH (*MM/DD/YY*) 07/11/56	SEX/GENDER
SOCIAL SECURITY NUMBER (last 4 digits only) XXX-XX- 9333	☒ Female ☐ Male

ETHNICITY
1. Do you consider yourself to be Hispanic or Latino? (See definition below.) Select one.

> *Hispanic or Latino.* A person of Mexican, Puerto Rican, Cuban, South or Central American, or other Spanish culture or origin, regardless of race. The term, "Spanish origin," can be used in addition to "Hispanic or Latino."

☐   **Hispanic or Latino**

☒   **Not Hispanic or Latino**

RACE
2. What race do you consider yourself to be? Select one or more of the following.

☐   *American Indian or Alaska Native.* A person having origins in any of the original peoples of North, Central, **or** South America, and who maintains tribal affiliation or community attachment.

☐   *Asian.* A person having origins in any of the original peoples of the Far East, Southeast Asia, or the Indian **subcontinent**, including, for example, Cambodia, China, India, Japan, Korea, Malaysia, Pakistan, the Philippine Islands, Thailand, and Vietnam. (Note: Individuals from the Philippine Islands have been recorded as Pacific Islanders in previous data collection strategies.)

☐   *Black or African American.* A person having origins in any of the black racial groups of Africa. Terms such as "Haitian" or "Negro" can be used in addition to "Black" or African American."

☐   *Native Hawaiian or Other Pacific Islander.* A person having origins in any of the original peoples of Hawaii, Guam, Samoa, or **other** Pacific Islands.

☒   *White.* A **person** having origins in any of the original peoples of Europe, the Middle East, or North Africa.

☐   Check here if you do not wish to provide some or all of the above information.

PHS 398 (Rev. 11/07)   DO NOT PAGE NUMBER THIS FORM   **Personal Data Form Page**

Section 2. Specific Aims

According to the U.S. Census Bureau, in September, 2007, there were 198,400 active duty women in the military (http://www.infoplease.com/spot/womencensus1.html). This number represents 15% of the total Armed Forces. Fifteen percent of the total number of officers are women (33,500) and 15% of the enlisted corps (164,900). Women represent approximately 21% of the reserve component with 78,339 serving as officers or in the enlisted corps (http://www.womensmemorial.org/PDFs/StatsonWIM.pdf). In addition, there are 63,831 women in the National Guard representing 14.3% of the total National Guard Forces. About half of the active duty women are married and out of that total 22% are married to other active duty service members and 22.8% of those in the Reserve component are married to other reservists. On the active duty side, 22,745 women are single mothers while a similar number of reservists are also single parents (22,595). (DOD, 2006). The Defense Manpower Center reports that in the four main service branches, as of 2008, there are 70,969 women with children on active duty and 54,611 in the selected reserve (Personal communication, Defense Manpower Data Center, February, 2009). Forty percent of active duty women have children as compared to 44% of the men on active duty (U.S. Senate, Joint Economic Committee, 2007).

With the large mobilization that occurred during Desert Shield/Desert Storm, women in great numbers were included in a mass deployment. According to Pierce, Vinokur, and Burns (1998), a total of 40,793 women served in the Persian Gulf by

Table 1 • The No. of Female Military Members With Children By Service/Component and Year		
Service/Component	*2006*	*2008*
Active Duty		
Army	27,041	29,409
Navy	16,226	15,857
Marine Corps	2,784	3,271
Air Force	23,273	22,432
Coast Guard	1,239	1,398
Total	70,563	72,367
Selected Reserve		
Army National Guard	14,383	16,787
Army Reserve	14,665	16,359
Navy Reserve	6,466	6,104
Marine Corps Reserve	406	422
Air National Guard	7,587	8,184
Air Force Reserve	7,090	6,755
Coast Guard Reserve	298	313
Total	50,895	54,924

the end of the war. Most notably during this period, for the first time, many women with dependent children were included in the deployment (Vogt, Pless, King & King, 2005). While in previous wars, father separations were the predominant model, the Desert Shield/Desert Storm deployment was dubbed by the media as the "Mommy's War". Pierce, Vinokur, and Burns (1998) noted that at least 32% of Air Force women deployed for the Gulf War left dependent children to be cared for at home.

According to a report prepared by the joint Economic Committee by Senator Shumer and Representative Maloney, as of May 11, 2007, 160,500 female soldiers have served in Iraq, Afghanistan, and the Middle East since the start of the "war on terror"; 474 military women have been wounded in Iraq; and 85 female soldiers have died (U.S. Senate, Joint Economic Committee, 2007). Additionally, as noted in the report, "nearly half of all women in [the] active duty force have been deployed to Iraq or Afghanistan, and according to the Department of Defense in February 2007, 24,475 women are currently deployed to Iraq or Afghanistan" (U.S. Senate, Joint Economic Committee, 2007, p. 1).

Women are serving in more dangerous and frequent deployments than ever before. With the repeal of Title 10 U.S.Code, section 6015, women are now assigned to "any combat unit, classes of combat vessels, and combat platforms" (Bunch, Eastman, & Snow, 2007, pg 2). As a result, women represent 1 in 7 total troops assigned in Iraq, with additional women assigned in Afghanistan. With the increased numbers, women, and in particular, military mothers, are not only potentially separated from their children for deployments more often, but also for longer periods and in more dangerous environments. To date, however, research has been deficient in describing the experience of such deployments for military mothers specifically and the effects upon the mothers and their relationship with their children. The purpose of this study is to describe the perceptions of military mothers regarding separation from their children over the trajectory of the wartime deployment experience (preparation through reunion and reintegration).

Employing grounded theory methods, this study will answer the following research questions:

1. What is the process of managing a deployment for military mothers and their children?
2. How do military mothers describe the effects of a deployment upon themselves and their children?
3. How do military mothers prepare themselves and their children for deployment?
4. How do military mothers manage the separation from their children during deployment?
5. How do military mothers manage their relationship with their children during and following deployment?
6. What strategies were effective in maintaining relationship with children during deployment?

Section 3. Background and Significance

Separation as a cause for family reorganization has most often been studied in relation to wartime or deployment for military duties. These have primarily considered father separations from the family and the effects upon the remaining non-military spouse (Black, 1993; Knapp & Newman, 1993; Rosen, Teitelbaum, & Westhuis, 1994) and children (Amen, Jellen, Merves, & Lee, 1988; Rosen, Teitelbaum, & Westhuis, 1993; Yeatman, 1981). More recently however, in conjunction with Operation Desert Storm/Desert Shield, studies have considered the effects of mother separations upon children (Birgenheier, 1993).

Literature review in grounded theory has been debated by its originators, Glaser and Strauss (1967), as well as other grounded theorists, and has most often been advocated to occur following data analysis and development of theory so as not to bias the emergence of the theory from the data. However, realistically, in order to justify the need for the study, a critique of existing literature is presented in order to delineate gaps in knowledge regarding specifically military mothers and strengthen the argument that this project will add to understanding and identify supportive interventions to facilitate positive deployment experiences and separations.

Research has shown that "a soldier's family problems can affect his duty or combat performance, increase his absence without leave (AWOL) risk, and lead to retention difficulties. The well being of the family unit directly impacts upon the soldiers' readiness, retention, and overall effectiveness" (Amen, Jellen, Merves, & Lee, 1988, p. 441). With the increased operation tempo (optempo) over the past years since the beginning of Operation Enduring Freedom in Afghanistan in response to the 2001 9/11 attacks followed by Operation Iraqi Freedom with the invasion of Iraq in 2003, deployments have occurred more frequently and for longer periods of time which have affected both military members and their families (Newby et al, 2005). Newby and others (2005) queried 951 male and female soldiers who had returned from deployments in Bosnia about the positive and negative consequences. Married soldiers most notably mentioned that being away from family and missing family events was the second most frequently mentioned consequence followed by "'deterioration of marital/significant other relationships'" (p. 817). While this study included both single and married men and women, it did not specifically consider military women. It was evident from the findings, however, that deployments can affect family relationships which, in turn, could affect the military member's decision to remain in the service thus impacting retention. Women may feel more pressure in this regard, as noted by Roper (2007), since women are traditionally more often primary caregivers, "factors involved in deploying may impact the mother's decision to stay or leave the military" (p. 38) . She further states that since "studies show that retention of military personnel is vital to maintaining a quality force. . . . [military mothers] must find ways to address the goals of the mission that sometime directly conflict with the needs of her family" (p. 40). Now is a good time to elucidate the process of deployment from the view of military mothers to increase understanding from the maternal perspective thus perhaps affecting policy initiatives to more specifically support the military mothers' deployment and increase retention.

Stages of Family Deployment: Conceptual Orientation

Stages define the process for families preparing for a separation for deployment: preparation, survival, and reunion. Each stage represents different stressors and adjustments for the military member and family members left behind. First described by Logan (1987), and refined by Peebles-Kleiger and Kleiger (1994), and more recently Pincus, House, Cristenson, and Adler (2005) the cycle of deployment incorporates stages modeled upon those of Kubler-Ross of the emotional cycle for families and the military member experiencing deployment. As the family learns of an impending deployment, the first stage, pre-deployment, occurs over a one to two week period marked by tension, protest, and anger. During this stage, preparations are made for deployment; family members feel "on edge" and may exhibit some emotional and physical withdrawal in anticipation of the separation while the service member experiences prolonged absences during the preparation. As departure becomes imminent, the family may experience more Detachment and Withdrawal, as family members feel increasingly frightened by the impending loss of the military member and increased emotional detachment as a protective mechanism. The second stage, Deployment is marked by Emotional Disorganization occurring during the first 6 weeks following departure, and is marked by symptoms of sadness, despair, tension, depression, and sometimes even relief that the deployment has finally occurred after such a busy time of preparation. Wives usually remark upon feeling overwhelmed by having all the responsibility for parenting and household management during this initial adjustment period. As the remaining spouse learns to cope, the third stage, referred to as Sustainment, begins around the first month of the deployment until about a month before redeployment. During the actual deployment families learn how to adjust to the separation and communication lines are established. As the deployment nears an end, the service member and family again experience turmoil in the Redeployment stages marked by Anticipation of Homecoming as activity becomes focused upon reuniting the military member with the family and preparations are focused upon preparing themselves and the home.

The stage of Reunion/post deployment begins upon arrival of the military member home and then up to six weeks following as the family becomes a family again becoming reacquainted with each other, negotiating changes in roles, reestablishing intimacy, and responding to perceived changes in each other over the course of the deployment. Most families, according to Peebles-Kleiger and Kleiger (1994), have stabilized again about 12 weeks out from the deployment. They note that separations under wartime deployments represent more of a stressor and conflict for the families. Stages take much longer to move through and represent more difficult adjustments for family members since danger is more imminent for the military member, less may be known about the environment or circumstances of the deployment, and information about, or communication with the military member may be more difficult. Most of the research upon which the stages are based have been elicited from the heretofore more common deployment of male military members away from their non-military wives and dependent children. However the stages span the trajectory of the experience from notification through return. The stages as proposed by Pincus, House, Cristenson, and Adler (2005) will serve as the conceptual orientation for this study as a framework in which to structure the initial focused interview questions in order to be inclusive of the entire deployment period.

Research on Military Separations

In general most research on military deployment has focused upon normal rotations incurring separations for overseas assignments, peacekeeping operations, and more recently during wartime. Primarily these studies have focused upon the reaction of the military member, in most cases father separations, and effects upon those left behind. For example, Blount, Curry, and Lubin (1992) described the adjustments that are required of the remaining spouse, who has usually been the wife. These include decision making, new responsibilities such as "mechanical repairs, dealing with financial matters, cooking, child care, or housekeeping once done by the deployed spouse . . . [and] may entail learning new skills" (p. 77); changes in relationships with children; and some isolation from support systems. Black (1993) suggests that military families are more vulnerable to crisis as a result of the pile-up of stress inherent in military life. These include "frequent moves, the potential for being deployed into hostile environments, frequent periods of family separation, geographic isolation from extended family support systems, low pay, young age as compared to the general civilian population, and a high incidence of young children living in the home" (p. 273). Knapp and Newman (1993) similarly found a vulnerability to psychological distress associated with separation in military wives who reported an accumulation of stressors.

Of note, most of the research that has looked at families and deployment experiences has used the model of the traditional family. These studies have primarily considered father separations from a nuclear family structure. Mothers stay at home and care for any dependent children. Dual military, maternal separations, and single parent family separations have not been considered in as much detail. Are the stages and adjustments different when the mother is the deployed family member? What happens when single mothers deploy and must leave children with extended family, ex-spouses, or friends?

Other researchers have looked at the stressors experienced by the deployed member in relation to family concerns. For example, Kleigher and Kennedy (1993) documented military parent concerns as they provided support services to Navy staff aboard the USNS Comfort during DS/DS. While the family adjusts at home, they found that deployed parents also have concerns to include how children are functioning at home, school and elsewhere; how the spouse is functioning as single parent; sometimes envy and concern about special relationships developing between children and the at-home parent; and worries of "Will they remember me? Will I recognize them?" (Kleigher & Kennedy, 1993).

In general, research on military women has been more problem focused in nature. In a MEDLINE literature review, search terms of *military women*, *military mothers*, *deployment*, and *war* located research dealing with active duty and reserve component/ National Guard women. The majority of these articles were concerned with military women's reproductive health (Brunader, Brunader, & Kugler, 1991; Guenter & Estela, 1971; Messersmith-Heroman, Heroman, & Moore, 1994;) risk factors such as HIV and sexually transmitted diseases (Gerrard, Gibbons, & Warner, 1991; Nishimoto, 1990); training issues (Allnutt, 1988; Protzman, 1979; Protzman & Griffis, 1977); nutrition and weight control (Bathalon et al, 1995; Friedl et al, 1995; King, Fridlund, & Askew, 1993) health promotion (Agazio Ephraim, Flaherty, & Gurney, 2002); and specific illnesses (Bohan, 1983). There has been limited research published on military mother deployments. Davis and Woods (1999) noted "much work remains in addressing the multitude and variety of military women's needs."

Pierce, Vinokur, and Buck (1998) conducted the most comprehensive study considering the effects of deployment upon mothers and children. They used a quantitative survey design measuring strains in major life domains to include job strain, financial strain, parenting strain, depression, ability to provide for children during deployment, anxiety symptoms, children's adjustment problems and life changes as major variables in the study. The sample included active duty Air Force mothers participating in the study approximately two years after the Gulf War. Mothers reported difficulty providing comprehensive care for their children. Of the children with married mothers, 77% stayed with fathers or stepfathers, 21% stayed with mother's parents or siblings, and 2% stayed with paternal grandparents. For children who stayed with extended family, 67% changed residence at the time of the separation; 73% changed schools, and 7% were separated from one or more siblings. Mothers in the reserves or guard forces and officers reported greater difficulties in finding care for their children during the deployment. Interestingly, the mothers "who had experienced more difficulty in finding care, scored lower in their role and emotional functioning and reported more symptoms of depression and anxiety" two years following the deployment (Pierce & Buck, 1998, p. 3).

Effects of Military Maternal Separation on Children

About 2 million children are living with military families, ether active duty or reserve component (Chartrand & Siegel, 2007). While military children become accustomed to the peacetime routine of frequent moves and temporary absences of parents, less is known about their responses to parental separation during wartime. As noted by Chartrand and Siegel (2007), children may have different experiences depending on whether the parent is active duty or reserve component. Reserve troops are often located in communities outside and away from military bases. These children would remain in a familiar community perhaps closer to extended family and friends. They however may lack support provided on military posts such as family support networks and families may face "pay cuts, job loss, and changes in medical insurance" (p. 2) not experienced by active duty families. Active duty families on the other hand may be stationed far away from family support systems leaving wives (or husbands) feeling isolated and alone during separations. Lincoln, Swift, and Shorteno-Fraser (2008) described the reactions and response to separation based on age and developmental level. They note that infant response is related to the stress and anxiety displayed by the remaining caregivers. The infant may react "by becoming more irritable and unresponsive, vulnerable to sleep disruption, eating problems, and increased periods of crying" (p. 987). Toddlers may display more resistive behaviors and perhaps become more clingy. Preschoolers may regress "to behaviors that they have previously outgrown" (p. 987). School aged children have more awareness of what is happening and the potential danger faced by the deploying parent. Consequently most studies of military children's reaction to deployment has focused upon school aged or older (Huebner et al, 2007; Shamai & Kimhi, 2007).

Related to research with military mothers, Vinokur, and Buck (1998) found that the strongest predictor of adjustment problems for children during a mother deployment was related to the number of life changes experienced as a result of the separation. They noted "children with older mothers and the children who were younger or who had a very young sibling experienced greater adjustment problems than did children of younger mother and children who were older" (p. 1300). Children whose mothers were away longer or stationed in the combat theater demonstrated greater stress. Of note, despite finding war-related behavior problems, two years after the deployment these problems did not predict subsequent behavior problems and the children did not "demonstrate more symptoms of stress than children whose mothers were not deployed" (Pierce & Buck, 1998, p. 3). These findings were similar to those of Kelley and others (2001) who studied children of deployed Navy mothers post-Desert Shield/Desert Storm deployment. They also found younger children more susceptible to depression and sadness as well as more behavior problems in general compared to children whose mothers were not deployed. Despite these findings, in general, "group differences were modest and overall mean scores were in the normal range" (p. 464) indicating no lasting pathology for the children with a deployed mother.

In comparison to other studies of children whose fathers were deployed for war or humanitarian missions, research has shown these experiences pose unique stressors for them and for their families (Amen et al, 1988; Black 1993; Blount, Curry, & Lubin, 1992; Jensen, Martin, & Watanabe, 1996, Zeft, Lewis, & Hirsch, 1997). According to Kelley and others (2001), the degree to which the children experience stress depends upon several factors to include previous experience with separations; the nature of the deployment; the parent's emotional development, satisfaction with the military, and stability of the marriage; and most importantly the developmental level of the child. Interestingly, Jensen, Martin, & Watanabe (1996) found not only younger children experiencing higher depression, but also a marked increase for boys making them especially vulnerable to deployment effects. This study was particularly valuable as the researchers had previously collected data on the children prior to the war's beginning, so they were able to "prospectively evaluate the impact of wartime deployment by comparing follow up ratings" (Cozza, Chun, & Polo, 2005, pg 373). Considering that this study primarily considered the effects of father deployments, would the reverse hold true for children of deployed mothers?

On a more positive note, Ryan-Wenger (2001) demonstrated the resilience of military children in comparison with a group of civilian children. Her findings showed no difference in levels of anxiety or psychopathology when considering the threat of war. Comparably, Applewhite and Mays (1996) demonstrated that psychosocial functioning in military children did not differ based upon maternal or paternal separations. In his study, 55 fathers and 55 mothers completed survey packets to identify predictors of child psychosocial functioning. While the authors noted the contradictory nature of their findings regarding maternal versus paternal separation, the study was limited by a convenience sample dependent on recall of the child's first extended separation. There was also a potential bias in a response rate of 52% as "families whose experiences with separation may be significantly different from those who were included in the study" (p. 36). More recently, Chartrand, Frank, White, and Shope (2008) in their cross-sectional study found "that children aged 3 years or older with a deployed parent exhibit[ed] increased behavioral symptoms compared with peers without a deployed parent after controlling for caregiver's stress and depressive symptoms" (p. 1094). Obviously, contradictory evidence continues to emerge regarding effects of deployment on children.

Of special note in the Gulf War and in the current conflict, military mothers have been deployed shortly after returning from maternity leave or during the first year of their child's life. According to regulation, military mothers could request a 4 month deferment of mobilization following birth of the child, however, anecdotally, in the PI's experience, deferments are not universally granted depending on the mission and unit needs. More recently, deferments have been extended to up to 6 months following birth, however that still means mothers can be separated during the infant's first year of life. Concerns have been raised in the literature regarding the effects of maternal separations from the child upon attachment, a particularly important process during infancy (Schen, 2005). Studies have considered separations as they occur for maternal incarceration; mothers leaving children in home countries to immigrate for work or education; homelessness; hospitalization for mental illness; and during evacuation in war-torn areas. Some of this literature may be applied in theory to processes that may be operative for military maternal separations. Studies have also focused primarily upon school aged children and adolescents in military related research, and less often on younger children (Huebner, Mancini, Wilcox, Grass, & Grass, 2007), so that in this project, the focus will be upon school-aged or younger children. In families with multiple children, as in the study by Kelley and others (2001;2002), mothers will be asked to comment especially about the youngest child or children in responding to interview questions.

For example, a recent dissertation considered communication between parents and children before, during, and after a parental absence for 2 months or longer. Pollom (2005) compared absences due to incarceration or deployment. While only 9 of the 54 participants included distal mothers and stay at home fathers, Pollom noted that in particular, more research was indicated to focus upon maternal absence. She found that parents employed a "mix of communication strategies and emotional climate management to maintain relationships" (p. 175). She noted that "parent/child distal relationships used maintenance strategies that were different from those of other relationships" (p. 176). Even though the main focus was primarily on communication, Pollom's work was particularly relevant in grounding the methodology of this study to focus on the process of how military mothers maintain relationship over the trajectory of the deployment. Pollom's study highlighted how this process can vary at different time points, however her small number of military women, aggregated with military men and incarcerated individuals, does not provide depth of understanding for military mothers and their children. Furthermore, her focus primarily elicited communication strategies, a significant component, but perhaps not the only, process involved in maintaining relationship during the deployment.

Current Research on the Deployment of Military Mothers

Most recently, with the advent of Operation Enduring Freedom in Afghanistan and Operation Iraqi Freedom, military mothers are receiving more attention in the lay press and in research. Recent articles in *The Washington Post* (Tyson, 2008) and *NPR* (Mann, 2009) detail accounts of single parent soldiers who have lost custody of their children to their ex-husbands while deployed related to an "unstable home life" despite having been awarded full custody in their divorce proceedings. As noted by the *Post*, "female troops may be particularly at risk because mothers are more likely to have custody of children after a divorce. 'For them to go away for 15–18 months, it opens the door to these challenges.'" (Tyson, 2008, p. A01). In a report of the Congressional Joint Economic Committee, it was noted that "women in the military are more likely to be a single parent or married to another member of the military and thus face the possibility of a dual deployment. Issues such as child care access, adequacy of medical leave and access to appropriate health care services are often heightened in importance during period of deployment and when faced with the uncertainty of being redeployed" (U.S. Senate, 2007, p. 4). Certainly at a minimum, military mothers are faced with multiple stressors between work and home responsibilities exacerbated with the increased operational tempo and frequency of deployment since the war began in 2001. The concerns most often translate into recruitment, retention, and possible health issues for military women committed to a military career.

Research on military women and military mothers in particular has begun to appear with more frequency in the literature. There appears to be two waves of studies: those emerging after the first Gulf War and now those emerging in response to the current wars in Iraq and Afghanistan. Following the first Gulf War, Angrist and Johnson (2000) documented effects of female separations as compared to their male counterparts. They found that military women who deploy appear to experience more divorces as compared to the deployed males. Similarly, Wynd and Dziedzicki (1992) found that women experienced more separation anxiety than men during deployments in Desert Shield/Desert Storm related to not being able to parent their children. Vogt and her colleagues (2005) similarly have documented the mental health effects associated with deployment stressors differentiating by gender, but not with a primary focus upon military women with children.

Michelle Kelley and her colleagues have built a program of research focused upon military mothers. She compared Navy mothers deployed for sea duty to those with shore duty to determine predictors of retention. Those who indicated intent to stay were most often those committed to a career in the military, satisfied with the benefits, and felt that children benefited from work-day separations. Those who expressed concerns about balancing work and family responsibilities and a high commitment to the mothering role were less likely to remain on active duty (Kelley, 2001). She notes that her findings support those of Pierce and her colleagues. Her studies, while focused on military mothers, did not include women deployed for wartime missions, the sample, while representative of Navy women, was small, and "findings must be considered exploratory" (p. 69). In her follow-on study (Kelley et al, 2002), she found that commitment to mothering could act as a protective factor for depression and other psychological symptoms during and following deployment. Because her sample participated in routine sea duty deployments, the team found that the "length of the most recent separation, rather than time away from the child the previous year, predicted mothers reports of psychological adjustment" (p. 211). Other protective factors for mother reaction to the deployment included time in service, being married, greater perceived support from the child's father and friends, and older children (Kelley, 2002). Kelley's work highlighted the need in this study to describe stress, health, and other psychological effects that the deployment may elicit in the mothers and children before, during, and after a wartime deployment as opposed to the peacetime duty deployment rotations studied in her research. The findings also supported the need in this study to consider deployment away from younger children.

Somewhat contradictory findings emerged from Roper's (2005) study of Air Force single parent mothers who were scheduled for deployment. She found that the mothers "experienced a greater level of separation anxiety and employment related concerns than Army single fathers, but there were not significant differences in separation effects. The study also suggested that Air Force single parent mothers and Army military fathers had similar emotions and concerns when balancing a career and family during deployment and separation" (p. ii).

Godwin (1996) focused her dissertation research on an ethnographic study of military women's deployments tracing the experience from pre-deployment through reunion. She was able to articulate some of the strategies military women in general use to make sense of the experience and how they manage the long separation from family and loved ones. Her study did not specifically consider only deployed mothers and in fact only had 3 mothers in her sample, but the study provides support for this project in terms of viewing the experience across the trajectory of stages articulated in previous research. Hopkins-Chadwick (2005) explored stress, role strain, and health in young Air Force women with and without preschool children. Hopkins-Chadwick did not find significant differences between the two groups, but unfortunately did not report the absolute levels of role strain and stress of the two groups, but only noted that "multiple role strain (measured as frequency and severity of daily hassles) was an important variable" in the study and that role strain was evident for both groups of women (p. 69).

While the military support network has been very adept at providing services for spouses and families during deployment, what if there are unique needs for families whose deployed military member is the mother rather than the father? What has yet to be documented is the trajectory of the deployment experience for the military mother and her perceptions of what works and what does not work in providing support for herself and for her children during the separation. This study will fill an important niche in the research literature by querying military women who have been separated from their children as to how they prepared themselves and their children for the experience; how they managed the actual deployment experience for themselves and their children; and identifying perceived effects on their health and their relationship with their children as a result of the deployment experience.

Definitions

1. <u>Military mother</u>: a female officer or enlisted woman on either active duty or in the reserve component of the U.S. Army, Navy, Air Force or Marines who has one or more dependent children
2. <u>Deployment</u>: Previously serving at least 3 months in either Iraq or Afghanistan as part of Operation Iraqi Freedom after 2003 or Operation Enduring Freedom after 2001

3. Maintain relationship: a process whereby women provide mothering behavior to their dependent children

4. Children: dependent family members of military women who normally live with their mother and are under the age of 12 years.

Assumptions

The following assumptions undergird this proposal:

1. Deployment separations are experienced differently by military mothers than military fathers
2. Deployments are stressful for both children and mothers
3. Mothers desire to reduce the stressful nature of deployments for their children and themselves.

Section 4. Preliminary Studies/Progress Report

The topic of this proposal emerged from two previous studies completed by the principal investigator and from recent reports in popular media and press. Most recently, the PI completed a study of nursing practice in Operations other than War and in wartime. Serendipitous findings in the study elicited data from female active duty and reserve component participants regarding the effects of the deployment for them personally. Several mentioned the hardships associated with separation from their children during deployments. One in particular recounted "my daughter has never forgiven me for leaving her to go to Bosnia." Another described how distracted some of the women with children were during the deployment, "We could always tell one of our friends, a head nurse, and we could tell whenever her moods would change we knew what was going on with her. She just missed her family; she wanted to see her kids. She was not tolerating the slightest bit of change or the slightest anything would bother her."

Additionally, studies conducted by the PI of health promotion in military women, medics' experiences during Desert Shield/Desert Storm, and in readiness issues have revealed some serendipitous findings of unique adjustments required by active duty mothers during deployment. However, rather than taking a problem-oriented approach as evidenced by some of the research literature of effects of separation upon children, this project will describe the trajectory of the experience beginning with preparation and moving through the deployment and reunion. Participants will be asked to share both successful and unsuccessful strategies they, as military mothers, used to maintain relationship with their child(ren) to offer a grounding for intervention and support for other military women and their families experiencing this type of deployment. This project represents a continuation of the PI's program of research focusing upon military women and military mothers. Long term plans would be to use the results of this project to continue research in this area. Gaps in the literature indicate a need for a prospective study of deploying military mothers longitudinally through the separation with some concurrent study of the children left behind. Other future studies may be indicated by the emerging findings.

The research team assembled to conduct this study brings a strong background in readiness and deployment issues. Dr. Agazio brings her military and research background in readiness issues to this project along with prior experience in qualitative research. She has previous grounded theory experience as co-investigator on MAJ Catrina Lasome's study on computer-mediated communication and teaches the method in the PhD-level qualitative and advanced qualitative methods courses at CUA. Additionally she has presented the method at a variety of conferences, classes, and grant writing workshops for TSNRP. She will be providing mentorship to the military co-investigators and the RA in qualitative and grounded theory methods, interview techniques, qualitative analysis procedures, and use of NVIVO software as an adjunct in qualitative analysis. Each of the team members will be involved in the project throughout data collection and analysis, interviewer training; pilot study; participant interviews; interview coding; and preparation of reports and final manuscript for publication and presentation. They will be mentored in grounded theory qualitative methods and will participate in all phases of the research project. Team meetings will be held frequently and detailed notes will be made in order to track coding decisions and theory development.

Dr Padden similarly is building a program of research in military family issues. Her dissertation focused upon the effects of perceived stress, coping and health promoting behaviors on general well being in military spouses during deployment separation. She has recently extended her work in a current study to identify determinants of health-promoting lifestyle in spouses of active duty military that has merged her work with the previous health promotion study of Dr. Agazio. Her research interests include stress and coping as well as health promotion and health prevention in primary care especially in their effects on female spouses and female military members.

COL Ricciardi will bring military and research experience to assist in ongoing study, analysis, and interpretation of the findings. As a practicing Pediatric and Adult Nurse Practitioner caring for military families for over 27 years, Colonel Ricciardi brings both a clinical and research perspective to the study team. In addition, he is an associate investigator on a TSNRP funded qualitative study entitled "Clinical Knowledge Development: Continuity of Care for War Injured Service Members." He will serve as site PI's at Walter Reed and LTC Ray Coe will be the site PI Womack Army Medical Center and they will facilitate IRB approval and recruitment at those sites. LTC Coe, while not able to serve as a research team member, was interested in the research topic, and supportive of facilitating recruitment at Womack and in the Ft Bragg area.

Sr Mary Elizabeth O'Brien brings a wealth of qualitative methods and grounded theory experience to the project to provide oversight and guidance with grounded theory methods and analysis. She has completed numerous projects using the grounded theory method to include studies with migrant workers, HIV patients and their families, and most recently in development of her theory of spirituality in illness. Her most recent projects have been focused upon the expression of spirituality in nurses. Her research has resulted in multiple books detailing the qualitative findings from her many projects. She has been an ongoing mentor and consultant for the PI since her doctoral dissertation committee, and has collaborated on previous projects as a qualitative mentor. She is also a retired Lieutenant Commander in the Navy Nurse Corps reserves so will also bring an understanding of the military environment to the project.

Section 5. Research Design and Methods

This study will use a grounded theory qualitative research design guided by the deployment stages proposed by Peebles-Kleiger and Kleiger (1994). Since no other studies have considered the effect of deployments upon military mothers and their children, grounded theory methods will allow an exploration of the process by which military mothers maintain relationship with their children across the trajectory of the deployment experience and the effects of the deployment upon them and the children.

Grounded theory is a "qualitative research approach used to explore the social processes that present within human interactions"(Speziale and Carpenter, 2007, p. 133). Derived from symbolic interactionism, grounded theory seeks to elicit the perspective of those with shared experiences to inductively derive common themes which are then related to identify the basic social processes involved in a phenomenon or experience. The focus of this particular study will be on the interaction between military mothers and their children across the trajectory of the deployment experience. In symbolic interactionism theory, "people behave and interact based on how they interpret or give meaning to specific symbols in their lives" (p. 134). These symbols may include communication, both verbal and non-verbal expression, but also other means people use to make sense of, or order, their social interactions and/or world view. Grounded theory will allow the exploration of the basic social processes involved in this particular deployment experience. The significance of developing theory is that it can next be tested, or applied, deductively, based upon the general principles that emerge.

Subjects

The target population for this study will include a sample of military mothers with at least one child, who have been deployed for at least three months away from their children during wartime. This would include deployments in support of Operation Enduring Freedom and Operation Iraqi Freedom. Primary focus will be upon the relationship between the mothers and younger children defined as children under 12 years of age. The effects of deployment upon adolescents has been considered in previous research and developmental issues are different from those of younger children (Chartrand & Siegel, 2007). In order to address the gap regarding younger child relationships, the focus of recruitment will be ask mothers to relate their experience for this younger age group.

Subjects will be recruited and interviewed until theoretical saturation is obtained and no new codes or themes are emerging from the data. Efforts will be directed at recruiting military mothers from all four services, officers and enlisted, single and married, both deployment locations and different times of deployment during the conflict, and single and multiple children. A sampling grid will be used to track the demographics for sampling to elicit rich experiences with deployment as a military mother. Morse (1989) indicates that it is important that the researcher have control over the composition of the sample in order to ensure that the sample meets the criteria of appropriateness and adequacy. From previous studies conducted by the PI, recall of previous deployments has never been problematic. The deployment experience is one that seems indelibly imprinted and one perceived as significant by the participants. Indeed, Stanton, Dittmar, Jezewski, & Dickerson (1996) and Scannell-Desch (1996) interviewed nurses years post-Vietnam, post-Korean War, and post-WWII and elicited rich details about the experience despite the time elapsed since the experience.

The estimated sample size will be 35–40 participants to allow for theoretical sampling. The maximum sample size would be dependent upon the need for more interviews based on emerging data (Sandelowski, 1986). As stated by Patton (2002), in qualitative inquiry, final sample size is dependent upon "what you want to know, the purpose of the inquiry, what's at stake, what will be useful, what will have credibility, and what can be done with available time and resources" (p. 244). Creswell (1998) similarly emphasizes the open nature of sampling and warns researchers to avoid premature closure by using too small a sample. Likewise, Speziale and Carpenter (2007) note that in grounded theory, "sample size is determined by the generated data" (p. 140). Theoretical sampling is achieved with "saturation of conceptual information and no new codes emerge" (p. 113).

Marketing of the study for subject recruitment will include articles in various newsletters, websites, and at local military facilities in the DC and Womack Army Medical Center area. Flyers will be placed in women's and pediatric clinics at the recruitment sites. Appropriate procedures will be followed to obtain permission to advertise in these venues. Snowball sampling will also be used to identify additional women known to volunteers who may also be interested in participating. These individuals will be contacted either by the participant or by mail to invite their participation.

All subjects will be individuals who are willing share their experiences of separation during a deployment. A good "informant" is someone who is articulate and who is willing to share with the interviewer (Morse, 1989). Informants will need to speak English and be willing to be interviewed once for approximately 1–1½ hours, with the option to attend a presentation and validation discussion (approx. 2 hours) at the end of the study (subject to time and availability). Preliminary plans for sampling will include military women with children, both officers and enlisted who are active duty, reserve component, or National Guard. Demographics will be collected to describe the characteristics of the final sample.

Setting

Recruitment will take place in women's and pediatric clinics at Walter Reed Army Medical Center, Pentagon Health Clinic, and Womack Army Medical Center. Interviews will be set up for face-to-face whenever feasible. Phone interviews will be set up for those who are not available to meet in person, such as those who may respond to nationally-placed ads. To ensure privacy, all face-to-face interviews will be conducted in a private, quiet location of the participant's choosing. Telephone interviews were used in the PI's most recent study and were very successful in achieving rapport and open dialogue regarding the study topic. Phone cards will be used for placing the calls and these interviews will be conducted in the PI's private office with the door closed. In that study, and in this one, consent to participate and tape-record the interview will be elicited prior to turning on the recorder and verified once the recorder is turned on before beginning any of the telephone interviews.

Instrumentation

Demographic Data Sheet. Demographic data will be collected to include rank, specialty, years in the military, age, race, educational level, number of children, current age and age of children at time of deployment, and deployment history. These data will be collected to describe the characteristics of the sample.

Focused Interview Guide. Focused interview questions developed for this study will be used for beginning data collection. Individual interviews are expected to last no more than 1–1½ hours, although depending on the informant, could extend for a maximum of 2 hours. The interview guide will serve as a beginning topical outline for the initial interviews, however, it will be refined and modified as themes and categories emerge from the data. The guide has been reviewed by a content and a methods expert to insure inclusiveness of the areas of interest as specified by the research questions. Preliminary questions are structured as broad open ended inquiries to "allow unanticipated material to emerge during the interview" (Charmaz, 2006, p. 30), yet coupled with some possible probes to elicit a detailed description of the experience.

The interview guide will be piloted using two military women prior to the first scheduled interviews in order to facilitate administration and ease of understanding by participants. This pretesting will be used to eliminate or revise confusing or poorly phrased themes of inquiry. The pilot interviews will also be used by the team for critique and practice of interview style and pacing.

Participants will be asked to describe the nature of their deployment; how they prepared themselves and their families; what the deployment was like for them and the children; what did they do to stay in touch with their children; what issues came up during the deployment; how they prepared for the reunion; what the reunion period was like for them and their children; what is their relationship like with their children now and whether there were any effects from the deployment; and what suggestions or tips would they have for other active duty mothers who may deploy in the future and for any support services or policy to assist military mothers. As interviews progress, the use of theoretical sampling and constant comparison, hallmarks of grounded theory methods, will be directed toward filling emerging categories and defining and describing the basic core process(es) that emerge from the data (Charmaz, 2006).

Limitations

The use of a purposive sample will limit generalizability of this study to the larger population of all military women. However, the use of a broad sample of married/single; active duty/reserve/Guard; officer/enlisted; and differing numbers and ages of children will increase the amount of information which may demonstrate commonalties to provide a general base for understanding the processes involved in this experience.

Procedure

1. The proposal will be submitted for approval by the Catholic University of America, the Institutional Review and Human use committees at Walter Reed and Womack Army Medical Centers and the Uniformed Services University of the Health Sciences.

2. The guide will be piloted on two military women. Any needed revisions will be identified and made prior to the first interview.

3. Participants will begin to be recruited into the study. After obtaining any necessary permissions, flyers will be posted in women's and pediatric clinics at the medical centers and clinic; high-traffic areas at facilities in the local area (commissary, post, PX Bulletin boards) and ads/articles placed in military-related newsletters and Internet sites. Those interested in participating will be asked to either call or send an email message to the PI. Snowball sampling will be used to identify additional women known to volunteers who may also be interested in participating. These individuals will be contacted either by the participant or by mail to invite their participation.

4. Once initial contact is made, a follow up phone call will ascertain if the person is interested in participating and to set up a time for an interview. Participants in the local area will be interviewed in person at a site of their choice (for example home, office) or by phone if they aren't available to meet in person. Demographic and consent forms will be mailed in advance and returned (signed and witnessed) prior to the telephone interviews. Additionally, verbal consent will be obtained on the tape-recording before beginning any formal interview questions. Multiple sites are being used in order to recruit a diverse sample of military mothers.

5. For consistency, the principal investigator will conduct most interviews. Other research team members will initially review tapes and transcripts to familiarize with the flow of questions followed by observing and then conducting interviews with the PI. To provide effective mentorship, the co-investigators will have the opportunity to conduct interviews, but recognizing the necessity for consistency and adherence to grounded theory methods and role of researcher as instrument, the PI will be integrally involved in supervision and training prior to any other members of the team conducting interviews.

6. The interviewer will initially provide introductory comments, and then conduct the interview using the interview guide and appropriate probes or follow-up questions as indicated by the flow of the discussion. Initial probes during these first interviews will primarily direct the respondent to expand or explain some of her answers as appropriate to the flow of the interview. The PI will make memos, seek clarification, and use additional probes as indicated by the flow of the interview. All memos will be entered into QSR NVIVO 8™, a qualitative data management program, as memos attached to the interview (Wimpenny & Gass, 2000).

7. All interviews will be tape-recorded with two tape recorders to provide back up and prevent data loss. A conference microphone will be used to enhance tape clarity for transcription purposes. Signed informed consent and the demographic data sheet will be completed prior to beginning the formal interview. Time will be given at the end of the interview for the participant to add or clarify any information shared in the preceding discussion.

8. Participants will be informed that the PI may contact them at a later time to verify information from the interview. Swanson (1986) advises that closure of the interview should be tentative to "leave the door open to obtain additional information if needed" (p. 77). Interviews will be designed to take no

more than 1–1½ hours to complete. Immediately following the interview, the interviewer will make appropriate memos to reflect descriptions of impressions and ideas.

9. Memoing will begin after the first interview to track methods and analytical process. According to Corbin (1986), memos "allow the analyst to keep a record or and to order the results of the analysis" (p. 108). Charmaz (2006) encourages memoing to address all aspects of data collection method decisions and the data analysis stream. Memos will be used to define and describe categories; define characteristics; identify gaps in theoretical sampling and in analysis; delineate emerging patterns and relationships; and track emerging theory.

10. The initial interviews will be transcribed immediately following the interview and verified by the PI and members of the research team for accurate transcription. The first codes will be defined and entered into QSR NIVO 8™. These will be assessed in order to identify any probes that should be added to the focused interviews to address some of the emerging themes or issues. These will be placed into the interview guide as "validation" probes. All codes will be recorded and defined in the codebook.

11. The research team will work to control potential bias through informant validation, recruiting sample diversity in status, number and ages of children, and deployment experiences, and thick description (actual quotes) to illustrate each major theme and issue. Objectivity of interview data will be protected through ongoing review of interviews to insure neutral non-directional probes, consistent question administration, and naturalistic comfortable tone and style.

12. Subsequent interviews will be conducted. Data collection and data analysis will occur simultaneously in a cyclical manner in order to refine and add probes to address emerging codes and themes using the constant comparative method. Data collection will then continue until no new findings emerge from the data (i.e., theoretical saturation).

13. All data will be transcribed verbatim and maintained by the Principal Investigator indefinitely on media storage (zip disk or CD) and hard copy in a locked file cabinet. Once the study is completed, data will be removed from any hard drive storage. Audiotapes will be destroyed once data are checked with the transcript. Code numbers will be used on the transcripts and data sheets. Links with identifying information will be secured by the PI. Access to data and any identifying information will be restricted to the PI, members of the research team, and approved individuals from sponsoring agency and review boards.

14. As the interviews continue, validation probes will be added reflecting back codes and themes identified in the previous interviews. This step is added to further enhance credibility of the data verifying that emerging data are not an isolated occurrence or experience. The verification is added after the other sections in order to decrease the potential of prematurely introducing closure of other emerging themes, codes or issues. The team will identify the emerging core variable or basic social process(es) which will serve to organize the emerging theory.

15. Once theoretical saturation is obtained, the research team will invite previous interview participants to meet together or join in a conference call. The purpose of these final groups will be to offer a presentation of findings for validation of codes, categories, and proposed relationships. This would offer the opportunity for those participants in the early interviews to respond to themes and issues that may have emerged later which would strengthen the findings.
16. Once the final validation groups' transcriptions have been coded, the team will complete the analysis and development of the grounded theory, final reports, and prepare a manuscript.

Data Analysis

Demographic data will be summarized and presented using frequencies and descriptive statistics. Qualitative data will be analyzed using the constant comparative method developed by Glaser and Strauss (1967) and further described by Strauss and Corbin (1990). The purpose of grounded theory is to "develop an inductively grounded theory about a phenomenon. The research findings constitute a theoretical formulation of the reality under investigation . . . [whereby] the concepts and relationships are not only generated but provisionally tested" (Strauss & Corbin, 1990, p. 25). While the goal of this study is directed toward developing an abstract theory for testing, an additional goal includes knowledge building with proposed relationships to guide policy, preparation, and assist in the promotion of positive experiences for military mothers and their children during deployment.

Three basic coding procedures direct both sampling and analysis in grounded theory (Patton, 2002). Initially, the data will be broken down and categorized using open coding. In this phase, data are examined for salient categories that are named. This process reduces the data into a set of themes that characterize the process or experience being explored. Categories may have properties, which are subcategories that further define the category. Two processes are inherent in the coding process: the making of comparisons and the asking of questions (Strauss and Corbin, 1990). Once data are broken down, questions are used to open up the data, or, according to Strauss and Corbin (1990) map a path toward future data collection and analysis. Sampling is then directed at collecting data that confirm or refute the emerging categories.

Once an initial set of categories is developed, the next step is to identify central phenomenon or core categories. Axial coding is then used to explore interrelationships between the categories. According to Creswell (1998), these relationships could include causal conditions, "strategies addressing the phenomenon, the context and intervening conditions that shape the strategies, and the consequences of undertaking the strategies" (p. 151). Categories are compared to each other and new data are used to discover or confirm links and define the type of relationships (Stern, 1986). This process continues until all major categories that have evolved from the data are explored and no new categories emerge. At this point, theoretical saturation is achieved.

Finally, the data are further abstracted to create a coding paradigm that "visually portrays the interrelationship of the axial coding categories" (p. 151). This is achieved through selective coding where the core categories are systematically related to other categories, relationships are validated, and remaining categories are further refined and developed. The final abstraction is then presented through the development of hypotheses; a visual model; and/or a descriptive narrative about the central phenomenon of the study (Creswell, 1998; Strauss and Corbin, 1990). The intent of this analysis will be to contexualize the data (core processes) as they emerge and impact across the trajectory of the deployment experience. Attention will be paid to providing concrete, and helpful, strategies proven to be useful in maintaining relationship with children during the deployment and after reunion. In addition, the effects of the deployment will also be documented to note any health or psychological effects perhaps indicative of further study.

Trustworthiness: Reliability and Validity

Methodological rigor in qualitative research needs to answer four questions: truth value (credibility), applicability, consistency, and confirmability (Sandelowski, 1986). Strauss and Corbin (1990) similarly describe four criteria for judging truth value, or applicability to the phenomenon of interest: fit; understanding; generality; and control.

Confirmability (applicability) refers to neutrality and replicability of the study. Actions to be taken to support confirmability will include: memos and detailed records of the study's methods provided by detailed documentation and tracking of meeting minutes by the PI and research team. These sources will provide an audit trail for identification of potential biases and tracking of coding decisions.

Consistency (fit) is sometimes labeled external reliability in qualitative research and means that the process of the study has been "reasonably stable over time and across researchers and methods" (Miles and Huberman, 1994, p. 278). Consistency will be achieved through close adherence to the methods including the constant comparative method and theoretical sampling; reviewing interview transcriptions to refine probes, and reviewing tapes to insure interview technique consistency (Appleton, 1995).

Truth value (understanding) addresses the authenticity of the data and is equivalent to internal validity: do the findings of the study "make sense" to the people being studied? Actions to be taken to support truth value include: the iterative process of data collection being guided by simultaneous data analysis, validation of key points at the end of each interview; and presentation back to the original participants to insure accurate depictions of their experiences.

Transferability (generality) refers to whether the conclusions have any further import or generalizability to other contexts or groups. Participation by a diverse sample of military mothers who have participated in different deployment locations will avoid a deployment-specific picture of maternal deployment separations and purposive sampling will ensure participation of personnel with different backgrounds and experience. This representation will provide a "theoretically diverse" sample to encourage broader applicability. Thick description (actual quotes) will be provided in discussion of findings and themes so that readers can make their own comparisons with other settings.

Chiovitti and Piran (2003) made further recommendations to enhance rigor within grounded theory and their six principles will also be incorporated into this project: "1) let participants guide the inquiry process; 2) check the theoretical construction generated against participants' meanings of the phenomenon; 3) use participants' actual words in the theory; 4) articulate the researcher's personal views and insights about the phenomenon explained; 5) specify the criteria build into the researcher's thinking; . . . and 6) describe how the literature relates to each category that emerged in the theory" (p. 427).

Section 6. References

Allnutt, R.A. (1988). Comparison of metabolic responses of United States Military Academy men and women in acute military load bearing. *Aviation, Space, and Environmental Medicine, 59*(8), 787–788. PMID: 3178633

Amen, D.G., Jellen, L., Merves, E., & Lee, R.E. (1988). Mimimizing the impact of deployment separation on military children: Stages, current preventive efforts, and system recommendations. *Military Medicine, 153*, 441–446. PMID: 3141832

Agazio, J., Ephraim, P., Flaherty, N., and Gurney, C. (2001). Health promotion in active duty women with children. *Women and health, 35*(1), 65–82. PMID: 11942470

Angrist, J.D. & Johnson, JH (2000). Effects of work-related absences on families: Evidence from the Gulf War. *Industrial and Labor Relations Review, 54*(1), 41–58.

Appleton, J.V. (1995). Analyzing qualitative interview data: Addressing issues of validity and reliability. *Journal of Advanced Nursing, 22*, 993–997.

Applewhite, LW & Mays, RA (1996). Parent-child separation: A comparison of maternally and paternally separated children in military families. *Child and Adolescent Social Work Journal, 13*(1), 23–39.

Bathalon, G.P., Hughes, V.A., Campbell, W.W., Fiatarone, M.A., & Evans, W.J. (1995). Military body fat standards and equations applied to middle-aged women. *Medical Science and Sports Exercise, 27*(7), 1079–1085. PMID: 7564976

Birgenheier P. S. (1993). Parents and children, war and separation, *Pediatric Nursing, 19*, 471-476. PMID: 8233670

Black, WG (1993). Military-Induced Family Separation: A Stress Reduction Intervention. *Social Work. 38*(3), 273–80.

Blount, B.W., Curry, A., & Lubin, G.I. (1992). Family separations in the military. *Military Medicine, 157*, 76–80. PMID: 1603391

Bohan, J.S. (1983). A strategy for efficient diagnosis and treatment of dysuria in Women in the military setting. *Military Medicine, 148*(3), 245–247. PMID: 6408506

Brunader, R.E., Brunader, J.A., & Kugler, J.P. (1991). Prevalence of cocaine and marijuana use among pregnant women in a military health care setting. *Journal of the American Board of Family Practitioners, 4*(6), 395–398. PMID: 1767690

Bunch, SG, Eastman, RJ, & Moore, RR (2007). A profile of grandparents raising grandchildren as a result of parental military deployment. *Journal of Human Behavior in the social environment, 15*(4), 1–12. ISSN: 1091-1359 CINAHL AN: 2009766079

Charmaz, K (2006). *Constructing grounded theory*. Thousand Oaks, CA: Sage Publications.

Chartrand, MMD, Frank, DA, White, LF & Shope, TR (2008). Effect of parents' wartime deployment on the behavior of young children in military families. *Archives of Pediatric and Adolescent Medicine, 162* (11), 1094–1095. PMID: 18981347

Chartrand, MM & Siegel, B (2007). At war in Iraq and Afghanistan:Children in US in military families. *Ambulatory Pediatrics, 7*(1), 1–2. PMID: 17261472

Chiovitti, R & Piran, N (2003). Rigour and grounded theory research. *Journal of Advanced Nursing, 44* (4), 427–435. PMID: 14651715

Corbin, J. (1986). Coding, writing memos and diagramming. In In W. C. Chenitz & J. M. Swanson (Eds.), *From practice to grounded theory: Qualitative research in nursing* (pp. 102–120). Reading, MA: Addison-Wesley.

Cozza, SJ, Chun, RS, & Polo, JA (2005). Military families and children during Operation Iraqi Freedom. *Psychiatric Quarterly, 76*(4), 371–378. PMID: 18981347

Creswell, J. W. (1998). *Qualitative inquiry and research design: Choosing among five traditions.* Thousand Oaks, CA: Sage.

Davis, L.J. and A.B. Woods. 1999. Military Women's Research. *Military Medicine 164*: 6–10.

DOD 2006 Demographics. *Profile of the military community*. Office of the Deputy Under Secretary of Defense. Retrieved 30 January 2008 at

Friedl, K.E., Klicka, M.V., King, N., Marchitelli, L.J. & Askew, E.W. (1995). Effects of reduced fat intake on serum lipids in healthy young men and women at the U.S.Military Academy. *Military Medicine, 160* (10), 527–533. PMID: 7501204

Gerrard, M., Gibbons, F.X., & Warner, T.D. (1991). Effects of reviewing risk-relevant behavior on perceived vulnerability among women marines. *Health Psychology, 10*(3), 173–179. PMID: 1879389

Glaser, B. G., & Strauss, A. L. (1967). *The discovery of grounded theory: Strategies for qualitative research.* New York: Aldine de Gruyter.

Godwin, SA (1996). An ethnography of women's experience with military deployment. (Doctoral dissertation, United States International University, 1996). *Dissertation Abstracts International, 57/08*, 5359.

Guenter, K.E. & Estela, L.A. (1971). Rubella antibody determination among pregnant women in the US military communities in Europe. *Obstetrics and Gynecology, 37*(3), 343–347. PMID: 5101213

Hopkins-Chadwick, DL (2005). Stress, role strain, and health in young enlisted Air Force women with and without preschool children (Doctoral dissertation, The Ohio State University, 2005). *Dissertation Abstracts International*, 66/06), 3057.

Huebner, AJ, Mancini, JA, Wilcox, RM, Grass, SR, & Grass, GA (2007). Parental deployment and youth in military families: Exploring uncertainty and ambiguous loss. *Family Relations, 36*, 112–122.

Jensen, PS, Martin, D, & Watanabe, H (1996). Children's response to parental separation during Operation Desert Storm. *Journal of the American Academy of Child and Adolescent Psychiatry, 35*(4), 433–441. PMID: 8919705

Kelley, ML, Hock, E, Bonney, JF, Jarvis, M.S., Smith, K.M, & Gaffney, M.A. (2001). Navy mothers experiencing and not experiencing deployment: Reasons for staying in or leaving the military. *Military Psychology, 13*(1), 55–71. ISSN: 0899-5605 CINAHL AN: 2009436084

Kelley, ML, Hock, E, Jarvis, MS, Smith, K.M, Gaffney, MA & Bonney, JF, (2002). Psychological adjustment of Navy mothers experiencing deployment. *Military Psychology, 14*(3), 199–216. ISSN: 0899-5605 CINAHL AN: 2004014439

Kelley, M.L., Hock, E, Smith, K.M., Jarvis, M.S., Bonney, J.F., & Gaffney, M.A. (2001). Internalizing and externalizing behavior of children with enlisted Navy mothers experiencing military-induced separation. *Journal of the American Academy of Child and Adolescent Psychiatry, 40*(4), 464–471. PMID: 11314573

King, N., Fridlund, K.E., & Askew, E.W. (1993). Nutrition issues of military women. *Journal of the American College of Nutrition, 12*(4), 344–348. PMID: 8409093

Kleigher, J.H. & Kennedy, D. (1993). Children don't forget me: A resource and support group for deployed parents during Operations Desert Shield and Desert Storm. *Health and Social Work, 18* (3), 237–240. PMID: 8406229

Knapp, TS & Newman, SJ (1993). Variables related to the psychological well-being of Army wives during the stress of an extended military separation. Military Medicine, 158(2), 77–79. PMID: 8441501

Lincoln, A, Swift, E, Shorteno-Fraser, M (2008). Psychological adjustment and treatment of children and families with parents deployed in military combat. *Journal of Clinical Psychology, 64*(8), 984–992. PMID: 18612969

Logan, KV (1987). The emotional cycle of deployment. *U.S. Navy Proceedings, 113*, 43–47.

Mann, B. (2009). Military moms face tough choices. NPR. Retrieved February 14, 2009 at http://www.npr.org/templates/story/story.php?storyId=88501564.

Messersmith-Heroman, K., Heroman, W.M., & Moore, T.R. (1994). Pregnancy outcome in military and civilian women. *Military Medicine, 159*(8), 577–579. PMID: 7824152

Miles, M.B.& Huberman, A.M. (1994). *Qualitative data analysis (2nd ed)*. Newbury Park, CA: Sage Publications.

Military Family Resource Center, *Military families in the millennium*. March, 2000.

Miltary Women in Service for American Foundation (2007). Statistics on Women in the Military. Retrieved February 2, 2009, at http://www.womensmemorial.org/PDFs/StatsonWIM.pdf

Morse, J. M. (1989). Strategies for sampling. In J. M. Morse (Ed.), *Qualitative nursing research: A contemporary dialogue (pp. 117–131)*. Rockville, MD: Aspen Publishers, Inc.

Newby, JH, McCarroll, JE, Ursano, RJ, Fan, Z, Shigemura, J, Tucker-Harris, Y (2005). Positive and negative consequences of a military deployment. *Military Medicine, 170*(10), 815–819. PMID: 16435750

Nishimoto, P.W. (1990). HIV infection and women of the military. *NAACOGS Clinical Issues in Perinatal and Women's Health Nursing, 1(*1), 107–114. PMID: 2364027

Patton, M.Q. (2002). *Qualitative evaluation and research methods (3rd ed.)*. Newbury Park, CA: Sage Publications.

Peebles-Kleiger, M.J. & Kleiger, J.H. (1994). Re-integration stress for Desert Storm families: Wartime deployments and family trauma. *Journal of Traumatic stress, 7*(2), 173–193. PMID: 8012742

Pierce, P.F. & Buck, C.L. (1998). Wartime separation of mothers and children: Lessons from Operations Desert Shield and Desert Storm. *Military Family Issues: The research digest, 2* (2), 1–4. Retrieved February 24, 2009 at www.eustis.army.mil/7grp/grp7/familyreadiness/FAMILY_READINESS_04/.../Childrens%20reactions%20to%20deployment.doc

Pierce, P.R., Vinokur, A.D., & Buck, C.L. (1998). Effects of war-induced maternal separation on children's adjustment during the Gulf War and two years later. *Journal of Applied Social Psychology, 28*(14), 1286–1311.

Pincus, SH, House, R, Cristensen, J, & Adler, LE (2005). The emotional cycle of deployment: A military family perspective. *Journal of the Army Medical Department*, 615–623.

Polit, D. F., & Hungler, B. P. (1991). *Nursing research: Principles and methods (4th ed.)*. Philadelphia: J. B. Lippincott.

Pollom, LH (2005). Parent/child distal relationships: A look at communication used before, during and after a parental absence (Dissertation, University of Missouri-Columbia). *Dissertation Abstracts International*, 67/01, AAT 3204272.

Protzman, R.R. (1979). Physiologic performance of women compared to men. Observations of cadets at the United States Military Academy. *American Journal of Sports Medicine, 7*(3), 191–194. PMID: 464176

Protzman, R.R. & Griffis, C.G. (1977). Stress fractures in men and women undergoing military training. *Journal of Bone and Joint Surgery, 59*(6), 825. PMID: 908707

Roper, LL (2007). Air Force single parent mothers and maternal separation anxiety (Dissertation, Capella University). *Dissertation Abstracts International, 67*/11, AAT 3243582.

Rosen, L.N., Teitelbaum, J.M., & Westhuis, D.J. (1993). Children's reactions to the Desert Storm deployment: Initial findings from a survey of Army families. *Military Medicine, 158*, 465–469. PMID: 8351048

Ryan-Wenger, NA (2001). Impact of the threat of war on children in military families. *American Journal of Orthopsychiatry, 71*, 236–244. PMID: 11347364

Sandelowski, M. (1986). The problem of rigor in qualitative research. *Advances in Nursing Science, 8*(3), 27–37. PMID: 3083765

Schen, CR (2005). When mothers leave their children behind. *Harvard Review of Psychiatry, 13*(4), 233–243. PMID: 16126609

Scannell-Desch, EA (1996). The lived experience of women military nurses in Vietnam during the Vietnam War. *Image: Journal of Nursing Scholarship, 28*(2), 119–124. PMID: 8690427

Shamai, M. & Kimhi, S. (2007), Teenagers response to threat of war and terror: gender and the role of social systems. *Community Mental Health Journal. 43*(4):359–74. PMID: 17333347

Speziale, HJ & Carpenter, DR (2007). *Qualtitative Research in Nursing* (4th Ed). Philadelphia: Lippincott, Williams & Wilkins.

Stanton, MP, Dittmar, SS, Jezewski, MA, & Dickerson (1996). Shared experiences and meanings of military nurse veterans. *Image: Journal of Nursing Scholarship, 28*(4), 343–347. PMID: 8987282

Stern, P. N. (1986). Conflicting family culture: An impediment to integration in stepfather families. In W. C. Chenitz & J. M. Swanson (Eds.), *From practice to grounded theory: Qualitative research in nursing* (pp. 168–180). Reading, MA: Addison-Wesley.

Strauss, A., & Corbin, J. (1990). *Basics of qualitative research.* Newbury Park, CA: Sage Publications.

Swanson, J. M. (1986). The formal qualitative interview for grounded theory. In W. C. Chenitz & J. M. Swanson (Eds.), *From practice to grounded theory: Qualitative research in nursing (pp. 66–78).* Reading, MA: Addison-Wesley.

Tyson, A. (2008). Fighting War—and for Custody. *The Washington Post,* December 30, 2008. Retrieved 2 February 2008 at *http://www.washingtonpost.com/wp-dyn/content/article/2008/ 12/29/AR2008122902611.html*

U.S. Census Bureau (2007). Women by the numbers. Retrieved 2 February 2009 at http://www.infoplease.com/spot/womencensus1.html

U.S. Senate, Joint Economic Committee (2007). *Helping military moms balance family and longer deployments.* Retrieved February 7, 2009 at http://jec.senate.gov/archive/Documents/Reports/MilitaryMoms05.11.07Final.pdf

Vogt, D.S., Pless, A.P., King, L.A., & King, D.W. (2005). Deployment stressors, gender, and mental health outcomes among Gulf War I veterans. *Journal of Traumatic Stress, 18*(2), 115–127. PMID: 16281203

Wimpenny, P. & Gass, J. (2000). Interviewing in phenomenology and grounded theory: Is there a difference? *Journal of Advanced Nursing, 31* (6), 1485–92.

Wynd, C.A. & Dziedzicki, R.E. (1992). Heightened anxiety in Army reserve nurses anticipating mobilization during Operation Desert Storm. *Military Medicine, 157,* 630–634. PMID: 1470371

Zeff, K.N., Lewis, S.J., & Hirsch, K.A. (1997). Military family adaptation to United Nations Operations in Somalia. *Military Medicine, 162,* 384–387. PMID: 9183158

Section 7. Protection of Human Subjects

The initial approach to prospective participants will be through flyer, newsletter and email advertisements, and/or a personal invitation to participate via someone known to the individual (snowball sample). If the individual is interested in participating, then the PI or research team member will explain the study's purpose and methods in more detail and schedule an interview. Prior to the interview, participants will provide and sign an informed consent. Participants will be assured of their freedom to withdraw consent at any time. Interviews will be audio taped to preserve the integrity of the data. Before each phone interview, additional verbal consent will be obtained plus acknowledgement that they understand the interview is being tape-recorded. Military IRB's will require institution-specific HIPAA authorization forms to be included with the consent in case the participant reveals any medical information.

Confidentiality will be assured by assigning identification numbers to each individual, using these numbers in the tape transcriptions, avoiding the use of last names in the validation groups, and destroying the tapes after transcription and analysis are complete. Tapes will be destroyed by crushing the cassettes and shredding the tape. Any identifying information will be kept separate from interview tapes or transcriptions and all data will be reported in the aggregate. Cited quotes will be carefully screened to avoid identifying characteristics. Any names mentioned during interviews will be replaced with a pseudonym. All data will be secured and only the PI and research team will have access. Code numbers will be assigned to each demographic form so the PI can match transcriptions to the appropriate individuals. The PI will control all access to any identifying data on the participants. All findings will be reported in aggregate and no identifying information will be published in any format.

Audio recordings will be transcribed by either a court reporter transcription agency used in the past by the PI (the Carol J Thomas Agency in Fairfax, VA) or another similar service that provides confidential transcription services. After delivery of each transcript to the study Principal Investigator, Dr. Janice Agazio, the Carol J. Thomas Agency or comparable agency will destroy all files associated with the transcripts.

All transcribed data and demographic databases will be stored without identifiers and only code numbers. Files will be stored on the portable hard drive to which the PI will have the only access. Thumbdrives used by the research team will contain interview transcripts without identifiers and cleaned for identifying information (locations, unit names, etc). Thumbdrives will not be used on federal computers. The research team will store them securely in locked drawers or files when not being used for data analysis. The dedicated laptop used for the project will be password protected and has a security firewall. All paper copies of study files and data will be stored in the locked filing cabinet purchased for the project and located in the PI's office at CUA. This office is locked and has limited access by master key (Dean and her designees only). Data will not be transmitted electronically or placed on any shared drive.

Section 8. Inclusion of Children

No children will be included in this study

Section 9. Vertebrate Animals

N/A

Section 10. Consortium/Contractual Arrangements

None

Section 11. Letters of Support

Please see appendix

Informed Consent Document for the Research Study Entitled

Deployment of Military Mothers

I. Introduction

You are being asked to voluntarily take part in a research study. Before you decide to take part in this study, you need to understand the risks and benefits so that you can make an informed decision. This is known as informed consent.

This consent form provides information about the research study that will be explained to you. Once you understand the study, you will be asked to sign this form if you want to take part in the study.

II. Purpose and Procedures

You are being asked to participate in this study because you are a military woman with child(ren) and have served during a deployment for a wartime mission in Iraq or Afghanistan. There has been little research regarding the experience of military mothers separated from their children during a deployment. The purpose of this study is to describe the experience of being deployed as a military mother. Approximately 40 active duty or reserve component mothers will participate in the study.

If you agree to participate, you will be asked to take part in an interview and complete a demographic data sheet. In the interview, you will be asked about your experiences during your deployment; how you prepared yourself and your child(ren) for the deployment; how you managed your separation during the deployment; what the deployment was like for you and your child(ren); what you did to stay in touch with your child(ren); what issues came up during the deployment; how did you prepare for reunion; what the reunion period was like for you and your child(ren); what is your relationship like with your child(ren) now and were there any effects from the deployment; and what suggestions or tips would you have for other active duty mothers who may deploy in the future and for any support services or policy to assist military mothers. The data sheet will ask you for demographic information about yourself, such as your age, gender rank, current position, assignment and deployment experiences, and the number and age of your children at the time of your deployment.

The interview is an individual interview with you only, either in person or via telephone. *The interview will be recorded by audiotape and will be fully transcribed.* The interview will take up to 1–1½ hours time.

You will also be invited to take part in a final group interview with up to ten participants at the end of the study to verify the information learned in this study. This may be in person or through a phone conference call. *The group discussion will be recorded by audiotape and fully transcribed.* The discussion may take up to 2 hours time. During this discussion, participants will be presented preliminary findings from the study and asked to provide their feedback and opinions. *You are not required to participate in this group discussion in order to volunteer for the study.* You will be asked at the end of this informed consent form to indicate whether or not you are interested in participating in the group discussion. If you change your mind regarding

USU G161CE   Expires   Subject Initials ____ Date ____ Witness Initials ____ Date ____ participation in the group discussion, you may inform the Principal Investigator Dr. Janice Agazio at 202-319-5719 or using the contact information provided below.

Information that you provide will be used to prepare reports and briefings that will be presented to Department of Defense leaders, at military and scientific conferences, and in the scientific and lay literatures. You will not be identified in any report or presentation.Quotes from the interview may be used in publications or presentations, but you will not be able to be identified.

III. Right to Withdraw from the Study

You may decide to stop taking part in this study at any time. Refusal to participate in this study will involve no penalty or loss of benefits to which you are otherwise entitled. If you withdraw from the study you will be asked whether you wish for you data to be destroyed or retained for analysis and use in the study If you decide to withdraw from the study, please contact Dr. Janice Agazio at 202-319-5719 or using the contact information provided below.

IV. Risks Associated with the Study

There are no anticipated individual health or injury risks associated with this study. There are no anticipated risks to psychological health, although some subjects may find discussion of experiences during peacekeeping missions to be stressful. No clinical services are provided in this study. Treatment for any health problems experienced by subjects enrolled in this study are the responsibility of the subject.

If you have been feeling generally worse than you normally do, you may wish to contact a health care provider in your area. If you are active duty military, contact your local medical treatment facility. Otherwise, consult your regular doctor or refer to listings under "physicians" in your local phone book. For referral to a mental health professional in your area you may call the American Psychiatric Association at **1-888-357-7924** and selection option "0" for an answer center coordinator. The coordinator will provide referral information for a psychiatrist in your area.

V. Benefits

There are no benefits to you for participating in this study. You will not be compensated for participation in the study. The results will not help you personally but may assist military leaders and other miltary mothers who are planning or involved in deployments.

VI. Privacy/Confidentiality

Confidentiality of your information will be maintained to the extent possible under existing regulations and laws. Your name will not appear in any published paper or presentation related to this study. The Institutional Review Board of The Catholic University of America, Walter Reed Army Medical Center, Womack Army Medical Center, and the Uniformed Services University of the Health Sciences, Bethesda, MD; and other Federal agencies that provide oversight for human subject protection may see your records.

USU G161CE   Expires   Subject Initials ____ Date ____ Witness Initials ____ Date ____

Audio recordings will be transcribed by **Carol J. Thomas Agency (Court Reporters)** in Fairfax, Virginia. **The Carol J. Thomas Agency** provides confidential transcription services for the U.S. government and will hold materials from this study only during the period that specific transcripts are being prepared. After delivery of each transcript to the study Principal Investigator, Dr. Janice Agazio, **the Carol J. Thomas Agency** will destroy all files associated with the transcripts.

Transcripts of interviews in which you participate will be kept in unmodified form and will be retained indefinitely as confidential research data. Your social security number will not be associated with these interviews. Tapes used during interviews will be destroyed or erased after the interviews are transcribed.

VII. Points of Contact

Please call Dr. Janice Agazio, School of Nursing, The Catholic University of America, at 202-319-5719, with any questions or concerns. If you have questions regarding your rights as a research participant, you should call the Director of Human Research Protections Programs in the Office of Research at the Uniformed Services University of the Health Sciences (301) 295-3303. This person is your representative and is not involved with the researchers conducting this study.

PLEASE FEEL FREE TO ASK ANY QUESTIONS YOU MAY HAVE

PLEASE INDICATE YOUR PREFERENCES REGARDING THE GROUP DISCUSSION

I DO/DO NOT wish to participate in the group discussion. SUBJECT INITIALS: _____

SIGNATURE BLOCKS:

PRINTED NAME:

SIGNATURE: DATE

WITNESS: DATE

PRINCIPAL INVESTIGATOR: DATE

Focused Interview Questions

Could you tell me about your deployment? Where were you assigned, when, and for how long?

Was this your first time deployed away from your children?
    Possible probes to ask where and for how long; preparations made then; experience being away from children during previous deployments

How did you prepare yourself and your children for your deployment?

What were some of their concerns? What were some of your concerns prior to the deployment?

How were you able to stay in touch with your children during the deployment? How often was it possible to talk with them?

What, if any, concerns or issues came up during the deployment related to being away from your children? How were you able to handle these?

What was the hardest part of being separated? For you? For them? Were there any effects on your health related to the separation?

What seemed to help you and your children cope with the separation? Helpful strategies? Not helpful strategies?

Is there anything you would differently if you were to be deployed again?

When you were ready to redeploy, how did you and your children prepare for the reunion?

What was it like the first few weeks to be back together?

Did you notice any differences in your relationship with your children after the deployment?

Did you notice any effects on your children from the deployment separation? On yourself as a mother?

What suggestions or tips would you have for other active duty mothers who may deploy in the future?

Were there any support services or policy changes that you think are needed to assist military mothers?

16 April 2010

Dear Military Mother,

Thank you so much for your interest in this study. The purpose of the study is to describe the experience of military mothers separated from their children during a deployment. This study will fill an important gap by understanding the strategies women use to manage this separation experience to assist other women preparing for deployment. If you are interested in participating, you will be asked to take part in an interview to discuss how you prepared yourself and your children for the deployment; how you managed the actual deployment separation for yourself and your children; and what effects the deployment may have had upon your relationship with your children.

The process of participation is very easy. This packet contains several items: (1) a personal data information sheet; (2) two consent forms; and (3) a self-addressed stamped envelope. Since this is a research study, we need to have a consent form filled out to make sure all participants understand the purpose of the study and how we are conducting our research. One copy of the consent needs to be signed on the last page and returned to us. We will confirm your signature at the beginning of the interview. The other consent form is for you to keep. When we receive the packet back from you, we separate the consent form from the data sheet and keep confidential the names of all participants. We will use the information from the consent (name and address) to send you a copy of the study's results at the end.

The personal data sheet will be used to summarize information regarding our participants. None of this information will be reported specific to you and will only be grouped with information from all participants. We will label this form and your interview with code numbers so that they will no longer be able to be identified as your information. All information regarding our participants and the information they provide will be secured in a locked filing cabinet with access granted only to the research team members.

After completing the consent form and data sheet, please return them in the enclosed envelope. Once I receive the signed consent form, I will call or email you and we can set up a time to talk about your deployment experience. We can decide at that time whether to talk by phone or in person.

If you have additional questions, please call me directly at (202) 319-5719 or email me at agazio@cua.edu. Thank you again for your time, interest, and participation.

Sincerely,

Janice G. Agazio, PhD, CRNP, RN
LTC (Ret), U.S. Army
Principal Investigator

Proposed Newsletter/Bulletin Board/ Clinic Advertisement

Active Duty or Reserve Component Mothers needed as volunterrs for Deployment Study

If you are an active duty or reserve component woman who has been separated from your children during a deployment to Iraq or Afghanistan, you are being invited to participate in a research study to describe the experience of being deployed as an active duty mother. The knowledge you have from your experiences will help us to understand what this experience is like for mothers and their children and what their needs are for support during deployments.

If you are interested in participating, you will be asked to take part in an interview. In the interview, you will be asked about your experiences during your deployment. You may be interviewed in person or by telephone. You may also be asked to take part in a final presentation at the end of the study to verify the information learned in this study.

If you would like to participate in this study, please contact the Principal Investigator, Janice B. Agazio, LTC (ret), AN,PhD. RN, Assistant Professor, The Catholic University of America, at 202-319-5719 or by email at agazio@cua.edu

Miltary Times Advertisement

Military Mother Research

If you are an active duty or reserve component woman who has been separated from your children during a deployment to Iraq or Afghanistan, you are being invited to participate in a research study to describe the experience of being deployed as an active duty mother. Please contact Janice Agazio, LTC (ret), USA at agazio@cua.edu

Critique of Funded Grant

TriService Nursing Research Program
FY 2009 Scientific Review Discussion Summary

Proposal Number: N09-P02   **SRP Score:** 1.1

PI: LTC (ret) Janice B. Agazio

Title: Deployment of Military Mothers during Wartime

Discussion

Primary: The primary reviewer had a high level of enthusiasm for this proposal. The principal investigator (PI) did an outstanding job of developing the methodology and explaining it accurately and thoroughly. The literature review is strong and shows the need for the proposed research. The research questions correlate well with the instrument. The qualitative format is appropriate for developing the substantive knowledge that is critical to understanding the topic. The PI and her team are strong. The PI has had several prior grants and publications, and she has published and presented the results of all of her prior TSNRP grants. The institutional resources are appropriate. The only minor concern is that the study participants are very vulnerable and the PI should plan to follow up with some of the mothers based on what the data show.

Secondary: The secondary reviewer had a high level of enthusiasm for this well-crafted proposal. The study's findings will provide valuable information for future interventions. The few minor weaknesses include the lack of clarity about whether the recruitment sites will generate a sample that represents all of the military branches, as proposed. In addition to the demographic variables that the PI plans to measure, she should consider length of deployment, relationship status, and child care arrangements during the mother's deployment. These factors might shed light on variances in participant responses.

Military: The military reviewer had a high level of enthusiasm for this proposal, which addresses an important issue. The team is well qualified, with experience completing military studies. The timeframe is feasible. The study has the potential to make an exceptional contribution to military health care. The team is stable. However, the proposal does not specify LTC Cole's time commitment.

Budget: No specific budget recommendations were made.

Brief Summary: This study is clearly related to the welfare of military families and is likely to make an exceptional contribution to the military nursing field. The PI summarized the methodology accurately and thoroughly. The PI has a history of completing funded studies and has successfully published all of her funded research. The resources are clearly listed. The proposal addresses an important topic and the PI makes a good case for the study's significance. This study will inform future interventions. However, the PI needs to take into account the vulnerability of the study population, and she might need to follow up with some of the mothers, depending on what the data show. In addition, it is not clear if the recruitment plans will generate the number of participants needed. The committee recommended that the PI also measure length of deployment, child care arrangements, and relationship status.

TriService Nursing Research Program Format for Primary Reviewer's Evaluative Comments

Proposal Number:	N09-P02
Principal Investigator:	LTC (ret) Janice B. Agazio
Title of Proposal:	Deployment of Military Mothers during Wartime

ABSTRACT

Military women with children are being deployed in greater numbers than ever before in support of wartime missions. With the current wartime missions in Iraq and Afghanistan, more women are deploying and leaving children at home. Further, these women are being exposed to higher threat levels as they have integrated into all but actual combat units. Critical gaps remain in the literature concerning the process of how women and children experience separation during wartime. **The purpose of this study is to describe perceptions of military mothers regarding separation from their children over the trajectory of the deployment experience during wartime.** *This study will answer the following research questions:*

1. *What is the process of managing a deployment for military mothers and their children?*
2. *How do military mothers describe the effects of a deployment upon themselves and their children?*
3. *How do military mothers prepare themselves and their children for deployment?*
4. *How do military mothers manage the separation from their children during deployment?*
5. *How do military mothers manage their relationship with their children during and following deployment?*
6. *What strategies were effective in maintaining relationships with children during deployment?*

Using a grounded theory design, approximately 35–40 active duty and reserve component women with children who have been deployed to Iraq or Afghanistan will participate in an interview structured around the stages of deployment to explore the process of maintaining relationships. Interviews will be transcribed verbatim and the constant comparative method will be used to analyze the data in order to identify core processes through a combination of open, axial, and selective coding in order to construct a theoretical model of their deployment separation. Participants will be recruited from clinics at two military medical centers and through media such as military publications, websites, and post newspapers. Women with at least one child under the age of 12 years will participate in a tape recorded face to face or telephone focused interview following completion of a signed informed consent and demographic data sheet.

Employing theoretical sampling, all interviews will be transcribed verbatim and analyzed using the constant comparative method. QSR NVIVO 8 software. The significance of this study will be to: 1. Add to the body of knowledge regarding separation during military deployments; 2. Increase understanding of how this experience is unique for mothers and their children; 3. Identify successful strategies women use to maintain relationships with their children during deployment separation 4. Provide evidence based indications for policy development and support networks to use with stay-behind families with children, and 5. Develop theory for further testing and research regarding deployment separations particularly for military mothers.

Evaluation Criteria

Scientific Approach and Technical Merit

The purpose of this project is to describe deployment of military mothers during wartime. This is an original, descriptive study that lends itself appropriately to a qualitative investigation. The literature review is comprehensive, clearly articulated and well synthesized. The author notes that completion of the literature review for qualitative investigations is often postponed to prevent misinterpretation of the results. However in grounded theory the literature review is generally ongoing. That is, as new thematic elements emerge the researcher often needs to return to the literature to ensure comprehensive synthesis of all related information. The background section provides a very solid justification for the methodology and is relevant to the research question. Most important to note is the clear and accurate identification of a missing piece of information related to military deployment. More specifically, the author has identified a need to further develop the theoretical understanding of military deployment as it relates to mothers. The research team has multiple strengths and provides convincing evidence that the team can conduct this study. Findings from this study will be useful and will contribute to the development of a substantive body of nursing knowledge. The research design and methods section is also well developed. There is a solid description of grounded theory that demonstrates expertise with the method. Justification provided for all methodological decisions.

Research Design: Grounded theory is a qualitative research approach used to explore the social processes that present within human interactions. As a research approach, the primary purpose of this methodology is to develop theory about dominant social processes rather than to describe a particular phenomenon. Through application of the approach, the researcher develops explanations of key social processes or structures that are derived from or grounded in the data. The goal of grounded theory is to discover theoretically complete explanations about particular phenomena. Given this understanding of grounded theory method, the approach is appropriate to studying deployment of military mothers during wartime and makes sense in terms of its potential to contribute to the overall wellbeing of the family unit. As the research develops descriptions of the social processes that emerge in understanding deployment of military mothers and a theory emerges, the significance of the study becomes evident.

Problem and Purpose: The research question identifies the phenomenon or problem to be studied. Further the research question allows the PI to have some flexibility and freedom to explore the phenomenon in depth. This is important to a grounded theory investigation since new concepts may emerge throughout the process of data collection and will require additional investigation. The researcher has made clear that the concepts pertaining to deployment of military mothers during wartime have not been fully identified and the relationships between the concepts are poorly understood and conceptually undeveloped. Because the nature of grounded theory requires that investigators refine the research question as they generate and analyze the study data the original research question is not only clear but also has the flexibility to be modified depending on the data generated. Finally, the researcher has made clear the rationale for a qualitative study by noting that substantive information related to the deployment of women is missing from the literature. Therefore a qualitative approach is most relevant to build this body. The purpose of the study is clearly stated and is as follows:

> *"The purpose of this study is to describe perceptions of military mothers regarding separation from their children over the trajectory of the deployment experience during wartime"*

Sampling: Theoretical Sampling is appropriate for grounded theory methodology. In theoretical sampling, the sample size is determined by generated data. The researcher simultaneously collects codes and analyzes the data. Although the researcher is anticipating 35 to 40 participants, limits should not be determined a priori with regard to participants and sources of data. The author does note that "subjects will be recruited and interviewed until theoretical saturation is obtained and no new codes or themes are emerging from the data. Tape recording interviews and transcribing them verbatim is appropriate and allows for the collection of comprehensive, rich, thick data.

Ethics: Ethical considerations have been fully addressed along with issues related to informed consent. IRB approval will be secured from Catholic University of America, and the Institutional Review and Human use committees at Walter Reed and Womack Army Medical Centers and the uniformed Services University of the Health Sciences. A system is in place for secure storage of data to maintain confidentiality. *One concern may be related to topics that might emerge during data collection. The sample should be considered a vulnerable population and follow-up for some participants may be needed depending on what is revealed in the interviews.*

Appropriateness: When individuals choose to conduct a grounded theory investigation, usually they have decided there is some observed social process requiring description and explanation. In this instance it is the deployment of military mothers. Given that military women with children are being deployed in greater numbers and that they are being exposed to higher threat levels it seems critical to support this investigation. The project seems feasible in terms of the ability to complete the work in two years and adequate resources and equipment are or will be available to support the study. There are no adjustments required to the budget.

Originality and Innovative Nature of the Proposal; Applicability of Previous Findings

This grounded theory study speaks to an important gap in the research related to military deployment. The primary investigator has clearly articulated a major gap in the literature related to military deployment of mothers and notes that prior research has focused on the military deployment of fathers. The study is innovative, and closely linked to the research agenda of the primary investigator and will contribute to nursing's substantive body of knowledge. Given the absence of significant research in this area, this project is perfectly suited to a grounded theory approach.

Qualifications, Expertise and Research Experience of the Principal Investigator and Staff

Individuals Name, Title and Degree	Field of Training or Experience	Publication Record	Strengths	Weaknesses
LTC (Ret) Janice Agazio, PhD, RN **Principal Investigator** Assistant Professor, Catholic University of America	Dr. Agazio has been assistant professor at CUA since 2004 with previous experience teaching at the Uniformed Services University of the Health Sciences for four years. Her research proposal clearly builds on content and methods of her research program.	14 peer reviewed journal articles, six of which she is first author. Prior grants through Triservice Nursing Research Program, all successfully completed published and presented. Co Author on 2 book chapters. Multiple scholarly presentations	• 31 years of Nursing experience, 22 of which were military related. • Proven track record of high quality research experience.	None
Sr. Mary Elizabeth O'Brian **Associate Investigator** Ordinary Professor, School of Nursing, at the Catholic University of America.	Extensive experience in grounded theory methodology. Sr. O'Brian has completed numerous studies using grounded theory methodology and is an expert in the use of qualitative data management software. Sr. O'Brian is also a retired Navy Reserve Officer and therefore brings additional understanding regarding military issues.	7 peer reviewed journal articles, three of which she is first author. Multiple scholarly presentations	• 51 years of Nursing experience. • Proven track record of high quality research experience. • Expert in qualitative research and qualitative data management software.	None

(Continued)

423

Qualifications, Expertise and Research Experience of the Principal Investigator and Staff (*continued*)				
Individuals Name, Title and Degree	*Field of Training or Experience*	*Publication Record*	*Strengths*	*Weaknesses*
Dr. Diane Padden, Associate Investigator Chair of the Department of Health, Injury and disease Management and educator at the Uniformed services University of the health s/sciences graduate school of Nursing.	Dr. Padden role as a Nurse practitioner at the Kimbrough Ambulatory Care Center makes her acutely aware of the health issues facing both active duty service members as well as military families. Her doctoral dissertation is related to the current project and focused on the effects of perceived stress, coping and health promoting behaviors on the general well being in military spouses during deployment separation. Dr. Padden also brings a background in descriptive qualitative methods.	Peer reviewed publications and multiple scholarly presentations.	• Has a background in qualitative research	Requires mentoring in grounded theory methods

Richard Ricciardi, COL Associate Investigator Chief nursing Research service at Walter Reed Army Medical Center	Dr. Ricciardi has experience with deployment issues.	Peer reviewed publications and multiple scholarly presentations.	• Extensive experience in quantitative design.	Limited experience in qualitative research methods. Retiring in 2010
Research Assistant: First year of study only. Graduate student	Military nurses or a graduate student at CUA.			Dissemination of recruitment and survey materials Data checking Formatting of qualitative data for entry into NVIVO Participate in analysis of data Update Study records Prepare reports and Manuscripts Transcription rechecking

Overall, this team is well formulated. The team reflects expertise in the method as well as the substantive area. In addition the consultation identified is appropriate. It is quite likely this team can accomplish the project aims in a credible fashion. The following table highlights key information related to each member of the research team.

Availability of Institutional Resources and Adequacy of the Environment to Support the Project	
Institutional Resources	*Adequacy of Environment*
The Catholic University of America	• The Catholic University of America, situated on 144 landscaped acres in Washington, D.C., offers a traditional, medium-size college campus, the resources of a major research university and the excitement of the nation's capital.
	• CUA has its own university press. Among the journals it publishes are *Anthropological Quarterly* and *The Catholic Historical Review.* Among other works published or edited on campus are *Review of Religious Research, Law and Policy, The New Catholic Encyclopedia* and *The Journal of Chinese Philosophy.*
	• CUA hosts a number of research centers and facilities. Among them is the Center for Advanced Training in Cell and Molecular Biology, the Center for Irish Studies, the Institute for Communications Law Studies and the Institute for Social Justice.
	• The School of Nursing, established in 1932, has long provided outstanding nursing education that clearly emphasizes the role of ethics, values and spirituality in health care and faculty with extensive research backgrounds. Currently all faculty have private offices equipped with computers, telephones, internet connections and private printers.
Information Technology	• The Center for Planning and Information [CUA] Technology (CPIT) provides computing and network facilities to students and faculty for their educational and research activities, supports the university's management information systems, manages the campus network and provides telecommunication services and leadership on the ethical use of computing.
	• General purpose software available to students and faculty include the Microsoft Office 2003 suite (Access, Word, PowerPoint, Excel, and Publisher), SPSS, Internet Explorer, email, Mozilla Firefox and Netscape Navigator.

Availability of Institutional Resources and Adequacy of the Environment to Support the Project (*continued*)	
Institutional Resources	*Adequacy of Environment*
Library Services [CUA]	• The library system of CUA offers academic resources and services to support student, faculty and staff research. The John K. Mullen of Denver Memorial Library is the main campus library and maintains collections in the humanities, social sciences, library science, chemistry, religious studies, philosophy, and canon law.
	• The Nursing-Biology Library occupies one full wing (2 floors) on the second and third floor of the SON building, Gowan Hall. The Nursing-Biology Library currently has on site about 34,000 items, approximately two-thirds of the space and collection is designated for the nursing portion of the library.
Walter Reed Army Medical Center	• Walter Reed Army Medical Center (WRAMC) is a 350 bed tertiary care medical facility located in Washington, DC serving active and retired military beneficiaries as well as Congressionally designated beneficiaries.
	• It is the US Army's leading center of support to meet three critical goals to provide the best in patient care, to encourage the education and training of tomorrow's health professionals, and to expand the field of healthcare knowledge through research.
The Nurse Research Service	• Provides a superb environment for research and scholarly interchange. Staffed usually by 2–3 doctorally-prepared nurse researchers, it serves as a bustling nerve center for a variety of active and ongoing studies as well as other research.
	• The NRS fosters an open atmosphere of formal and informal consultation based upon their methodological, theoretical, and clinical strengths.
Womack Army Medical Center	• The Army Medical Department is committed to providing quality, cost-efficient care for "The Total Army Family." Womack Army Medical Center is proud to serve the more than 160,000 eligible beneficiaries in the region, the largest beneficiary population in the Army.
DiLorenzo Tricare health Clinic	• The DiLorenzo Tricare Health Clinic is located inside the north face of the Pentagon offering on-site care to eligible beneficiaries and their dependents stationed at the Pentagon.

Availability of institutional resources is satisfactory.

Significance and Relevance to Nursing Research

This investigator makes some very important points about the effects of separation on moms and children. Identifying ways to ameliorate some of these effects and better prepare moms and children can

Reasonableness of the Budget and Duration of the Project in Relation to the Proposed Research

There doesn't appear to be anything out of line in the budget and for the most part justification is adequate. One question with regard to the budget might be the need for a graduate assistant. Much of the work assigned to this individual should probably be done by the PI to ensure authenticity and trustworthiness of the data. However, since the PI will be doing the majority of data collection and analysis a RA may be useful for task oriented work.

Summary

Part One, Summary

This grounded theory research study will focus on development of substantive theory related to the perceptions of military mothers regarding separation from their children over the trajectory of the deployment experience during wartime. Thirty five to forty participant will participate in tape recorded interviews organized around focus group questions. Data will be transcribed verbatim for analysis. The design reflect grounded theory approach and is appropriate for the study. This research will add important descriptive information to nursing's substantive body of knowledge and has implications for how military mothers and their families handle separation during wartime. The principal investigator is qualified. She has successfully fulfilled other grant requirements, published manuscripts and presented on prior funded projects, and has experience in qualitative research methods.

Part Two, Strengths and Weaknesses

Strengths

- This study is grounded in a solid review of the literature related to military nursing and parental separation.
- The literature review is complete, well synthesized and clearly articulated making it easy to follow and enjoyable to read.
- The author provides clear justification for the use of grounded theory methods and each step of the research process is clearly linked.
- The preliminary studies section addresses the strengths and experiences of the research team and provides convincing evidence that the team can conduct this study.
- Findings from this study will be useful and contribute to improving nursing practice.
- The research design and methods section are well developed.
- The description of grounded theory is accurate and demonstrates knowledge as well as experience with the methodology.
- There are rational for all methodological decisions.

- Careful attention is paid to the 'science' of the project and appropriate attention is paid to issues related to authenticity and trustworthiness.
- Careful attention is given to ethical issues related to the project.
- The study is original an innovative.
- The study has the potential to contribute to our understanding about militarily nursing.
- The resources appear adequate to support this project.

Weaknesses

Part Three

Please list your conclusions and indicate your level of enthusiasm for this proposal.

Level of Enthusiasm (circle one): **High**   Moderate   Low Score: _____

Part Four

Please rank how closely the Title of the proposals reflects the actual proposal (circle one).

1. **Good match** 2. Matches 3. Neutral 4. Partially matches 5. Does not match

Primary Reviewer_____X_____ Secondary Reviewer_____

TriService Nursing Research Program Format for Secondary Reviewer's Evaluative Comments

Proposal Number: N09-P02
Principal Investigator: LTC (ret) Janice B. Agazio
Title of Proposal: Deployment of Military Mothers during Wartime

---

Evaluation Criteria

Scientific Approach and Technical Merit

The proposed qualitative research is focused on a description of the trajectory of the wartime deployment experiences of military women with children. The research will focus on previously identified phases of deployment ranging from predeployment preparation through reunion and reintegration. The research will address six specific questions related to the deployment experience: 1) What is the process of managing a deployment for military deployment and their children; 2) How do military mothers describe the effects of a deployment upon themselves and their children; 3) How do military mothers prepare themselves and their children for deployment; 4) How do military mothers manage the separation from their children during deployment; 5) How do military mothers manage their relationships with their children during and following deployment; 6) What strategies are effective in maintaining relationship with children during deployment. The research will used grounded theory methodology for data collection and analysis. Standard qualitative methods are used including in-depth individual interviews with a sample f approximately 35 to 40 women from all services and inclusive of officers and enlisted personnel. Recruitment will be conducted through three military health clinics including WRAMC, Womack Army Medical Center, and DiLorenzo Tri-Care Health Clinic. Recruitment will continue until data saturation and all facets of the phenomenon of interest have been fully explored. The sample is limited to women who deployed for a minimum of three months and who also have a child under the age of 12 during deployment.

This is a well crafted application. The investigators' expertise in qualitative research in general and grounded theory in particular is evidence in the crafting of the proposal. The study aims and research questions are well integrated with the study methods which are an appropriate fit. The problem being addressed is well-documented in the literature review as is the study's focus as a major gap in the research. The procedures are described in detail and are well justified.

There are a few minor issues identified. It is not clear whether or not the recruitment sites will generate a sample that represents all military branches. This needs to be clarified and the choices of sites needs to be justified. A number of demographic variables will be measured to provide a description of the sample; however it appears that some important characteristics will not be measured as they are not noted in the application. For example, length of deployment, marital status, and arrangements that were made for care f the children during deployment are important factors that should be documented. These issues, however, are minor and are probably just omissions.

Originality and Innovative Nature of the Proposal; Applicability of Previous Findings

The research is quite innovative in terms of its focus. The investigators have identified a clear gap in the research of the experience of deployment that is of increasing importance. The research questions are particularly innovative in that if the research questions are answered, the findings of the study will not only provide a description of the issues that impact mothers and their children during deployment, but it will go a long way toward documenting strategies that mothers have used to deal with deployment. Undoubtedly some of these strategies would have been effective and their identification will provide a foundation for intervention development.

Qualifications, Expertise and Research Experience of the Principal Investigator and Staff

The PI, Dr. Agazio, is well qualified to lead the research team toward completion of this research. She has a strong track record of funded research upon which the current research is based. She has successfully published the findings from each of these studies. She is clearly expert in qualitative research methods and the grounded theory approach. The team is further strengthened by another qualitative research expert from USUSH (Dr. Padden), and Dr. Ricciardi is knowledgeable of the effects of deployment through his role at WRAMC and will be able to take the lead in recruitment of study participants. Additionally, it is noteworthy plans to mentor Drs. O'Brien and Ricciardi in grounded theory methods. There is also a history of collaboration among research team members that should contribute to the effectiveness of the team and increase their potential for success.

Availability of Institutional Resources and Adequacy of the Environment to Support the Project

The resources available to the research team through CAU and the military medical facilities are sufficient to ensure successful completion of the research. Of note at the letters of support for the research provided by all involved organizations.

Significance and Relevance to Nursing Research

The research addresses a problem of high significance and relevance and is positioned to shed light on an important issue for military women and their families that could have a significant impact on retention in the military.

Reasonableness of the Budget and Duration of the Project in Relation to the Proposed Research

The budget is very reasonable.

Summary

This is a very strong and well crafted application with high significance and relevance. I am very enthusiastic about this application.

Part Three: Please list your conclusions and indicate your level of enthusiasm for this proposal.

Level of Enthusiasm (circle one): <u>**High**</u>   Moderate   Low Score: **1.2**

Part Four: Please rank how closely the Title of the proposals reflects the actual proposal (circle one).

1. <u>**good match**</u> 2. matches 3. neutral 4. partially matches 5. does not match

Please indicate whether you are primary or secondary reviewer.

Primary Reviewer_____ Secondary Reviewer_____X_____

TriService Nursing Research Program Format for Military Reviewers' Evaluative Comments

Proposal Number: N09-P02
Principal Investigator: LTC (ret) Janice B. Agazio
Title of Proposal: Deployment of Military Mothers during Wartime

Evaluation Criteria

Military Feasibility

The strengths of this proposed study, in terms of military feasibility, are that the study relates directly to the welfare of the military family and that the investigators have military experience. The primary research team members are highly qualified qualitative researchers with prior military studies completed and published, as well as experience with completion of funded research.

The proposed timeline should allow the specific aims to be met.

Military Relevance

The strength of the proposed study, in terms of military relevance, is the critical need to assist mothers, who are at particular risk, to adjust to deployments.

Stress in Army families is most relevant today and studies such as this may define relationship strategies that can be facilitated in families for the future deploying soldiers.

The potential contribution or applicability of the proposed research to military healthcare is exceptional. The importance of the research problem to military trauma care is clearly presented.

No weaknesses for military relevance are noted.

Stability of the Research Team

The PI and the research team's ability to carry out the study is well established by the track record of their previous research. Military deployments, reassignments, and temporary duty orders are not a factor in the stability of the primary research team members, except Col Ricciardi. Support letters indicating the commitment of the research team are presented. The time dedicated by LTC Coe is unclear.

Summary

Please provide a summary using the **TWO-PART FORMAT** described below.

Part One: Please list, <u>in bullet format,</u> first the strengths and then the weaknesses of the proposal relative to military feasibility, military relevance, and stability of the research team.

Military Feasibility

Strengths
- All of the investigators have military experience.
- The study is feasible and practical.

Weaknesses
  None

Military Relevance

Strengths
- The study has direct relevance to the healthy relationship of mothers and children and the stability of the military family.
- The aims of the study related to identification of strategies is most relevant to immediate application to military family support systems.

Weaknesses
  None

Stability of the Research Team

Strengths
- There is minimal risk of deployment delaying the study since the majority of the research team are not at risk of deployment.

Weaknesses
- No back-up for COL Riccardi who will site PI, is identified.
- LTC Coe's time commitment is not described.

Part Two: Please list your conclusions and indicate your level of enthusiasm for this proposal.

Level of Enthusiasm (circle one): **High**   Moderate   Low

Part Three: Please rank how closely the Title of the proposals reflects the actual proposal (circle one).

1. good match 2. **matches** 3. neutral 4. partially matches 5. does not match

TriService Nursing Research Program FY 2009 Programmatic Review Discussion Summary

Proposal Number: N09-P02
Principal Investigator: LTC (ret) Janice B. Agazio
Title: Deployment of Military Mothers during Wartime
Programmatic Review Score: 1.5

Discussion: This proposal is well written and the study is feasible. The proposal addresses a deployment health programmatic priority. The research team has the expertise needed to complete the proposed study, and the PI has produced publications and presentations from all of her funded studies. The study's minor weaknesses can be easily addressed.

Recommendation: Fund after the PI addresses the minor weaknesses identified by the Scientific Review Committee.

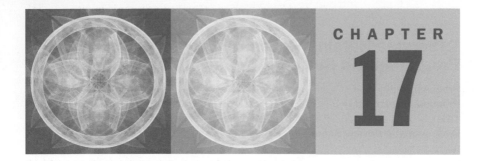

A Practical Guide for Sharing Qualitative Research Results

*T*he completion of a qualitative research study is only the beginning of the nurse investigator's work. The value of the research will never be fully appreciated unless it is shared. Dissemination of qualitative research can be invigorating, particularly when the investigator has the opportunity to share the richness of the data. Telling the story of participants invites a dialogue between professional colleagues. It also provides the researcher with the privilege of offering insights into previously unknown areas of participants' lives. Sharing the results of a qualitative research study is an exciting opportunity to provide insights, receive thoughtful critiques, and learn from others who have related experiences.

Once qualitative researchers develop a degree of comfort with research activities involved in the conduct of a qualitative project, they may become interested in developing a grant proposal using qualitative approaches. Grant writing requires qualitative researchers to develop additional skills, an effort well worth the time, especially when researchers' ideas are validated through the receipt of grant funds.

This chapter informs qualitative researchers about the differences in presentation style when a researcher submits a qualitative manuscript for publication, offers suggestions on how to submit a qualitative proposal for grant funding, and shares creative strategies for presenting qualitative research findings.

PUBLICATION PREPARATION

f a research study invites the opportunity to share the
rofessional audience. The findings of an inquiry have
hey are offered to the larger nursing community.
ways that researchers can disseminate the results of
ul in sharing one's research, the qualitative inves-
or the nuances of publishing qualitative research.
offered as a guide to those who are interested in
form of a journal article.

nce

hers begin their work, they should have an idea of
the results at the conclusion of the investigation. A
erally is shared. To prepare a report in the form of a
s must be aware of their audience. If the audience is
f qualitative researchers, the manuscript will read dif-
udience is made up of nurse clinicians, educators, or
administrators without expertise in qualitative methodologies. Identify the
audience clearly from the start. By reviewing current journals, the researcher
can begin to identify which journals support the publication of qualitative
research and which do not. Some nursing journals include more qualitative
research studies on average than others. Regular review of major research
journals will alert investigators to these journals. Journals that publish qualitative studies on a regular basis include: *Advances in Nursing Science, Nursing
Inquiry, Journal of Nursing Scholarship, Nursing Science Quarterly, Journal of
Advanced Nursing, Qualitative Health Research, Research in Nursing and Health,*
and *Western Journal of Nursing Research*. There are also specialty journals
such as *Action Research* and *Journal of Contemporary Ethnography*. Although
these are not nursing journals, they publish from a wide range of fields.
They are available as a resource as well as a potential publisher. This list is
not exhaustive, nor is it offered to suggest that other journals do not publish
qualitative studies. The purpose is to share the names of journals that have
demonstrated a sustained and ongoing commitment to the publication of
qualitative research.

In addition to identifying a journal that will be receptive to qualitative
research approaches, it is essential to identify a journal with a focus on the
content area of the study. For instance, the purpose of *Qualitative Health
Research* is to disseminate qualitative research; however, the journal focuses
on practice issues in health care and does not usually publish nursing
education research articles. Therefore, an education study that utilizes qualitative methods would best be reported in an education journal such as the
Journal of Nursing Education or *Nurse Educator*.

Once researchers have identified the potential journal, it is essential that
they obtain a copy of the journal's guidelines for authors. This document

assists researchers to develop a manuscript that meets the editorial expectations of the selected journal. Most guidelines for authors do not offer specific recommendations for the presentation of qualitative findings. Reading qualitative studies published in journals is the best way to develop an understanding of how to meet editorial guidelines when submitting results of a qualitative study for publication. Regardless of the journal in which the findings will be published, qualitative researchers should follow certain guidelines.

Each journal's readership has a specific purpose in reading a particular journal. Therefore, researchers must speak to the important facets of the research as they relate to the audience. These facets should reflect the purpose of the journal. For example, if researchers are writing for a scientific journal such as *Nursing Research*, detailing methods and data analysis will be as important as sharing the findings. In contrast, if they plan to publish in *Home Health Care Nurse*, the findings and implications for practice will be more important to the readership than the actual methods for conducting the study.

A phone call or e-mail to the journal will confirm whether the topic you wish to publish is of interest to the readership of a particular journal. Once the interest of the journal is confirmed and writing begins, pay particular attention to your writing. Poorly prepared manuscripts can set the stage for a rejection letter even if the study has significant merit.

Once researchers have submitted a manuscript, editorial staff will review the submission and decide whether the content reflects the journal's purpose and is well-written. If not, they will return the manuscript. Researchers are then responsible for identifying a more suitable periodical. Authors should expect to receive a postcard, letter, or e-mail within a few weeks of submission reporting on the status of the manuscript. The time from submission to publication may be more than 1 year. However, if, after 3 or 4 months, authors have not received a progress report on the disposition of the manuscript (i.e., whether it has been accepted or rejected), they should follow up with a phone call, e-mail, or letter.

Developing the Manuscript

The most difficult thing about writing is getting started. This statement is not intended to suggest that qualitative researchers have not been writing. However, documenting field notes and analyzing interviews are much different forms of writing than writing for publication. Documenting field notes or interviews is personal and these personal writings usually will not be read or analyzed by others. Researchers frequently learn through the implementation of their studies that it is easy and even fun to write notes for themselves, but it is more difficult to transfer those personal ideas to paper for others to read.

The very nature of data collection and analysis requires that researchers write. Documenting feelings, perceptions, observations, theoretical directions, or insights is part of the implementation of the qualitative research investigation. Transforming diaries, field notes, memos, or transcripts into a publishable manuscript requires rigor and determination, as well as keen synthesis, writing, and organizational abilities.

The most important point that a qualitative researcher must remember when beginning to write is to be clear. Qualitative research generates a large amount of raw data. In raw form, the data are interesting but unusable for research reporting. Qualitative researchers must condense, analyze, and synthesize for readers the importance of the research while not losing the richness of the findings. This effort can be a significant challenge because of the prolonged and intimate involvement of researchers with participants. It is also important to include evidence to support that the information included in the study was obtained from appropriates sources. In addition, it is essential to include relevant data to defend the interpretations made (Lambert, Lambert, & Tsukahara, 2002).

One way to focus on research for publication in a journal is to break the study into parts. Researchers often can develop more than one manuscript from a qualitative research study. Sandelowski (2006) suggests that there are ways to divide the volumes of data to be reported without "inappropriately multiplying the number of qualitative research reports or duplicating information" (p. 371). These divisions include temporal, thematic, events, and subjects (p. 371). A *temporal* focus has as its organizer the concept of time. For example, if a researcher is studying the experience of undergoing open heart surgery, he or she might choose to focus on reporting on the period just before being sedated for the surgery.

The researcher could choose to focus on theme. A *thematic* focus allows the researcher to expose varying points of interest. Using the open heart surgery example, the nurse researcher might discover that individuals either focus on the possibility of death or the new vitality that will result from the surgery. Exploiting these two mindsets can provide important insight into the personalities of individuals undergoing open heart surgery which very well might have an impact on recovery. Reporting either of these themes in separate journal articles is appropriate as long as the researcher can justify the reason for doing so.

The third way to focus the research report according to Sandelowski (2006) is by event. In the example of studying the experience of open heart surgery, clearly there are specific events that lead up to or are part of the experience. For example, the researcher might choose to focus on the diagnosis or the observation of the surgical site. Reporting specifically on these events may provide valuable information which can improve patient outcomes.

Another way to focus the report is by *subject*. Participants in the study may provide data which is interesting from particular subject characteristics such as gender, age, or ethnicity. Using subject as the organizing theme can provide the opportunity for reporting variations in the study subjects.

Regardless of how the researcher chooses to focus the study for publication, preservation of the integrity of the findings (Sandelowski, 2006) and a clear understanding of why they are being reported separately are critical. In addition, when the findings are disaggregated for reporting, the articles should not duplicate previously reported information.

Given the voluminous amount of data that often results from a qualitative study, the ideal medium for reporting them is a book or several chapters of a book. As Morse and Field (1995) point out, a book-length manuscript is best when researchers wish to share a description of the research process. However, time, commitment, and opportunity may limit publication in this format.

If researchers are uninterested in publishing the study in parts, then they can certainly develop the report so that it will be of greatest interest to readers. For instance, using the open heart surgery unit example, the researcher can present findings in the context of practice implications in critical care journals. A manuscript for publication in a practice journal would not require a great deal of emphasis on method or analysis but would require significant attention to findings and implications.

The most difficult obstacle to overcome in developing a qualitative manuscript for publication is the need to report the study in 12 to 15 pages, as required by most journals. With this limitation, it is critically important to be concise, focused, and logical rather than to try to report the entire study.

Once researchers have identified the journal and determined the focus, the next step is to logically develop the ideas they wish to convey. "An outline provides guidance in writing" (Field & Morse, 1985, p. 130). The purpose of the outline is to keep the writer focused. It is easy to drift away from the focus of the manuscript without an outline. Depending on the preference of the author, the outline may be more or less detailed.

When beginning to write, the author should be clear about the research questions and the audience for whom the publication is being prepared (Devers & Frankel, 2001). In addition to reporting on the steps of the qualitative research process, it is important to tell the story by using the participant's own words. It is equally important to be "cognizant of the differences between description and interpretations" (Choudhuri, Glauser, & Peregoy, 2004, p. 445). Interpretation moves beyond description to address what is going on in the setting.

On completion of the manuscript, authors should ask colleagues to critique the ideas presented. Too often, novice qualitative researchers make the mistake of believing that, because they have spent much time immersed in the data, writing about the data is straightforward. Qualitative research manuscripts are subjected to rigorous review. It is essential that the ideas be clear and demonstrate important findings to the nursing community. Review by knowledgeable colleagues will assist in ensuring the logic, organization, consistency, and importance of the findings.

Once the manuscript is submitted, researchers should be ready to revise as requested by the reviewers. Few manuscripts, qualitative or quantitative, sustain juried review without requests for revision. Morse (1996b) further suggests that, if researchers receive a request for revision in which reviewers' recommendations are contradictory, the researchers' responsibility is to attend to the most meaningful comments. Investigators should indicate why they did not use all of the reviewers' comments; however, when the comments do not reflect the truth of the study, researchers should not revise to attend to those particular comments. Never be naive, though, to the point of not considering reviewers' comments. Researchers have a great deal to gain in positive and negative comments. They need to ask, Why did someone read this in a particular way?

When asked to revise, researchers must work quickly. The sooner they return the revised manuscript, the sooner the acceptance, and the earlier the manuscript will be queued for publication (Morse, 1996b).

If the unfortunate circumstance occurs—receipt of a rejection letter—do not throw away the manuscript. Look carefully at the critique, use the comments to improve the manuscript, and try another journal. It is acceptable also to use the comments, revise the manuscript, and resubmit it to the same journal. Quality research should be published. Sometimes, it takes a fair amount of tenacity to see ideas through to publication. But once published, researchers will enjoy the thrill of having the work available in print for readers interested in the topic and particular research approach.

Qualitative research that is considered for publication should meet the following minimal standards: (1) the approach (phenomenology, grounded theory, etc.) must be clearly identified; (2) the research question and the approach are congruent and specified; (3) "the approach is clearly situated in a specific research paradigm and philosophical tradition as evidenced by congruence with the explicitly stated or implied underpinnings throughout the manuscript" (p. 320); (4) all elements of the design are consistent with the philosophical underpinnings; (5) the methodology is defined and the steps are followed; (6) rigor is demonstrated; (7) findings of the study are useful; and (8) they exhibit the versatility and sensitivity to meaning and context (Nelson, 2008, p. 320).

CONFERENCE PRESENTATION

Satisfaction results from the publication of a manuscript that shares the results of intensive investigation. Manuscript publication is just one of researchers' responsibilities in their dissemination of the findings. In addition to getting ideas in print, which may take between 10 and 18 months, researchers should present the findings to the scholarly community using other forums. One way to share results in an efficient and effective way is through a formal conference presentation as a paper or poster presentation.

Whether presenting findings in a paper or poster, qualitative researchers need to address important guidelines for sharing results in public forums.

Most formal presentations result from a *call for abstracts*, which requires investigators to submit a synopsis of the research in a few paragraphs, with an average limit of between 150 and 500 words. Guidelines for abstract submissions generally are available from the group sponsoring the research conference or workshop. It is essential that responses to the call reflect the theme of the conference and meet the criteria for presentation. The guidelines for abstract submission usually include the study purpose, the method the researcher used to conduct the inquiry, the sample, the findings, and the significance of the findings to nursing. Inclusion of the information requested will greatly improve the chances for abstract acceptance. However, because the results of a qualitative study are rich and dense, the question becomes, How do I demonstrate the richness of my work and the significance in 150 to 500 words when I have trouble writing it in 15 pages?

When submitting an abstract, be convincing. Illustrate for the reviewers that the work has been done well, will be interesting, and is significant to the profession. It is impossible to share the richness of the research in an abstract. What researchers should be striving for is to whet the reviewers' appetites so that they want to know more about the study.

A call for abstracts generally asks researchers to indicate the format in which they prefer to present: poster or paper. Novice qualitative researchers would be wise to indicate both. Podium presenters of a paper often have demonstrated their ability to successfully engage a group in their work through their ability to clearly articulate their ideas in the abstract. For individuals who have their abstracts rejected for podium presentation, poster presentations offer the opportunity to share the findings in a comfortable, relaxed atmosphere. A poster presentation provides new qualitative researchers with the chance to develop skill and confidence in presenting research findings. More important, in some conference formats, posters are the only opportunity to present findings because podium presentations may be reserved for invited keynote speakers.

Preparing for an Oral Presentation

If accepted for an oral presentation, researchers must keep in mind important aspects of sharing the results. They should present qualitative research so that they engage the conference participants in the work. Because the average length of podium presentation is between 20 and 30 minutes, be careful not to spend too much time discussing the method used to conduct the inquiry. Although the method is essential information, the audience will be most interested in the findings. Inform the audience about the method to give them the context and direction of the study, but do not share so much information that presentation of the findings is rushed. Presenters should not be hurried through the presentation of quotations from informants or the analysis of findings because these elements *are* the study results. Share the quotations and analysis thoughtfully, giving the audience time to absorb the words. Slides, overheads, or a computerized multimedia presentation can be used to provide a visual representation of the quotes, giving the audience additional time to assimilate the meaning of the words. Photographs and illustrations add to the presentation as well. Be sure to leave adequate time for questions. If the research has been presented well, the audience will want to know more because its interest has been aroused. During the question-and-answer period, a unique opportunity is available to share additional findings and anecdotal information.

Be aware that not all questions will be easy or fun to answer. At times, the audience can demonstrate interest in the trustworthiness or ethical considerations in the study. If you have executed a well-designed study, you can handle these questions. If you have not been insightful enough to predict questions and do not have ready answers, be honest. Use the critique questions shared in this text as a developmental learning experience. In this way, you, too, will have learned from sharing your results.

Preparing for a Poster Presentation

Presenting qualitative research in poster format is a unique challenge, but certainly one that researchers can meet successfully. Many good articles are available on the mechanics of preparing and presenting a poster. Display poster presentations so that, in a glance, interested individuals can determine whether they want to know more or whether they prefer to move to the next poster. Anyone who has ever attended a poster session knows that the sheer volume of posters available limits interested parties from spending time with each poster presenter. Therefore, the poster must immediately capture attention. The title, color of the poster, size of print, and content should catch the passerby's interest first. However, the most important part of the poster is the title. The title immediately informs readers of the topic and research approach. For instance, the title "Living in Fear" would attract individuals interested in the topic. Because the title is brief, passersby can decide in a moment whether they want to know more. Similarly, a title such as "Living with AIDS: A Cultural Examination" quickly informs people about the subject matter and research approach. Also of importance is the author's name and affiliation. There are situations in which the poster presenter may not be available to answer questions related to the research. If the consumer can jot down the presenter's name and affiliation or pick up a business card, then he or she can contact the poster author at a later time.

In addition, researchers should present the content in a visually appealing way. At a minimum, the poster should include the title of the research, the researcher's name, the purpose, the sample, the method used, the findings, a summary, and the implications. Not all of this information will fit on the poster, depending on the space provided. Therefore, it is up to the researcher to illustrate as much as possible and then indicate to the viewer the availability of additional information either on a handout or in a note-book on the table. Pictures and illustrations capture the passerby's attention and give presenters the ability to verbally share results. For qualitative researchers, there is benefit in providing interested individuals with a handout of the abstract or handouts highlighting the important research findings or offering an exhaustive description, if appropriate. On the printed handouts, researchers can include their names and addresses so that nurses interested in the findings or the method may contact them for additional information. Russell, Gregory, and Gates (1996) suggest that researchers place a notebook on the table with the poster. In the notebook, the researcher can insert additional information, including narrative, pictures, and illustrations that are too cumbersome to place on the poster. The note-book provides people interested in additional information about the study an opportunity to get it "on the spot."

As well as using a matted poster format, some qualitative researchers have used audiovisual materials such as a multimedia projection system to give an added dimension to their presentations. The inclusion of sound and changing visuals connects consumers to the work. Presenting a poster using a multimedia system, however, requires access to electricity and additional space. Researchers interested in presenting a poster in this format need to contact the conference planners to see whether there is accessible electricity and adequate space.

Creativity is the key to the successful presentation of ideas. The nature of qualitative research supports creativity in presentation. Because of the type of data collected, the strategies used, and the rich narrative that results, researchers have much more to draw from in developing their poster. Nurses presenting a poster illustrating a qualitative research approach should take advantage of the possibilities open to sharing their findings and exploit those possibilities. However, remember to do so in a logical and appealing manner.

GRANT WRITING

Although some graduate students are successful in submitting proposals for funding of their dissertation work before they have a publication history, the more frequent scenario is for a researcher to submit a grant pro-posal after having had one or more research studies published. The develop-ment of a competitive research proposal requires researchers to construct the project so that they convince a panel of reviewers that they have the nec-essary knowledge, experience, and commitment to complete the proposed project. Reviewers will be looking at a researcher's credentials, the scientific merit of the project, and the potential contribution of the project to the profession.

Identifying Funding Sources

One of the first steps in developing a competitive proposal is to identify potential funding sources, a number of which are available to nurses interested in conducting a qualitative inquiry. Different organizations offer materials on the types of projects they fund and their submission guidelines. For researchers seeking their first funding dollars, small grants are the most useful and are generally easier to access. Examples of small grant programs include college or university funds, which are accessible through small grant proposals available on a competitive basis within institutions. The monies generally come from allocations to faculty development budgets, foundations, or alumni gifts.

In addition to college or university funding, several nursing organizations offer small grants. These organizations, among others, include Sigma Theta Tau International (STTI), National League for Nursing (NLN), American Nurses Foundation (ANF), American Association of Critical Care Nurses (AACN), and Association of Rehabilitation Nurses (ANA). Many corporations also offer small grants, including product companies such as infant formula manufacturers or durable medical equipment firms. Health care organizations, such as hospitals and community health organizations, frequently fund research as well.

Nurses interested in receiving funding need to identify the available resources. This effort will require a moderate amount of time to first determine the available funding sources and then select the source that will most likely be interested in funding the project. Nurses might use resource libraries found in universities that have established nursing research centers to identity potential funding sources. If a nursing research center is not available in your institution, within your academic affairs or advancement units you will find grant writers who are experts at locating corporate, government, and foundation funding sources. Using these resources, you will find a plethora of diverse materials and experienced staff to assist in locating the appropriate resources and developing the proposal. In addition, it is no longer necessary for potential grant writers to spend hours in the library: the Internet is a great source for identifying potential grant funds. If university-based nursing research centers are unavailable, researchers may log onto the web sites of organizations such as the AACN, NLN, STTI, and ANA, which have resource materials on their sites, as well as links to other sites to help focus the search. In addition, sites such as http://fdncenter.org offer a starting point. This is a more general site and is not specific to nursing. It does, however, reference large foundations that provide funds for health-related projects, such as Kellogg and Coca Cola. If you choose to consider a nonnursing organization, look for the eligibility requirements, the organization's purpose and mission statement, and the compatibility with your project (Carey & Swanson, 2003).

Individuals interested in developing larger projects should have completed and published results of small, funded projects before seeking monies from organizations that offer larger funding support. Such organizations include the National Institute of Nursing Research (NINR), National Institutes of Health (NIH), American Educational Research Association (AERA), Kellogg Foundation, Robert Wood Johnson Foundation, and National Science Foundation (NSF). In addition, many nonprofit organizations such as the American Heart Association, National Arthritis Foundation, and American Cancer Society provide moderate to large funding for projects. Critical to receiving larger sums of money and submitting a well-developed project is experience. Organizations that make large awards do not do so unless single researchers or research teams demonstrate significant, documented experience.

Developing the Proposal

Because Chapter 16 focuses on proposal development and grant writing, this section will not address the specific mechanics of developing a research proposal for funding. Instead, the section gives qualitative researchers' ideas about the challenges and potential pitfalls in developing qualitative grant proposals. In 1991, Morse stated, "In comparison to the WYSIWYG (what you see is what you get) presentation of the quantitative application, the qualitative proposal is vague, obscure, and may even be viewed as a blatant request for a blank check" (p. 148). Although this was written almost 20 years ago, many qualitative grant writers continue to experience a more difficult time convincing reviewers of the rigor of their work. The idea of developing a proposal for funding, knowing beforehand that the ambiguities cannot be written out of the grant, presents a unique but not insurmountable challenge. Researchers interested in receiving funding for a qualitative study must convince reviewers not only of the merits of the project, which may seem obscure and undirected, but also of the researcher's experience. Carey and Swanson (2003) report that "the three major areas in common across most applications are identifying appropriate funding sources, developing a work plan and a team and writing the application" (p. 852). These should be carefully considered before moving forward.

There is inconsistency in the literature as to whether a pilot study is important for qualitative research funding. Clearly, quantitative research proposals require pilot work to demonstrate the potential design strengths and weaknesses. Connelly and Yoder (2000) offer that conducting pilot work enhances the qualitative researcher's chances for funding. Given the inconsistencies in the literature and strong possibility of review by quantitative researchers, qualitative researchers are well-served to state why they did or did not conduct a pilot study.

In qualitative proposals, the number of participants is determined by data saturation, which can include as few as 5 or more than 50 people. In a quantitative study, the number of participants is determined by the design, projected outcome, and number of variables under study. Based on these parameters, researchers can establish a precise number of participants for inclusion in a study. In qualitative studies, data collection and analysis require flexibility. In quantitative studies, data collection and analysis are largely objective. The preceding comparisons focus on the precise and often predictable nature of a quantitative research proposal versus the often imprecise and unpredictable nature of a qualitative proposal.

Morse (1998) recommends, "the first principle of grantsmanship is to recognize that a good proposal is an argument—a fair and balanced one" (p. 68). Therefore, qualitative researchers must clearly and persuasively present evidence that will convince grant reviewers the proposal is worth funding. To facilitate a clear understanding of the researchers' ideas, proposal authors have the responsibility of explaining everything.

The second principle of grant writing offered by Morse (1998) "is that one should think and plan before starting to write" (p. 70). Planning before writing will give proposal authors an opportunity to clearly delineate the research plan, beginning with development of the research question and ending with the distribution of research results. In addition to assisting with writing the actual proposal document, planning conclusively before beginning to write allows authors time to draft a complete budget. Because the budget is the part of the proposal that provides researchers with the resources to fully operationalize a project, it is essential that researchers develop a strong budget detailing all expenses. Items to include in the budget are personnel, such as research assistants, transcription services, secretaries, and consultants; equipment, such as a computer, printer, video camera, and data analysis program; supplies, such as tape recorders, paper, printer cartridges, audiotapes or videotapes, and photocopies; and travel, including mileage between research sites, conference travel, presentation fees, and consultant travel. Carefully laying out the project will assist greatly in developing a proposal that is clear and succinct and can be funded.

Identifying Investigator Qualifications

The challenge in obtaining larger sums for qualitative research is for prospective grant recipients to convince reviewers they are a risk worth taking. Proposal authors need to illustrate for reviewers a track record in scholarly publication, presentation, consultation, and success in acquiring small awards. "Granting bodies must [be made to] recognize the process nature of the research and that they are funding the *investigator* rather than the *proposal* per se" (Morse, 1991, p. 149). Morse adds that "for major grant applications, evaluation of the *investigator* is critical and should be most heavily weighted" (p. 149). This is not to say that the research project does not need to have scientific merit and be described as fully as possible; rather, it illuminates the nature of the process that is decidedly imprecise when compared with a quantitative proposal.

Morse (1996a) points out that funding agencies have given the distinct impression that qualitative research is not an end but rather a means to an end. Based on the literature, qualitative researchers are led to believe that qualitative inquiry is a prelude to "good" quantitative design. This assumption does not demonstrate knowledge of qualitative research. Researchers must make clear to funding agencies the project goal(s) and clearly describe how the method selected is appropriate. This will help to insure that the study being conducted is properly evaluated.

Adding a qualitative dimension to a large quantitative study is one way that a researcher can increase the possibility of funding for qualitative research. However, it is up to the principal investigator to determine whether the study will be enhanced by the addition of a strong team with varied philosophical beliefs and interests. Based on experience with funded projects, grant reviewers are frequently viewing research teams more favorably, particularly if the teams are multidisciplinary.

A very serious problem identified by Morse (2003) is that many reviews of qualitative research proposals are not valid. She argues that rejection of proposals is often based on the inexperience of the reviewers with qualitative studies. Currently, the procedures for ensuring a meaningful evaluation of qualitative projects need to be strengthened. An alternative model for review described by Morse includes the addition of an external reviewer with qualitative expertise. Depending on the reviewing agency, this can be in person or by phone. In some cases, the reviewer is permitted to be part of the discussion, and in others, the external reviewer is dismissed for the discussion. In another model, a token qualitative reviewer is added to the review panel (Morse, 2003, p. 741). Although this might at first glance seem a more responsible way to conduct the review, Morse explains that "proposals are funded using the average score obtained from the entire committee, not just the input from one advocate" (p. 741). It is important for qualitative researchers to be aware of the review process so that they can attempt to manage some of the ongoing questions relative to their work.

Identifying Mechanisms for Ensuring Participant Protection

Not only must qualitative researchers clearly demonstrate their expertise and qualifications, it is also essential that their qualitative research proposals conclusively identify the mechanisms for ensuring the protection of participants. One of the strengths of qualitative approaches is the unique opportunity to get to know individuals, groups, or communities over a long period. This strength creates its own potential hazards for participants' protection because the nature of the data—personal descriptions—precludes qualitative researchers from maintaining confidentiality, particularly when they publish quotes or use them as references in publications (Munhall, 1991). Nevertheless, qualitative researchers can ensure anonymity. It is important that they demonstrate how they will protect informants' identities. In some cases, such as in ethnography or action research, participant identification may actually contribute significantly to the position of groups or their ability to access resources. In such cases, qualitative researchers should document that participants have agreed that researchers may make the informants' identities public. Audiotaping interviews and taking photographs are additional examples of potential violations of participants' rights. Researchers must document informants' permission for such activities.

Although developing mechanisms for ensuring confidentiality and anonymity contributes significantly to a grant proposal, it is also important to clarify for institutional review boards and funding agencies that mechanisms are in place to deal with potentially sensitive outcomes. For example, if a researcher is living with a community and discovers that one of the group rituals involves physically isolating and abusing children who do not excel in academics, the researcher must be able to clearly define steps he or she will take to protect the vulnerable group (i.e., the children). It is necessary to try to identify all the potentially sensitive situations and develop mechanisms to intervene or to have intervention available.

Qualitative research is unpredictable in its implementation. Often, the study moves in directions not originally planned. For this reason, it is important to describe for review panels the concept of process consent. "In process consent, researchers continuously renegotiate the consent, allowing participants to play a collaborative role in the decision-making process regarding their ongoing participation" (Polit & Beck, 2006, p. 93). Fully describing the necessity of process consent and the conditions under which it will be used gives reviewers a better understanding of the attention paid to protecting participants.

Other Considerations

Connelly and Yoder (2000) identify a number of common problems with qualitative research proposals that are worth noting. These authors share that researchers should clearly demonstrate an understanding of the assumptions of the research approach they are using. "It is critical to write from the perspective of the appropriate assumptions" (p. 70). Often the proposal author will slip from qualitative terminology to quantitative terminology, which is the second common problem identified. Qualitative researchers must be very careful to fully understand the philosophical foundations of qualitative research in general as well as the specifics of the particular method selected. Sharing methodological information is important. It is especially important when the reviewer is unfamiliar with the assumptions of the method, terminology, and techniques used to collect and analyze data. Connelly and Yoder (2000) state that qualitative researchers have a responsibility to respond to the outline presented for funding, albeit quantitative in orientation. It is the qualitative researcher's responsibility to explain why it is not possible to provide specific requested information.

Other common problems identified include no logical argument for why a qualitative research approach is warranted, no discussion of how data collectors will be trained, a little or no discussion of methodological rigor, inadequate description of the unique nature of the researcher–informant relationship and its impact on human subjects' protection, inadequately developed significance of the research, inexperienced researcher without adequate consultation, and underestimating budget requirements (Connelly & Yoder, 2000). Any one or more of these common problems can lead to an unsuccessful grant proposal.

SUMMARY

Qualitative research is an exciting opportunity to create meaningful nursing knowledge from individuals' lives and experiences. To make the knowledge accessible, researchers must share the findings in a significant way. Presenting a qualitative project in an article, poster, speech, or grant proposal requires imagination and refined presentation skills. Qualitative researchers have a responsibility to their consumers and to developing qualitative scholars to present their ideas in a clear and meaningful manner. They should share their research in a way that illustrates the richness and value of conducting research using the approaches described in this text.

The development of qualitative research projects and the refinement of social sciences approaches to human inquiry that are appropriate to nursing science establish a major research focus for the profession. Nurses interested in these projects have a unique opportunity to be on the cutting edge of the developments. It is an exciting time for nurses and for research. There is a vast and expansive qualitative research landscape waiting for interested nurse researchers. This is a landscape of imagination that is colored by the lives and experiences of the individuals with whom nurses interact: clients, students, and other nurses. It is essential to document these unique experiences and share them to fully explore and describe the human experience. The challenge awaits those nurses who are willing to participate.

References

Carey, M. A., & Swanson, J. (2003). Funding for qualitative research. *Qualitative Health Research, 13*(6), 852–856.

Choudhuri, D., Glauser, A., & Peregoy, J. (2004). Guidelines for writing a qualitative manuscript for the Journal of Counseling and Development. *Journal of Counseling and Development, 82*, 443–446.

Connelly, M. L., & Yoder, L. H. (2000). Improving qualitative proposals: Common problem areas. *Clinical Nurse Specialist, 14*(2), 69–74.

Devers, K. J., & Frankel, R. M. (2001). Getting qualitative research published. *Education for Health, 14*(1), 109–117.

Field, P. A., & Morse, J. M. (1985). *Nursing research: The application of qualitative approaches.* Rockville, MD: Aspen.

Lambert, C. E., Lambert, V. A., & Tsukahara, M. (2002). Editorial: The review process. *Nursing and Health Science, 4,* 139–140.

Morse, J. (1991). On the evaluation of qualitative proposals [Editorial]. *Qualitative Health Research, 1*(2), 147–151.

Morse, J. M. (1996a). Is qualitative research complete? [Editorial]. *Qualitative Health Research, 6*(1), 3–5.

Morse, J. (1996b). "Revise and resubmit": Responding to reviewers' reports [Editorial]. *Qualitative Health Research, 6*(2), 149–151.

Morse, J. M. (1998). Designing funded qualitative research. In N. K. Denzin & Y. S. Lincoln (Eds.), *Strategies of qualitative inquiry* (pp. 56–85). Thousand Oaks, CA: Sage.

Morse, J. M. (2003). Editorial: The adjudication of qualitative proposals. *Qualitative Health Research, 13*(6), 739–742.

Morse, J. M., & Field, P. A. (1995). *Qualitative research methods for health professionals* (2nd ed.). Thousand Oaks, CA: Sage.

Munhall, P. L. (1991). Institutional review of qualitative research proposals: A task of no small consequence. In J. M. Morse (Ed.), *Qualitative nursing research: A contemporary dialogue* (rev. ed., pp. 258–272). Newbury Park, CA: Sage.

Nelson, A. M. (2008). Addressing the threat of evidence-based practice to qualitative inquiry through increasing attention to quality: A discussion paper. *International Journal of Nursing Studies, 45,* 316–322.

Polit, D. F., & Beck, C. T. (2006). *Essentials of nursing research: Methods, appraisal, and utilization* (6th ed.). Philadelphia, PA: Lippincott Williams & Wilkins.

Russell, C. K., Gregory, D. M., & Gates, M. F. (1996). Aesthetics and substance in qualitative research posters. *Qualitative Health Research, 6*(4), 542–552.

Sandelowski, M. (2006). Divide and conquer: Avoiding duplication in reporting of qualitative research. *Research in Nursing and Health, 29,* 371–373.

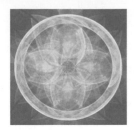

Glossary

A

Action Research A research method characterized by the systematic study of the implementation of a planned change to a system.

Actors Individuals within a particular cultural group who are studied by ethnographic researchers.

Analytic Induction A method of qualitative data analysis wherein the researcher seeks to refine a theory through the identification of negative cases.

A *Priori* Form of deductive thinking in which theoretical formulations and propositions precede and guide systematic observation.

Archives Contain unpublished materials that often are used as primary source materials.

Auditability The ability of another researcher to follow the methods and conclusion of the original researcher.

Authenticity Term used to describe the mechanism by which the qualitative researcher ensures that the findings of the study are real, true, or authentic. In historical research refers to assuring that a primary source document provides the truthful reporting of a subject.

B

Biographical History Studies the life of a person within the context of the period in which that person lives.

Bracketing A methodological device of phenomenological inquiry that requires deliberate identification and suspension of all judgments or ideas about the phenomenon under investigation or what one already knows about the subject prior to and throughout the phenomenological investigation.

C

Category Classification of concepts into broader categories following comparison of one category to another. Broader categories serve as an umbrella under which related concepts are grouped.

Coding The process of data analysis in grounded theory whereby statements are grouped and given a code for ease of identification later in the study.

Conceptual Density Data generation that is exhaustive and comprehensive and provides the researcher with evidence that all possible data to support a conceptual framework has been generated.

Confirmability This is considered a neutral criterion for measuring the trustworthiness of qualitative research. If a study demonstrates credibility, auditability, and fittingness, the study is also said to possess confirmability.

Constant Comparative Method of Data Analysis A form of qualitative data analysis wherein the researcher makes sense of textual data by categorizing units of measuring through a process of comparing new units with previously identified units.

Core Variable The central phenomenon in grounded theory around which all the other categories are integrated.

Covert Participant Observation A method of data collection that

452

involves observing participants however, the individuals are unaware that they are being observed.

Credibility A term that relates to the trustworthiness of findings in a qualitative research study. Credibility is demonstrated when participants recognize the reported research findings as their own experiences.

Critical Theory A philosophy of science based on a belief that revealing the unrecognized forces that control human behavior will liberate and empower individuals.

Cultural Scene An anthropological term for culture. It includes the actors, the artifacts, and the actions of the actors in social situations.

D

Deductive The process of moving from generalizations to specific conclusions.

Dependability This is a criterion used to measure trustworthiness in qualitative research. Dependability is met through securing credibility of the findings.

Dialectic A form of logic based on the belief that reality is represented by contradiction and the reconciliation of contradiction.

Dialectical Critique A form of qualitative data analysis wherein the researcher engages in dialogue with research participants to reveal the internal contradictions within a particular phenomenon.

Discipline of History Both a science and an art that studies the interrelationship of social, economic, political, and psychological factors that influence ideas, events, institutions, and people.

Dwelling A term used to demonstrate the degree of dedication a researcher commits to reading, intuiting, analyzing, synthesizing, and coming to a description or conclusion(s) about the data collected during a qualitative study. Also called immersion.

E

Eidetic Intuiting Accurate interpretations of what is meant in the description.

Embodiment (or Being in the World) The belief that all arts are constructed on foundation of perception, or original awareness of some phenomenon (Merleau-Ponty, 1956).

Epistemology The branch of philosophy concerned with how individuals determine what is true.

Essences Elements related to the ideal or true meaning of something that gives common understanding to the phenomenon under investigation.

External Criticism Questions the genuineness of primary sources and assures that the document is what it claims to be.

F

Field Notes Notes recorded about the people, places, and things that are part of the ethnographer's study of a culture.

Fittingness A term used in qualitative research to demonstrate the probability that the research findings have meaning to others in similar situations. Fittingness is also called transferability.

Free Imaginative Variation A technique used to apprehend essential relations between essences and involves careful study of concrete examples supplied by the participant's experience and systematic variation of these examples in the imagination.

G

Genuine When a primary source is what it purports to be and is not a forgery.

Grand Tour Question(s) General opening question(s) that offer(s) overview insights of a particular person, place, object, or situation.

H

History Webster's New International Dictionary defines history as "a narrative of events connected with a real or imaginary object, person, or career . . . devoted to the exposition of the natural unfolding and interdependence of the events treated." History is a branch of knowledge that "records and explains past events as steps in human progress . . ." [it is] "the study of the character and significance of events." Barzen and Graff (1985) describe history as an "invention" and as an "art."

Historiography Historiography requires that historiographers study and critique sources and develop history by systematically presenting their findings in a narrative. Historiography provides a way of knowing the past.

Historian/Historiographer Balances the rigors of scientific inquiry and the understanding of human behavior; develops the skill of speculation and interpretation to narrate the story.

Historical Method Application of method or steps to study history systematically.

Holism A belief that wholes are more than the mere sum of their parts.

I

Immersion A term used to demonstrate the degree of dedication a researcher commits to reading, intuiting, analyzing, synthesizing, and coming to a description or conclusion(s) about the data collected during a qualitative study. Also called dwelling.

Induction The process of moving from specific observations to generalizations.

Inductive Theory Building Theory derived from observation of phenomena.

Informed Consent When engaging participants in a research study, ensuring that they have complete information, that they understand the information, and that they have freely chosen to either accept or decline participation in the investigation.

Intellectual History Studies ideas and thoughts over time of a person believed to be an intellectual thinker, or the ideas of a period, or the attitudes of people.

Intentionality Consciousness is always consciousness of something. One does not hear without hearing something or believe without believing something.

Internal Criticism Concerns itself with the authenticity or truthfulness of the content.

Interpretive Phenomenology/Hermeneutics The interpretation of phenomena appearing in text or written word.

Intuiting A process of thinking through the data so that a true comprehension or accurate interpretation of what is meant in a particular description is achieved.

L

Life History A research method wherein the researcher listens to the telling of life story for the purpose of understanding a particular aspect of the individual's life.

Local Theory A theory that describes a particular group or sample that cannot be generalized to a larger population.

N

Narrative Picturing A data collection method whereby participants are asked to imagine or picture an event or sequence of events as a method of describing an experience.

Naturalistic Inquiry A research methodology based on a belief in investigating phenomena in their natural setting free of manipulation.

P

Participant Observation The direct observation and recording of data that require the researcher to become a part of the culture being studied.

Phenomenological Reduction A term meaning recovery of original awareness.

Present-Mindedness Use of a contemporary perspective when analyzing data collected from an earlier period of time.

Primary Sources Firsthand account of a person's experience, an institution, or of an event and may lack critical analysis; examples include private journals, letters, records.

Process Informed Consent Requires the same criteria as informed consent; however, is differentiated by the fact that this type of consent requires the researcher to reevaluate the participants' consent to be involved in the study at varying points throughout the investigation.

R

Reflexive This term refers to being both researcher and participant and capitalizing on the duality as a source of insight.

Reflexive Critique A form of qualitative data analysis wherein the researcher engages in dialogue with research participants to reveal each individual's interpretation for the meanings influencing behavior.

Reliability The consistency of an instrument to measure an attribute or concept that it was designed to measure.

S

Saturation Repetition of data obtained during the course of a qualitative study. Signifies completion of data collection on a particular culture or phenomenon.

Secondary Sources Materials that cite opinions and present interpretations from the period being studied such as newspaper accounts, journal articles, and textbooks.

Selective Sampling In a grounded theory investigation, selecting from the generated data those critical pieces of information relevant to the current investigation, and avoiding incorporation of material that is not connected to the current investigation.

Situated A term that reflects the position of the researcher within the context of the group under study.

Social History Explores a particular period of time and attempts to understand the prevailing values and beliefs through the everyday events of that period.

Social Situation The activities carried out by actors (members of a cultural group) in a specific place.

Symbolic Interactionism A philosophic belief system based on the assumption that humans learn about and define their world through interaction with others.

T

Tacit Knowledge Information known by members of a culture but not verbalized or openly discussed.

Theme Used to describe a structural meaning unit of data that is essential in presenting qualitative findings.

Theoretical Sampling Sampling on the basis of concepts that have proven theoretical relevance to the evolving theory (Strauss & Corbin, 1990).

Theoretical Sensitivity Personal quality of the researcher that is reflected in an awareness of the subtleties of meaning of data (Strauss & Corbin, 1990).

Transferability A term used in qualitative research to demonstrate the probability that the research findings have meaning to others in similar situations. Transferability is also called fittingness.

Triangulation Method of using multiple research approaches in the same study to answer research questions.

Triangulation of Data Generation Techniques The use of three different methods of data generation in a single research study for the purpose of generating meaningful data.

Trustworthiness Establishing validity and reliability of qualitative research. Qualitative research is trustworthy when it accurately represents the experience of the study participants.

V

Validity The degree to which an instrument measures what it was designed to measure.

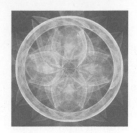

Index

Note: Page numbers followed by *f* indicate figures; those followed by *t* indicate tables; those followed by *b* indicate boxed material.

LIBRARY, UNIVERSITY OF CHESTER

LIBRARY, UNIVERSITY OF CHESTER